Practical Management of Liver Diseases

Practical Management of Liver Diseases is an easy-to-use reference for clinicians and trainees involved in the care of patients with liver diseases. It is designed to ensure that healthcare professionals are up-to-date on recent advances and can detect and treat these diseases rapidly and efficiently for maximum patient benefit. Each chapter is written by an international expert in the field of hepatology and presents a review of the disease or problem and a systematic approach to diagnosis and treatment. With clear illustrations, algorithms, and tables for easy access to key information, this helpful guide is an essential resource for the day-to-day management of patients with liver disease and its complications.

Zobair M. Younossi, MD, MPH, FACG, FACP, is Executive Director of Research for Inova Health System and Executive Director of the Center for Liver Diseases at Inova Fairfax Hospital, Falls Church, VA. He is also Professor of Medicine, Virginia Commonwealth University, Inova Campus and Affiliate Professor of Biomedical Sciences at George Mason University. Dr. Younossi has authored more than 150 articles and presented more than 150 abstracts at international meetings. He sits on multiple local and national committees and has served on the editorial boards of *Hepatology* and *World Journal of Gastroenterology* and as an associate editor of *Liver International* and *Evidence-Based Gastroenterology*. Over the past decade, Dr. Younossi has been actively involved with the American Liver Foundation. He is a member of the American Association for the Study of Liver Disease, American College of Gastroenterology, and the American Gastroenterological Association.

Practical Management of Liver Diseases

Zobair M. Younossi, MD, MPH, FACG, FACP

Executive Director, Center for Liver Diseases, Inova Fairfax Hospital

Executive Director of Research, Inova Health System

Professor of Medicine, Virginia Commonwealth University–Inova Campus

Affiliate Professor of Biomedical Sciences, George Mason University

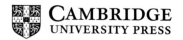

CAMBRIDGE UNIVERSITY PRESS
Cambridge, New York, Melbourne, Madrid, Cape Town, Singapore, São Paulo, Delhi

Cambridge University Press
32 Avenue of the Americas, New York, NY 10013-2473, USA

www.cambridge.org
Information on this title: www.cambridge.org/9780521684897

First published 2008

Printed in the United States of America

A catalog record for this publication is available from the British Library.

Library of Congress Cataloging in Publication Data

Practical management of liver diseases / edited by Zobair M. Younossi.
   p. ; cm.
Includes bibliographical references and index.
ISBN 978-0-521-68489-7 (hardback)
1. Liver – Diseases – Handbooks, manuals, etc.   I. Younossi, Zobair M.   II. Title.
[DNLM: 1. Liver Diseases – therapy. 2. Liver Diseases – diagnosis. WI 700 P8952 2008]
RC846.P73   2008
616.3'6 – dc22   2008000516

ISBN   978-0-521-68489-7 hardback

Dedicated to the unconditional love and support of my wife, Sanya, and my two sons, Issah and Youssef.

Contents

Preface   *page* ix
Contributors   xi

1. Acute Viral Hepatitis   1
    Janus P. Ong, MD, MPH

2. Chronic Hepatitis B and D   26
    Dimitrios Vassilopoulos, MD, and Stephanos J. Hadziyannis, MD

3. Chronic Hepatitis C   39
    Sam Galhenage, MD, and John G. McHutchison, MD

4. HIV and Viral Hepatitis   61
    Mark S. Sulkowski, MD

5. Nonalcoholic Fatty Liver Disease   77
    Poonam Mishra, MD, Nila Rafiq, MD, and
    Zobair M. Younossi, MD, MPH, FACG, FACP

6. Alcoholic Liver Disease   98
    Robert O'Shea, MD, Srinivasan Dasarathy, MD, and Arthur J.
    McCullough, MD

7. Genetic Hemochromatosis and Iron Overload   117
    Bruce R. Bacon, MD

8. Wilson's Disease   131
    Jamile Wakim-Fleming, MD, FACG, and Kevin D. Mullen,
    MD, FRCPI

9. Alpha-1 Antitrypsin Deficiency and the Liver   140
    Steven D. Nathan, MD, and James K. Stoller, MD, MS

10. Autoimmune Liver Disease   155
    Andrea A. Gossard, MS, CNP, and Keith D. Lindor, MD

11. Drug-Induced Liver Disease (DILI)   174
    Julie Polson, MD, and Naga Chalasani, MD

12. Benign and Malignant Tumors of the Liver   195
    Morris Sherman, MD, PhD

13. Complications of Cirrhosis   215
    Jorge L. Herrera, MD

14. Liver Transplantation   235
    Robert L. Carithers, Jr., MD

15. Novel Technologies in Studying Chronic Liver Disease   256
    Ancha Baranova, PhD, Emanuel Petricoin III, PhD, Lance Liotta,
    MD, PhD, and Zobair M. Younossi, MD, MPH, FACG, FACP

Index   277

Preface

Liver disease is increasingly recognized as an important chronic disease world-wide because of its potential impact on the patient's health and the entire society. The impact of chronic liver disease falls into three categories: clinical, quality-of-life, and economic. The clinical impact of chronic liver disease relates to its prevalence and potential for progression. Chronic liver disease is common and is considered one of the leading causes of death in the United States. Chronic viral hepatitis and nonalcoholic fatty liver disease are quite prevalent in the United States and the rest of the world. In general, 20–25% of patients with chronic viral hepatitis and probably other chronic liver diseases can develop advanced fibrosis and cirrhosis. The disease burden for viral hepatitis is significant, with hundreds of patients dying each year from acute liver failure and thousands of others succumbing to the sequelae of chronic hepatitis and cirrhosis. In addition to viral hepatitis, other liver diseases such as nonalcoholic fatty liver disease, alcoholic cirrhosis, autoimmune liver diseases, and others result in significant mortality and morbidity. Because complications of cirrhosis can be recognized early, liver transplantation has become the standard of care treatment modality for end-stage liver disease. However, as the number of patients on the liver transplant list grows, the median waiting time for a liver transplant has increased. This increase in the number of patients listed for liver transplantation, coupled with a shortage of available organs, has resulted in an increasing number of patients dying on the transplant list. In order to respond to this increase in demand for liver transplantation and shortage of organs, a number of alternative modalities are being considered (living-related transplantation, artificial liver support, hepatocyte transplantation, etc.).

In addition to its clinical impact, chronic liver disease impairs patient's health-related quality of life (HRQL), resulting in significant morbidity. These patients suffer from debilitating fatigue, pruritis, loss of self-esteem, depression, and complications of cirrhosis such as hepatic encephalopathy, ascites, spontaneous bacterial peritonitis, and recurrent variceal bleeding. These complications can have a profound negative impact on patient's HRQL and well-being. Although HRQL impairment can be detected early in the course of chronic liver disease, this impairment worsens with disease severity.

Finally, chronic liver disease has an important economic impact on society. The exact economic impact of liver disease and its complications remains unknown, but the direct medical expenditure from HCV, HBV, and NAFLD seems to be enormous. Additionally, the direct and indirect costs of early mortality and morbidity from other chronic liver diseases can cost society additional billions of dollars.

In addition to understanding the full impact of chronic liver disease, it is also important to point out the progress that has been achieved in the development of new therapies for patients with a variety of chronic liver diseases. The past century has witnessed the emergence of Hepatology as a thriving, full-fledged subspecialty. We now have effective therapies in our armamentarium for the treatment of autoimmune hepatitis, chronic hepatitis B, primary biliary cirrhosis, and chronic hepatitis C. Additionally, we have seen tremendous gains in treatment modalities available for complications of cirrhosis, such as Transjugular Intrahepatic Portosystemic Shunt (TIPS) for variceal bleeding, radiofrequency ablation (RFA) for hepatocellular carcinoma, and liver transplantation as the definitive therapy for decompensated liver disease. Whereas the one-year survival of decompensated liver disease is extremely low, orthotopic liver transplantation offers a five-year survival of approximately 75–80%. In addition to advances in the treatment of end-stage liver disease, newer treatment modalities for viral hepatitis and noninvasive markers for early disease detection (diagnostic biomarkers) have become increasingly available.

It is important to emphasize that if liver disease is recognized early, a variety of effective treatment modalities can be offered. Therefore, it is crucial that health care professionals are up-to-date in recent advances in our understanding of liver diseases and are familiar with strategies to detect and treat them early. Early detection and treatment can prevent the development of more advanced liver disease, which is accompanied by an increased risk of complications with the associated morbidity and mortality.

In the context of this newly gained knowledge, *Practical Management of Liver Diseases* is developed as an easy-to-use textbook for clinicians and trainees involved in the care of patients with liver diseases. Each chapter is written by an international expert in the field of Hepatology. The book is designed to deal with the most common causes of chronic liver disease in an efficient and user-friendly manner and to provide the reader with a practical resource for the care of their patients with liver disease.

Zobair M. Younossi, MD, MPH, FACG, FACP

Contributors

Bruce R. Bacon, MD
Saint Louis University
St. Louis, MO

Ancha Baranova, PhD
George Mason University
Manassas, VA

Robert L. Carithers, Jr., MD
University of Washington
Seattle, WA

Naga Chalasani, MD
Indiana University
Indianapolis, IN

Srinivasan Dasarathy, MD
Cleveland Clinic
Cleveland, OH

Sam Galhenage, MD
Duke University Medical Center
Durham, NC

Andrea A. Gossard, MS, CNP
Mayo Clinic
Rochester, MN

Stephanos J. Hadziyannis, MD
Henry Dunant Hospital
Athens, Greece

Jorge L. Herrera, MD
University of South Alabama
Mobile, AL

Keith D. Lindor, MD
Mayo Clinic
Rochester, MN

Lance Liotta, MD, PhD
George Mason University
Manassas, VA

Arthur J. McCullough, MD
Cleveland Clinic
Cleveland, OH

John G. McHutchison, MD
Duke University Medical Center
Durham, NC

Poonam Mishra, MD
Center for Liver Diseases
Inova Fairfax Hospital
Annandale, VA

Kevin D. Mullen, MD, FRCPI
Metro Health Medical Center
Case Western Reserve University
Cleveland, OH

Steven D. Nathan, MD
Inova Lung Transplant Program,
Inova Fairfax Hospital
Falls Church, VA

Janus P. Ong, MD, MPH
Center for Liver Diseases
Inova Fairfax Hospital
Annandale, VA

Robert O'Shea, MD
Cleveland Clinic
Cleveland, OH

Emanuel Petricoin III, PhD
George Mason University
Manassas, VA

Julie Polson, MD
University of Texas at South Western
Dallas, TX

Nila Rafiq, MD
Center for Liver Diseases
Inova Fairfax Hospital
Annandale, VA

Morris Sherman, MD, PhD
University of Toronto
Toronto, ON

James K. Stoller, MD, MS
Cleveland Clinic
Cleveland, OH

Mark S. Sulkowski, MD
Johns Hopkins University
Baltimore, MD

Dimitrios Vassilopoulos, MD
Hippokration General Hospital
Athens, Greece

Jamile Wakim-Fleming, MD, FACG
Metro Health Medical Center
Cleveland, OH

Zobair M. Younossi, MD, MPH,
FACG, FACP
Center for Liver Diseases
Inova Fairfax Hospital
Annandale, VA 22003

Acute Viral Hepatitis

Janus P. Ong, MD, MPH

BACKGROUND

Acute viral hepatitis is a term that is generally given to the disease condition attributed to a group of viruses that have the propensity to infect the liver and cause necroinflammation. Although these hepatotropic viruses share a common clinical presentation, they belong to different virus families, have different modes of transmission, and differ in their propensity to lead to chronic infection (Table 1.1). Even as acute viral hepatitis remains an important public health problem in the United States, it is noteworthy that there has been and continues to be a decline in the number of new infections of hepatitis A, B, and C (Table 1.2).[1]

It is important to keep in mind that there are a number of conditions that can have a clinical presentation consistent with an acute hepatitis – elevated serum aminotransferases with variable elevations in bilirubin levels. Aside from the hepatotropic viruses, other viruses such as the herpes viruses can also lead to acute hepatitis. The differential diagnoses for acute hepatitis include alcoholic hepatitis, acute Budd-Chiari syndrome, drug-induced liver injury, shock liver, autoimmune hepatitis, biliary obstruction, and Wilson's disease (Table 1.3). A careful history and physical examination can usually point the clinician to the appropriate diagnostic evaluation to arrive at a correct diagnosis. This chapter will review the hepatotropic viruses – hepatitis A to E.

ACUTE HEPATITIS A

In 1973, Feinstone and colleagues first identified the hepatitis A virus (HAV) in the stool samples of normal volunteers who were infected with HAV and had developed acute hepatitis.[2] HAV is a nonenveloped, icosahedral particle that measures 27 nm in diameter and belongs to the hepatovirus genus within the picornavirus family of viruses.[3] It is a positive-sense RNA virus and its genome measures 7.5 kilobases in length. HAV has a single open reading frame that transcribes a polyprotein, which is then cleaved into the structural and nonstructural proteins. Although there have been four genotypes of HAV identified, there is

Table 1.1. Hepatotropic Viruses that Cause Acute Viral Hepatitis

Virus	Genome	Virus Particle	Classification	Incubation Period	Mode of Transmission	Chronic Infection
HAV	7.5 kb single-stranded RNA	27 nm	Picornavirus	15–50 days	Fecal-Oral	None
HBV	3.2 kb partially double-stranded DNA	40–42 nm	Hepadnavirus	28–70 days	Parenteral	Present
HCV	9.4 kb single-stranded RNA	40–60 nm	Flavivirus	14–84 days	Parenteral	Present
HDV	1.7 kb single-stranded RNA	36–43 nm	Deltavirus	Variable	Parenteral	Present
HEV	7.5 kb single-stranded RNA	32–34 nm	Hepevirus	15–60 days	Fecal-Oral	None

HAV – Hepatitis A Virus; HBV – Hepatitis B Virus; HCV – Hepatitis C Virus; HDV – Hepatitis D Virus; HEV – Hepatitis E Virus; kb – kilobases– nm – nanometers

Table 1.2. Estimated Number of New Infections of HAV, HBV, and HCV in the United States

	2004	2003	2002	1990–1999*	1980–1989*
Hepatitis A	56,000	61,000	73,000	310,000	254,000
Hepatitis B	60,000	73,000	79,000	140,000	259,000
Hepatitis C	26,000	28,000	29,000	67,000	232,000

*mean (per year)
Data from the CDC[1]

Table 1.3. Conditions that Can Cause Acute Hepatitis

Condition	Characteristics
Infections (e.g., Epstein-Barr virus, Cytomegalovirus, Herpes Simplex virus, Yellow fever, Leptospirosis)	Appropriate serologic tests in the setting of negative serologies for the hepatotropic viruses
Alcoholic Hepatitis	History of alcohol abuse, serum aminotransferases generally less than 10x ULN, AST:ALT ratio usually > 2
Acute Budd-Chiari Syndrome	Abdominal pain, ascites, hypercoagulable state (e.g., inherited thrombophilic disorders such as protein C or S deficiency, malignancy)
Drug induced liver injury	Recent history of intake of hepatotoxic drugs such as acetaminophen, isoniazid, or herbal agents such as kava
"Shock" liver	Recent history of hypoperfusion or "shock" or severe right-sided heart failure
Autoimmune hepatitis	Positive antinuclear antibody, anti-smooth muscle antibody, elevated gamma globulin levels
Biliary obstruction	Dilated bile ducts on ultrasound
Wilson's disease	Hemolytic anemia, Kayser-Fleischer ring, low ceruloplasmin levels, low uric acid, low alkaline phosphatase

ULN – upper limits of normal

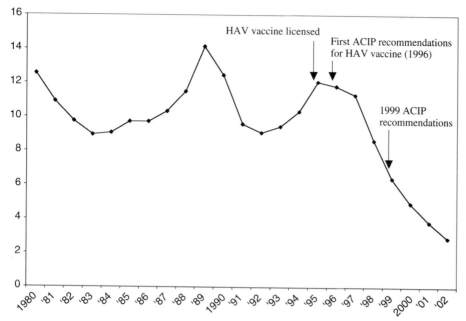

Figure 1.1. HAV Incidence, United States, 1980 to 2002. *Adapted from CDC.[1]

only one serotype and infection with one genotype confers immunity to the other genotypes.[4,5]

Epidemiology

HAV is distributed worldwide and is the most common cause of viral hepatitis. In high-prevalence areas, infection generally occurs in childhood, and immunity to HAV is almost universal in adulthood.[5] These high-prevalence areas include parts of Africa, Asia, South and Central America, and the Middle East.[6] In the United States, the incidence of HAV infection has been declining (Figure 1.1). In 2004, there were 5,683 reported cases of symptomatic HAV infection, the lowest recorded rate in four decades.[7] This corresponds to an estimated 56,000 cases of HAV infection after adjusting for underreporting and asymptomatic infection (Table 1.2). The decline in the incidence has been attributed to the availability and use of HAV vaccination (Figure 1.1).[8] Historically, the incidence of HAV infection was higher among children, men, and certain ethnic groups (e.g., American Indians); however, more recently, the rates have equalized due to the larger declines in incidence rates among children, men, and American Indians.[7]

The principal mode of transmission of HAV is through the fecal-oral route either through person-to-person contact (including sexual activity that involves contact with fecal material) or through the ingestion of contaminated food and water.[5,9] In the past, sexual or household contact with a HAV-infected person was the most frequently reported risk factor.[5,6] However, in 2004, the proportion of cases reporting this risk factor had decreased to 11% from about 20%.[7] The same trend was noted for homosexual activity as a risk factor that decreased from a high of 23% in the early 2000s to a low of 2.5% in 2004.[7] The proportion

Table 1.4. Serologic Diagnosis of Acute Viral Hepatitis

IgM Anti-HAV	HBsAg	IgM Anti-HBc	Anti-HCV	HCV-RNA	Anti-HDV	IgM Anti-HEV	Diagnosis
+	−	−	−	−	−	−	Acute HAV
−	+	+	−	−	−	−	Acute HBV
−	−	+	−	−	−	−	Acute HBV ("window period")
−	−	−	+	+	−	−	Acute HCV
−	−	−	−	+	−	−	Acute HCV, early infection
−	+	+	−	−	+	−	Acute HBV/HDV coinfection
−	+	−	−	−	+	−	Acute HDV superinfection on chronic HBV
−	−	−	−	−	−	+	Acute HEV

of cases reporting either international travel or injection drug use as a risk factor was increased in 2004 compared to previous years.[7]

Diagnosis

There are no biochemical test abnormalities that are specific for acute HAV. Significant elevations in serum aminotransferases are not uncommon in acute HAV. The height of the serum aminotransferases have no prognostic significance, however.[10] In those with the cholestatic variant and those with fulminant hepatitis, bilirubin levels are significantly elevated, often higher than 10 mg/dL.[11] Prolongation of the prothrombin time may signify severe hepatic injury and should alert the clinician to watch for signs of fulminant liver failure.

Serologic tests are available to assist in the diagnosis of acute HAV. A positive IgM anti-HAV in a patient with acute hepatitis is consistent with a diagnosis of acute HAV (Table 1.4). The IgM anti-HAV becomes detectable as early as a week after exposure and can remain positive for up to six months. IgG anti-HAV becomes detectable soon after IgM anti-HAV becomes positive. This persists indefinitely and is consistent with lifelong immunity. A positive total anti-HAV with a negative IgM anti-HAV is consistent with immunity to HAV as a result of either prior exposure to HAV or vaccination. Tests for HAV-RNA in serum and stool during HAV infection as well as genotyping of HAV are performed principally for research purposes.

Clinical Presentation

HAV causes acute hepatitis. There is no chronic infection phase in HAV infection. The clinical presentation can range from subclinical infection, where patients present with asymptomatic elevations in serum aminotransferases, to clinically symptomatic hepatitis including fulminant hepatic failure with coagulopathy and hepatic encephalopathy. The severity of clinical presentation depends on the patient's age. Children generally have asymptomatic or minimally symptomatic hepatitis whereas the majority of adults will present with symptomatic disease.[7,12] Among cases of acute HAV reported to the CDC in 2004, 72% of cases had jaundice with 33% requiring hospitalization. The mortality rate was 0.6%.[7]

In patients with typical symptomatic acute HAV infection, there is an incubation period, a preicteric phase, an icteric phase, and a convalescent phase. The incubation period averages 25 days (range 15–50 days). This is followed by the preicteric phase where patients report fever, malaise, anorexia, diarrhea, nausea and vomiting, and abdominal pain. The icteric phase is characterized by the development of jaundice and the disappearance of the prodromal symptoms. The convalescent phase is marked by the resolution of jaundice and generally occurs within 8–12 weeks of illness onset.[10]

Acute HAV accounted for 4% of 308 cases of acute liver failure in a multicenter NIH-sponsored study in the United States.[13] Among cases with HAV-related acute liver failure, 31% required liver transplantation, and 14% died.[14] A prognostic model incorporating serum ALT, creatinine, intubation, and pressors was found to have better predictive value for either transplantation or death than the King's College Criteria or the Model for Endstage Liver Disease (MELD) score.[14]

Atypical presentations of acute HAV can occur in about 10% of patients. These include an evanescent skin rash, transient arthralgias, and cutaneous vasculitis.[11] Two forms of atypical manifestations of HAV infection are important to mention to avoid diagnostic confusion and unnecessary and potentially invasive procedures. The first is a cholestatic variant of HAV infection, where patients have a prolonged period of jaundice with bilirubin levels reaching 10 mg/dL or higher accompanied by pruritus, fever, diarrhea, and weight loss.[15] In these patients, IgM anti-HAV is positive and serum aminotransferases may have returned to normal levels.[10,15] Complete resolution is the norm in this variant. Corticosteroids have been used in these patients, resulting in relief of pruritus and a more rapid decline in bilirubin levels.[15] Another variant presentation is that of relapsing hepatitis. These patients have often recovered from acute HAV only to redevelop symptoms and liver test abnormalities consistent with acute hepatitis.[16] The disease is often milder during relapse. The IgM anti-HAV is positive during the relapse.[16] Multiple relapses have been observed in some patients. Prognosis is very good, with complete recovery. The role of steroids is unclear in relapsing hepatitis A.

Liver biopsies have very little, if any, additional diagnostic value and are often not done in acute HAV. When they are available, they are usually performed in the process of investigating atypical presentations of acute HAV. In those with cholestatic hepatitis A, marked centrilobular cholestasis with bile thrombi and a periportal inflammatory infiltrate that resembles chronic hepatitis have been observed on their liver biopsy.[15,17]

Pathogenesis

After oral ingestion, the HAV virus is transported across the intestinal epithelium to the liver via the portal circulation.[3] HAV replicates in the cytoplasm of the hepatocyte and newly assembled virus is secreted either into the bloodstream or into bile, subsequently being excreted into the small intestine.

The mechanism of liver injury in acute HAV infection appears to be immune-related as the virus is not directly cytopathic. HLA-restricted, virus-specific, cytotoxic T-cells appear in the liver during acute infection and are likely responsible for both viral clearance and hepatocyte injury.[6,18] These T-cells also release cytokines such as interferon-γ. These cytokines lead to recruitment of other nonspecific, inflammatory cells to the liver, contributing to liver injury. The humoral immune response in acute HAV is robust, and neutralizing antibodies are produced, which also contribute to viral elimination. These antibodies confer lifelong immunity to reinfection.

Management

Patients with acute HAV infection should receive supportive treatment. If the patient shows signs and symptoms indicating fulminant hepatic failure, admission and early referral to a liver transplant center is necessary. There is no specific treatment or antiviral agent for HAV. For patients with prolonged cholestasis, corticosteroids can be considered. This has been shown to lead to improvement in jaundice, pruritus, and fatigue soon after initiating therapy. Forty mg of prednisone daily can be given and tapered over a four-week period.

Effective and safe hepatitis A vaccines have been available since 1995. There are two inactivated hepatitis A vaccines and one combination vaccine with hepatitis A and hepatitis B vaccine components.[19] Both single-antigen vaccines are approved for use in children and adults, whereas the combination vaccine is approved for use in adults only. The vaccines are not approved for children younger than one year of age. The hepatitis A vaccines are highly immunogenic with 94% to 100% of vaccinated persons developing protective antibody levels a month after the first dose. The two single-antigen vaccines are interchangeable, and one can be given as a booster even if it was not the vaccine used for the initial dose. The Advisory Committee on Immunization Practices (ACIP) first came out with its recommendations for prevention of HAV through immunization in 1996.[20] At that time, the target groups were those who were at high risk of acquiring the infection. In 1999, these recommendations were expanded to include children living in states with HAV infection rates that were higher than the national average.[21] In 2006, the ACIP updated its recommendation to include routine vaccination of all children older than one year old and that hepatitis A vaccine be incorporated into the routine childhood immunization schedule.[22] Table 1.5 shows the current recommendations for hepatitis A vaccination. Persons with chronic liver disease do not necessarily have an increased risk for HAV infection; however, it is recommended that they receive routine vaccination because superimposed acute HAV infection has been associated with high morbidity and mortality rates in these patients.[23–25] Prevaccination testing for immunity to HAV might be considered in populations that are expected to have high rates of prior exposure to HAV, such as adults born in or who have lived in countries with intermediate or high endemicity for HAV and adults in certain population groups (e.g., Alaska natives, illicit drug users, persons with chronic liver disease). Prevaccination testing of children is generally not recommended because of the low prevalence of infection in this group.

Once acute HAV is confirmed in a patient, postexposure prophylaxis should be instituted for close contacts who do not have a prior history of hepatitis A

Table 1.5. Recommendations for Hepatitis A Vaccination

Men who have sex with men

Persons traveling to or working in areas that have intermediate or high endemicity of HAV

Users of illicit drugs

Persons who have an occupational risk for HAV infection such as those work with HAV in research settings

Persons with clotting factor disorders

Persons with chronic liver disease

All children at age 1 year (12–23 months). Children not vaccinated at the end of 2 years can be vaccinated at subsequent visits.

From Morbidity and Mortality Weekly Report[22]

vaccination. The CDC recommends HAV immune globulin at a dose 0.02 mL/kg via the intramuscular route.[22] This should be given within two weeks of exposure, as efficacy after two weeks has not been confirmed. Hepatitis A vaccine should be given to those contacts who also have an indication for vaccination.

ACUTE HEPATITIS B

Since the discovery of the Australia antigen in the 1960s, significant advances have been made in the understanding of the molecular virology, pathogenesis of liver disease and natural history, as well as management of hepatitis B virus (HBV) infection. In particular, the last decade has seen the evolution of antiviral therapy for HBV from the use of standard interferon to the development of safe and potent oral antiviral agents.[26]

HBV is an enveloped, DNA virus measuring 40–42 nm in diameter. Its genome is a circular and partially double-stranded DNA that is 3.2 kb long. The genome has four overlapping open reading frames. Unique features of HBV include the use of reverse transcription in its life cycle and the generation of covalently closed circular (ccc) DNA. The cccDNA serves as a template for all viral mRNAs and is responsible for viral persistence in chronic HBV infection.[27,28] There are eight genotypes of HBV – A through H.[29] The genotypes differ from each other by more than 8% of their nucleotide sequence. The genotypes have a varied geographic distribution worldwide. The most common genotypes in the United States are genotypes A and C.[30] There is a strong correlation between genotype and ethnicity, with genotype A being common among white and black patients and genotypes B and C among Asians patients. In chronic HBV, differences in genotypes may affect HBeAg seroconversion rates, severity of liver disease, likelihood of development of liver cancer, as well as treatment response rates.[31] It remains unclear if HBV genotype influences the outcome of acute HBV infection.[29,32,33]

Epidemiology

Hepatitis B is a major public health problem worldwide.[34] Nearly one-third of the world's population, or 2 billion people, have been infected with HBV, with 350 million people having chronic infection.[35] The prevalence of infection varies geographically. The highest prevalence of chronic HBV infection can be found in

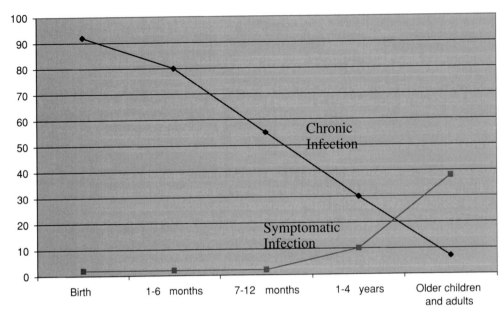

Figure 1.2. Outcome of HBV infection according to the age at infection. *Adapted from CDC.

sub-Saharan Africa, Asia, and the South Pacific region. Areas with intermediate rates of endemicity include North Africa, Southern and Eastern Europe, the Indian subcontinent, and the Amazon basin. Western Europe and the United States are considered low-prevalence regions. In the United States, the prevalence of HBV infection is 0.42%, with an estimated 1.25 million persons who are chronically infected.[1,36] The incidence of HBV infection has been declining in the United States. This has decreased from a peak of 287,000 infections per year in the 1980s to 51,000 in 2005.[1] Acute HBV infection rates are highest among persons 25–44 years old.[7] The rate of acute HBV is higher among men than women and non-Hispanic blacks have the highest rates among all racial and ethnic groups.

HBV is transmitted through contact with infected body fluids. Unlike the situation in endemic countries, where the primary mode of transmission of HBV is perinatal and close household contact, the primary modes of transmission in the United States are sexual transmission and via injecting drug abuse practices.[7,37] An important risk group in the United States is men who have sex with men.[35,37] Up to one-third of infected persons report no risk factors for HBV infection, although half of these persons have high-risk characteristics or behaviors that place them at risk for HBV infection.[37] The age at infection and the mode of transmission of HBV correlate with the likelihood of developing chronic infection. Infection in infancy and childhood, which is usually through perinatal or horizontal transmission, carries a high likelihood of developing chronic infection (60–95%) whereas infection during adulthood, which is usually through sexual transmission or injection drug use, is associated with a significantly lower risk of developing chronic infection (~5%) (Figure 1.2).[38]

The disease burden of HBV infection is significant and is mainly due to the consequences of chronic HBV infection such as liver failure and hepatocellular

carcinoma. The most catastrophic consequence of acute HBV infection is fulminant hepatitis. In the United States, HBV accounts for about 7% of all cases of
acute liver failure.[13] Among patients with HBV-related acute liver failure, 41%
went on to receive a liver transplant and 32% died.[33] Older age was the only
factor associated with a poor outcome. An interesting finding in a large series of
HBV-related acute liver failure was the association between genotype D infection
and HBV-related acute liver failure. This requires confirmation in other studies.

Diagnosis

The available serologic tests for acute HBV infection include hepatitis B surface
antigen (HBsAg), antibody to HBsAg (anti-HBs), antibody to HBcAg (anti-
HBc), and hepatitis B e antigen (HBeAg). The diagnosis of acute HBV infection
is based on the results of serologic testing performed in the appropriate clinical
scenario. In acute HBV infection, both HBsAg and IgM anti-HBc are positive
(Table 1.4). In some patients, HBsAg disappears before the development of anti-
HBs as the acute illness resolves. During this so-called window period, the IgM
anti-HBc remains positive (Table 1.4). A person with acute HBV can take one
of two clinical courses – recovery with viral clearance or persistent infection.
With viral clearance, anti-HBs appears as HBsAg disappears. Those who develop
persistent infection generally do not develop anti-HBs and have persistently
detectable HBsAg. HBeAg in acute HBV infection correlates with ongoing viral
replication. HBV-DNA testing is now available and is useful in chronic HBV
infection, especially in the monitoring of patients on antiviral therapy. In acute
HBV, HBV-DNA testing may be useful in cases with a protracted course of severe
acute hepatitis in whom antiviral therapy is being contemplated.

Clinical Presentation

The presentation of acute HBV infection can range from asymptomatic elevations in serum aminotransferases to icteric hepatitis to fulminant hepatitis.
Symptomatic infection is less likely among infants and children than in adults
(Figure 1.2). The incubation period for acute HBV infection is about 4–10 weeks.
HBsAg, the hallmark of HBV infection, becomes positive in the incubation
period. HBV-DNA is detectable at this time as well. This is followed by the
development of anti-HBc, generally coinciding with the onset of symptoms or
biochemical abnormalities with the IgM fraction appearing before IgG anti-HBc.
With clinical recovery, HBsAg disappears and anti-HBs becomes positive, con-
ferring immunity. In addition, the IgM anti-HBc becomes undetectable within
six months, whereas the IgG anti-HBc persists for life. Among acute HBV cases
reported to the CDC in 2004, 76% had jaundice and 39% were hospitalized.[7]
Clinical presentation was milder among children than in adults, with fewer
children presenting with jaundice and a lower proportion of children requiring
hospitalization. The mortality rate for acute HBV was 0.5%.

Pathogenesis

The hepatitis B virus is not directly cytotoxic. The liver injury in HBV infection is believed to be primarily the result of the immune response of the host
to the virus.[39] Virus-specific cytotoxic T lymphocytes recognize virally infected

hepatocytes and cause hepatocyte death through direct cell lysis. Other antigen-nonspecific inflammatory responses involving macrophages, NK cells, and neutrophils also contribute to the liver damage seen in acute infection.

In acute, self-limited hepatitis, studies have shown strong, polyclonal, and multispecific CD4+ and CD8+ T-cell responses to multiple epitopes of the HBV core, polymerase, and envelope proteins. On the other hand, the T-cell responses in persons with persistent infection are significantly diminished. These findings highlight the importance of cytotoxic T lymphocytes in viral clearance. Noncytolytic clearance of virus via the antiviral effects of inflammatory cytokines such as tumor necrosis factor and interferon-γ may also be important.

Management

Persons with symptomatic acute HBV infection should be provided supportive care. Prompt referral to a liver transplant center is necessary for those who develop fulminant hepatitis. Liver transplantation can be life-saving in these patients. Prevention of HBV infection is very important to decrease the burden of chronic liver disease, especially in regions of the world where the disease is endemic. Preventive measures include all the traditional activities for a parenterally transmitted agent such as screening of blood and blood products and risk reduction counseling. By far, however, immunization is the single most effective preventive measure for HBV infection. The use of hepatitis B vaccine has resulted in dramatic reductions in HBV infection rates and hepatocellular carcinoma among children in Taiwan, an achievement considered a "milestone in the annals of preventive medicine."[40,41] There are currently two licensed single-antigen hepatitis B vaccines and three licensed combination vaccines. Hepatitis B vaccine efficacy is as high as 95%. Several factors may affect vaccine response rates, including older age, obesity, male gender, smoking, and immunodeficiency.[19] At the present time, the immunization strategy to eliminate transmission of HBV in the United States includes (1) universal vaccination of infants beginning at birth, (2) prevention of perinatal HBV infection through routine screening of all pregnant women for HBsAg and immunoprophylaxis of infants born to HBsAg-positive women and to women whose HBsAg status is unknown, (3) routine vaccination of previously unvaccinated children and adolescents, and (4) vaccination of previously unvaccinated adults at increased risk for infection.[42] The ACIP recently updated its recommendations for hepatitis B vaccination of adults (Table 1.6).[43]

Immunoprophylaxis for children born to HBsAg-positive mothers should include hepatitis B vaccine and hepatitis B immune globulin (HBIG) within 12 hours of birth.[42] Those born to mothers whose HBsAg status is unknown should receive hepatitis B vaccine within 12 hours of birth. Testing for HBV should be done on the mother and HBIG should be given within seven days if the mother is found to be HBsAg-positive.[42]

Antiviral therapy for acute HBV has been undertaken in several studies either as a strategy to prevent fulminant hepatitis or death or to prevent the evolution to chronic HBV.[44] Most of the studies have been small, have lacked controls, and have heterogeneous patient populations.[44–46] A recent publication showed that of 17 patients with severe acute or fulminant hepatitis given lamivudine, 14, or 82%, recovered and did not need liver transplantation.[47] This compared

Table 1.6. Recommendations for Adults who Should Receive the HBV Vaccine

Persons at increased risk for infection by sexual exposure
- Sex partners of HBsAg-positive persons
- Sexually active persons who are not in a long-term, mutually monogamous relationship (e.g., persons with more than one sex partner during the previous 6 months)
- Persons seeking evaluation or treatment for a sexually transmitted disease
- Men who have sex with men

Persons at increased risk for infection by percutaneous or mucosal exposure to blood
- Current or recent injection-drug users
- Household contacts of HBsAg-positive persons
- Residents and staff of facilities for developmentally disabled persons
- Health care and public safety workers with reasonably anticipated risk for exposure to blood or blood-contaminated body fluids
- Persons with end-stage renal disease, including predialysis, hemodialysis, peritoneal dialysis, and home dialysis patients

Others
- International travelers to regions with high or intermediate levels of endemic HBV infection
- Persons with chronic liver disease
- Persons with HIV infection
- All other persons seeking protection from HBV infection

From Morbidity and Mortality Weekly Report[43]

very favorably against historical controls, among whom only 20% recovered. At this time, the utility of antiviral therapy in those with severe acute hepatitis needs further evaluation; however, it seems appropriate to recommend starting antiviral therapy in patients with fulminant hepatitis B as this may allow some patients to avoid liver transplantation and for those that eventually go on to need liver transplantation, antiviral therapy can decrease HBV viral load before transplant, thus decreasing the likelihood of post-transplant recurrence of HBV. Antiviral therapy with interferon in acute HBV was not shown to prevent the progression to chronic HBV in a placebo-controlled study; therefore the routine use of antiviral therapy in mild acute HBV is not recommended.[48]

ACUTE HEPATITIS C

Hepatitis C virus (HCV) infection is the most common blood-borne infection in the United States. Although the number of new infections has significantly decreased, the prevalence of chronic infection remains the same. More importantly, HCV remains the leading indication for liver transplantation in the United States today. The burden of chronic liver disease from HCV is expected to continue to rise in the next decade.[49]

The hepatitis C virus was discovered in 1989.[50] Its discovery has been hailed as a scientific tour de force as it marked the first time that an infectious agent was identified, using direct molecular cloning, despite very little knowledge of the nature of the agent. It is a small, enveloped single-stranded, positive-sense RNA virus.[51] There are at least six genotypes that differ from each other by about 30% of their nucleotide sequence. The most common genotypes in the United States are genotypes 1, 2, and 3.[52] HCV genotypes differ in their response to antiviral therapy with higher response rates observed with genotypes 2 and 3 than with genotype 1.

Epidemiology

HCV is endemic worldwide, although there is variability in its geographic distribution. There are an estimated 170 million persons infected worldwide. The highest prevalence of infection is seen in Africa and parts of Asia. In the United States, a recent report using data from the National Health and Nutrition Examination Survey (NHANES) 1999 to 2002 showed that 1.6% of Americans, or 4.1 million, are positive for antibodies to HCV.[53] Approximately 3.2 million persons are positive for HCV-RNA and are chronically infected with HCV. Because the NHANES does not include institutionalized persons, a population with a higher prevalence of HCV infection, the exact prevalence of HCV infection could actually be higher. More men than women are infected. The peak prevalence of infection was observed among those 40–49 years of age.[53]

The incidence of HCV infection is more difficult to determine because acute HCV infections are often asymptomatic. However, both mathematical modeling and surveillance program reports show that the number of new cases of HCV infection has been declining (Table 1.2).[54,55] The decline is largely attributed to the decline among injection drug users and the decline in cases of transfusion-associated hepatitis C.[56]

HCV is transmitted mainly through the parenteral route. In the United States, the leading risk factor for HCV infection remains injection drug use.[56] Blood transfusion has become a very uncommon source of HCV infection. Other risk factors include sex with an infected partner, multiple heterosexual partners, occupational exposure, and birth to an infected mother. In up to 10% of HCV-infected persons, a risk factor cannot be identified.[57] The relative importance of such percutaneous exposures as tattooing or body piercing as risk factors for HCV infection requires further study.

Diagnosis

Acute HCV is an uncommon diagnosis not only because the incidence has been on the decline but also because most patients with acute HCV are asymptomatic or have very mild symptoms and the illness will often run its course without the patient ever seeing a healthcare professional.[58]

The diagnosis of acute HCV should be considered in a patient who presents with signs and symptoms of acute hepatitis and a risk factor for HCV infection. Unlike acute HAV or HBV, where the detection of the IgM fraction of either anti-HAV or anti-HBc respectively indicates acute infection, there is no specific test for acute HCV. In the strictest sense, the diagnosis of acute HCV requires that a patient have undetectable HCV-RNA at the time of exposure with the subsequent development of viremia followed by antibody seroconversion.[59] However, the usual setting found in clinical practice is either a positive HCV-RNA or anti-HCV in a patient with clinical hepatitis and a recent history of exposure (Table 1.4).

The test that becomes positive earliest after acute HCV infection is the HCV-RNA. Viremia occurs within two weeks of infection.[58] Tests for viremia include commercially available sensitive PCR-based assays that have limits of detection as low as 50 IU/ml.[52,60] It is important to note that a characteristic of acute HCV infection is fluctuating as well as relatively low HCV-RNA levels compared to chronically infected persons.[60] A single negative HCV-RNA test therefore does not rule out HCV infection. Tests for antibodies to HCV become positive starting about eight weeks after infection.[60] A few patients never undergo antibody seroconversion during acute HCV infection (for more details regarding HCV testing, please see Chapter 3).

Clinical Presentation

The majority of patients with acute hepatitis C are asymptomatic. Those who present to the healthcare setting have symptoms and signs very similar to those with other forms of acute viral hepatitis. Fulminant hepatitis, however, is an uncommon occurrence.[61] There were no HCV-related cases of acute liver failure in 308 cases reported from the 17 centers in the United States Acute Liver Failure Study Group over a period of 41 months.[13]

In a typical case of acute HCV, the incubation period averages seven weeks with a range of 2–12 weeks.[50,62] The patients then develop nonspecific symptoms of malaise, nausea, right upper-quadrant pain, low-grade fever, and anorexia. This is followed by the development of jaundice and dark urine. The period of convalescence is marked by the gradual resolution of anorexia and jaundice. HCV-RNA, as noted earlier, becomes detectable within two weeks of infection as early as the preicteric phase of the acute illness. Anti-HCV by enzyme immunoassay becomes detectable at the time of onset of jaundice.

One of the features of acute HCV infection is the high proportion of cases that go on to develop persistent infection. Acute HCV progresses to chronic infection in 55–90% of patients. Younger age and female gender are associated with lower rates of chronic infection.[63] Immunodeficiency is associated with higher rates of chronic infection.[64] Patients who develop symptomatic disease during the acute infection have been observed to have a lower likelihood of developing chronic infection, suggesting that a robust immune response may a play a role in viral clearance in acute HCV.

Liver biopsies in patients with acute HCV have rarely been performed. Liver cell injury with ballooning degeneration, spotty necrosis, and apoptosis is found, which is similar to the acute injury noted in other forms of acute viral hepatitis. Confluent or bridging necrosis can be observed in more severe cases.

Pathogenesis

The development of persistent infection after acute HCV is a frequent occurrence, and the exact reasons are still being worked out. The likelihood of developing persistent infection may depend on viral dynamics as well as the host immune response during the acute phase of infection. Viral quasispecies and its evolution have been evaluated as a reason, and it appears that the development of persistent infection is associated with an increase in quasispecies diversity.[65] The host immune response to HCV infection is likely to play a role in determining between viral clearance or development of chronic infection. Persons with acute self-limited HCV infection display a vigorous and multispecific T-cell response to HCV antigens as well as a Th1 cytokine profile.[66]

Table 1.7. CDC Guidelines for Management of Occupational Exposure to HCV

Test source for HCV
Test a person exposed to HCV-positive source for:

- ALT and anti-HCV at baseline and,
- Follow-up ALT and anti-HCV at 4 to 6 months
- HCV-RNA testing may be performed at 4 weeks if earlier diagnosis is required

From Morbidity and Mortality Weekly Report[66]

Management

As with any patient with acute viral hepatitis, a patient with acute HCV should receive appropriate supportive care. In the United States, HCV transmission through either blood transfusion or organ transplantation has virtually been eliminated. Preventive efforts should now concentrate on reducing the risk of transmission of HCV in other high-risk groups such as injection drug users. Although nosocomial transmission is uncommon, the risk is finite, and thus infection-control procedures in healthcare settings should be in place. Occupational transmission of HCV is uncommon, with an incidence of 1.8%. The CDC recommends that each institution have its own policies in place for testing for HCV after percutaneous or permucosal exposures to HCV.[67] The management of persons exposed to HCV is shown in Table 1.7. Postexposure counseling should be given to exposed persons. There are no restrictions to activity, although exposed persons are advised to refrain from donating blood or tissue during the follow-up period. Antiviral agents and immune globulin are currently not recommended for post-exposure prophylaxis in persons exposed to HCV-positive blood. Patients diagnosed with acute HCV infection should be referred to an appropriate specialist for consideration for antiviral therapy.

Because HCV infection is common and most patients are asymptomatic, testing for HCV should be offered to persons who are likely to be infected and to those who express a desire to be tested. The CDC recommendations for screening for HCV are shown in Table 1.8. Those who test positive should be offered counseling and follow-up. This can prevent HCV transmission as well as identify persons who will need regular follow-up or consideration for antiviral therapy.

Specific therapy in the form of antiviral therapy has been advocated in acute HCV infection for the rationale of preventing the progression to persistent infection and its attendant liver-related complications. The National Institutes of Health Consensus Statement on HCV in 2002 stated that treatment of acute HCV is warranted.[68] However, the treatment of acute hepatitis C has remained a matter of debate. The evidence from clinical trials shows that treatment of acute HCV is associated with higher rates of viral clearance when compared with no treatment. This makes a persuasive argument for treatment in patients who do not otherwise have contraindications to antiviral therapy.

The main issues with antiviral therapy in acute HCV include the optimal timing of initiation of therapy, the antiviral regimen and dose to use, and the

---

Table 1.8. Persons for whom Routine HCV Testing is Recommended

Persons who ever injected illegal drugs, including those who injected even just once or a few times many years ago.

Persons who received a blood transfusion or organ transplant before July 1992.

Persons who received clotting factor concentrates before 1987.

Persons who were ever on long-term dialysis.

Children born to HCV-positive women*

Healthcare, emergency medical, and public safety workers after needlesticks, sharps, or mucosal exposures to HCV-positive blood.

Persons with evidence of chronic liver disease

*Testing of children born to HCV-positive mothers should be delayed until about 18 months of age to avoid confusion as passively transferred maternal anti-HCV may still be detectable if testing is done earlier.

From Morbidity and Mortality Weekly Report[66]

---

duration of treatment. With respect to the optimal timing of treatment initiation, twelve weeks after infection has been suggested by most experts as the ideal time to start antiviral therapy.[58] This permits the identification of those who will spontaneously clear the virus thus sparing them the cost and side effects of antiviral therapy without compromising antiviral efficacy.[69,70] A recent study using pegylated interferon alfa-2b for 12 weeks, initiation of treatment at 8–12 weeks resulted in higher response rates than initiation of treatment at week 20. The authors did note that patients with high viral load and genotype 1 infection might need to be treated at week 8 or earlier.[71]

The early trials on treatment of acute HCV employed the use of standard interferon. Several meta-analyses have shown that treatment with standard interferon resulted in higher rates of viral clearance compared to no treatment. These studies also showed that higher doses led to higher response rates. Pegylated interferons are now available that allow more convenient dosing and are the current standard of care in antiviral therapy for chronic hepatitis C in combination with ribavirin. Several studies have evaluated the use of pegylated interferon (1.5 µg/kg/week for 8–24 weeks) in acute HCV with sustained virologic response rates as high as 93–95%.[71–75] The addition of ribavirin to pegylated interferon does not appear to enhance response rates in acute HCV infection.[75]

Because of the costs and adverse effects associated with antiviral therapy for HCV, an important issue is the duration of therapy. Early studies used varying lengths of therapy ranging from 4–24 weeks. A recent study specifically addressed the issue of treatment duration using pegylated interferon monotherapy. This study found that optimal duration of therapy appears to be dependent on genotype. A treatment duration of 8–12 weeks may be appropriate for genotype non-1 patients whereas genotype 1 patients would require at least 24 weeks of treatment.[74]

The recent practice guideline on the diagnosis, management, and treatment of HCV from the American Association for the Study of Liver Diseases considers it appropriate to treat acute HCV with pegylated interferon initiated 8–16 weeks after onset of infection and continued for 24 weeks.[76] The guideline also suggested that a shorter duration of treatment might be appropriate for genotype non-1 patients although this requires confirmation.

ACUTE HEPATITIS D

Hepatitis D virus (HDV) is unique among the hepatitis viruses as it is totally dependent on the presence of another hepatitis virus, the hepatitis B virus, for its assembly and propagation. HDV infection therefore requires either simultaneous infection or pre-existing infection with HBV.

The virus was discovered in 1977 when investigators noted a novel nuclear antigen by immunofluorescense in the liver biopsies of patients with chronic HBV.[77] This novel antigen was termed delta antigen and later turned out to be a specific marker for HDV. HDV is a small, enveloped virus measuring 36–43 nm in diameter. Within the nucleocapsid are the viral genome and the hepatitis delta antigen (HDAg). The HDV genome was successfully cloned and sequenced in 1986.[78] The HDV genome consists of a single, minus-strand circular RNA about 1.7 kilobases in length. There are at least three genotypes of HDV that have a varying worldwide distribution.[79] Genotype I is found in the United States and Europe, genotype II in Japan and Taiwan, and genotype III in South America. Genotype II has been associated with milder forms of liver disease whereas genotype I has been associated with more severe liver disease.

Epidemiology

HDV is found worldwide although its geographic distribution varies. HDV is endemic in the Mediterranean, some countries in Eastern Europe, Africa, and South America. It is estimated that 5% of the chronic HBV carriers worldwide are also infected with HDV amounting to about 15 million persons.[80] In some Mediterranean countries, it has been reported that there appears to be a decline in the prevalence of HDV infections.[81] This has been attributed to the combined effects of universal HBV vaccination, HIV control measures, and socioeconomic improvements.[82] Outbreaks of HDV however have been reported in some parts of the world with a high proportion of cases of fulminant hepatitis.[83,84]

The modes of transmission are very similar to those for HBV. The principal mode of transmission is percutaneous exposure. In the United States, HDV is confined to intravenous drug users and persons who have received multiple transfusions. Other modes of transmission include sexual transmission and intrafamilial spread.[85,86] Perinatal transmission is very uncommon.

Diagnosis

The diagnosis of HDV infection should be suspected in a patient with fulminant hepatitis and in a patient with chronic HBV who has rapidly progressive liver disease or has an acute flare in the absence of active HBV replication. With the advent of molecular techniques, the armamentarium of tests for HDV has also expanded. The most useful test is the test for the presence of HDV-RNA in serum by PCR. It is useful especially in cases where the infection is very early and antibody seroconversion has not occurred. This test is also useful in the monitoring of patients who are on antiviral therapy. The HDV-RNA test however may not be available in commercial laboratories and in that case, testing for antibodies to the HDAg can be used. In acute HDV infection, IgM anti-HDV becomes positive and disappears unless the infection becomes chronic. In chronic HDV infection, both IgM and IgG anti-HDV remain elevated. The titers of IgM anti-HDV correlate with HDV replication; in fact, the disappearance of IgM anti-HDV signifies resolution of chronic HDV infection.

Clinical Presentation

HDV infection requires the presence of HBV infection. Two patterns of acute HDV infection have been described. One pattern is HDV/HBV simultaneous coinfection and the other is superinfection with HDV in a patient with chronic HBV infection.[80] The two patterns of infection differ mainly in their propensity to result in chronic HDV infection. Chronic HDV infection is more commonly seen with superinfection.

Simultaneous HDV/HBV coinfection occurs in a patient who is naïve for both HDV and HBV. The presentation may range from a mild acute hepatitis to fulminant hepatitis. The clinical manifestations are similar to those with acute HBV infection and the majority of patients have complete recovery with only a very small proportion developing chronic infection. To make a diagnosis of simultaneous HDV/HBV coinfection, IgM anti-HBc should be positive together with a positive IgM anti-HDV (Table 1.4).

Superinfection with HDV in a patient with chronic HBV usually presents as a severe hepatitis flare. In some cases, the clinical course may be fulminant. Majority of chronic HBV patients with superimposed HDV develop chronic HDV and most will go on to have progressive liver disease. Diagnosis of super-infection is made when markers for HDV are positive and IgM anti-HBc is negative (Table 1.4). In some patients, superinfection can lead to clearance of HBsAg.

Patients who develop chronic HDV infection can develop rapidly progressive liver disease with reports of cirrhosis developing in up to 70% of patients. Patients with cirrhosis can develop liver failure or hepatocellular carcinoma.

Pathogenesis

At the present time, the pathogenesis of liver injury in HDV infection is not clearly understood. Studies have shown that HDV may be directly cytotoxic however, studies in transgenic mice showed that the expression of HDAg failed to elicit significant liver injury.[87,88] The contribution of the immune response to the pathogenesis of liver injury was evaluated in chronic HBV patients with HDV superinfection. In these patients, HDAg-specific T-cell responses in peripheral blood were noted among patients with inactive liver disease (i.e., normal ALT and undetectable IgM anti-HEV) and not in those with active liver disease. The authors postulated that in those with active liver disease, HDAg-specific T-cells could be compartmentalized in the liver and thus are not detectable in peripheral blood.[89]

Management

In patients with acute HDV infection, there is no specific therapy. Supportive care should be provided. Those with fulminant hepatitis should be managed in an intensive care setting and referral to a liver transplant center should be made. At the present time, the only effective treatment for chronic HDV is high dose interferon (9 MU thrice weekly or 5MU daily) for one year.[90,91] Nucleoside analogues, such as lamivudine, have not been shown to be effective.[92] Long-term treatment is recommended for responders to prevent relapse. Liver transplantation is the only option for those who have fulminant hepatitis or decompensated liver disease. After liver transplantation, reinfection with HBV/HDV can be prevented by hepatitis B immune globulin.

ACUTE HEPATITIS E

In the early 1980s, hepatitis E was known as enterically transmitted non-A, non-B hepatitis when testing of stored serum samples of persons affected during large waterborne epidemics of infectious hepatitis showed no serologic evidence for either hepatitis A or B.[93,94] Discovery of virus-like particles in the stool of a human volunteer who developed clinical acute hepatitis after ingesting a pooled extract of fecal material from patients with enterically transmitted non-A, non-B hepatitis suggested that a new viral hepatitis agent was responsible for the acute hepatitis.[95] The virus was successfully cloned and sequenced in the early 1990s and became known as hepatitis E virus (HEV).[96,97]

HEV is a small (32 to 34 nm in diameter) nonenveloped single-stranded, positive sense RNA virus. Its genome is ∼7.5 kilobases long and contains three overlapping reading frames.[98] Analysis of genomes of strains from different geographical regions reveal four genotypes of HEV.[99,100]

Epidemiology

HEV is endemic in developing countries where large outbreaks involving several thousand persons occur. Epidemics have occurred in India, Southeast and Central Asia, and Africa.[101] During epidemics, the highest attack rates occur in persons between the ages of 15–40 years. There is a lower attack rate among children who may have a higher frequency of subclinical infection. Men are more likely to be affected than women although high attack rates are seen among pregnant women. HEV causes sporadic hepatitis in both endemic and nonendemic areas. Sporadic hepatitis cases occur more frequently in endemic areas than in nonendemic areas. In nonendemic areas, cases of HEV are mainly limited to travelers to disease-endemic areas.[102]

Transmission of the virus is through the fecal-oral route usually via contaminated water. Person-to-person transmission can occur but is insignificant.[103] Vertical transmission of HEV has been reported.[104] There is no evidence of transmission of HEV through sexual contact or blood transfusion.[102] HEV can be isolated from animals such as swine and rodents and these isolates appear to be phylogenetically related to human HEV.[105] These data suggest that animals might act as reservoirs of HEV infection and that HEV may be a zoonotic disease especially in nonendemic countries. This hypothesis however still requires confirmation.[102]

Diagnosis

At present, the laboratory tests for the diagnosis of HEV infection include serologic assays for the detection of anti-HEV antibodies by enzyme immunoassay (EIA) and RT-PCR for the detection of virus in serum or stool.

There are currently no approved tests for HEV; however, serologic assays may be available through commercial laboratories. The presence of IgM anti-HEV during the icteric phase of acute hepatitis indicates acute infection with HEV (Table 1.4). The IgG anti-HEV appears soon after the appearance of the IgM anti-HEV and persists into the convalescent phase. The presence of IgG anti-HEV in the absence of IgM anti-HEV indicates either convalescence or past infection. Detection of genomic sequences of HEV in stool or serum can be performed by RT-PCR but these tests are limited to research laboratories at this time.

Clinical Presentation

HEV causes a self-limited, acute, icteric disease similar to hepatitis A and has a variable clinical presentation ranging from subclinical infection to fulminant hepatitis.[106] The incubation period ranges from 15–60 days with an average of 40 days. Acute icteric hepatitis starts with a prodrome of flu-like symptoms followed by the appearance of jaundice, dark-colored urine, and light-colored stools. During this time, patients may have hepatomegaly and splenomegaly in addition to jaundice and abnormal liver-associated tests, in particular marked elevations in serum aminotransferases as well as variable degree of hyperbilirubinemia. During the convalescent phase, jaundice dissipates and all the liver test abnormalities normalize in all patients.[106] The acute infection does not lead to chronic infection, cirrhosis, or liver cancer. A cholestatic variant, similar to that for HAV, has been described.[102]

A small proportion of patients with acute HEV develop fulminant hepatitis. This appears to be more common among pregnant women, especially those in the last trimester of pregnancy.[107] In addition, patients with underlying chronic liver disease can develop severe decompensation if they develop a superinfection with HEV which can lead to increased morbidity or mortality.[108]

HEV infection leads to histologic features characteristic of acute hepatitis such as lobular inflammation with ballooned hepatocytes and acidophilic bodies.[94] Portal tracts show a predominantly mononuclear inflammatory infiltrate. Those patients with cholestatic hepatitis may show striking canalicular stasis and glandlike transformation of hepatocytes whereas those with fulminant hepatitis may show panacinar necrosis with collapse of hepatic parenchyma.[94]

Pathogenesis

In acute HEV infection, HEV-RNA can be detected in both stool and serum samples before the onset of illness and can persist for several weeks. The development of antibodies to HEV coincides with the rise in serum aminotransferases and onset of symptoms suggesting that the hepatic injury in HEV is immune-mediated. IgM anti-HEV is detected first and IgG anti-HEV appears a few days after. IgG anti-HEV has been shown to persist for up to 14 years and is believed to offer protection against subsequent infection.[109] The pathogenetic basis for the severe disease among pregnant women is not currently known.

Management

There is no specific therapy for acute hepatitis E. Prevention of infection in endemic areas should include measures to provide a safe water supply and proper personal hygiene practices. Patients with symptomatic disease should be given supportive care. In an epidemic, it is important that steps be taken to prevent the development of new cases in particular by ensuring a clean water supply through proper sewage disposal. Because person-to-person transmission is uncommon, isolation of infected persons is not necessary. The role of immune serum globulin is unclear at this time. Studies have not shown significant decreases in cases with pre- and post-exposure prophylaxis.[110,111] Vaccines for HEV are not available but are currently under development.

REFERENCES

1. Centers for Disease Control. Disease Burden from Hepatitis A, B, and C in the Unites States. Volume 2006.
2. Feinstone SM, Kapikian AZ, Purceli RH. Hepatitis A: detection by immune electron microscopy of a viruslike antigen associated with acute illness. Science 1973;182: 1026–8.
3. Martin A, Lemon SM. Hepatitis A virus: from discovery to vaccines. Hepatology 2006;43:S164–72.
4. Costa-Mattioli M, Di Napoli A, Ferre V, Billaudel S, Perez-Bercoff R, Cristina J. Genetic variability of hepatitis A virus. J Gen Virol 2003;84:3191–201.
5. Koff RS. Hepatitis A. Lancet 1998;351:1643–9.
6. Kemmer NM, Miskovsky EP. Hepatitis A. Infect Dis Clin North Am 2000;14:605–15.
7. Centers for Disease Control. Hepatitis Surveillance. Volume 2006.
8. Wasley A, Fiore A, Bell BP. Hepatitis a in the era of vaccination. Epidemiol Rev 2006;28:101–11.
9. Brundage SC, Fitzpatrick AN. Hepatitis A. Am Fam Physician 2006;73:2162–8.
10. Tong MJ, el-Farra NS, Grew MI. Clinical manifestations of hepatitis A: recent experience in a community teaching hospital. J Infect Dis 1995;171 Suppl 1:S15–8.
11. Schiff ER. Atypical clinical manifestations of hepatitis A. Vaccine 1992;10 Suppl 1: S18–20.
12. Romero R, Lavine JE. Viral hepatitis in children. Semin Liver Dis 1994;14:289–302.
13. Ostapowicz G, Fontana RJ, Schiodt FV, Larson A, Davern TJ, Han SH, McCashland TM, Shakil AO, Hay JE, Hynan L, Crippin JS, Blei AT, Samuel G, Reisch J, Lee WM. Results of a prospective study of acute liver failure at 17 tertiary care centers in the United States. Ann Intern Med 2002;137:947–54.
14. Taylor RM, Davern T, Munoz S, Han SH, McGuire B, Larson AM, Hynan L, Lee WM, Fontana RJ. Fulminant hepatitis A virus infection in the United States: Incidence, prognosis, and outcomes. Hepatology 2006;44:1589–97.
15. Gordon SC, Reddy KR, Schiff L, Schiff ER. Prolonged intrahepatic cholestasis secondary to acute hepatitis A. Ann Intern Med 1984;101:635–7.
16. Glikson M, Galun E, Oren R, Tur-Kaspa R, Shouval D. Relapsing hepatitis A. Review of 14 cases and literature survey. Medicine (Baltimore) 1992;71:14–23.

17. Sciot R, Van Damme B, Desmet VJ. Cholestatic features in hepatitis A. J Hepatol 1986;3:172–81.
18. Vallbracht A, Maier K, Stierhof YD, Wiedmann KH, Flehmig B, Fleischer B. Liver-derived cytotoxic T cells in hepatitis A virus infection. J Infect Dis 1989;160:209–17.
19. Davis JP. Experience with hepatitis A and B vaccines. Am J Med 2005;118 Suppl 10A:7S-15S.
20. Prevention of hepatitis A through active or passive immunization: Recommendations of the Advisory Committee on Immunization Practices (ACIP). MMWR Recomm Rep 1996;45:1–30.
21. Prevention of hepatitis A through active or passive immunization: Recommendations of the Advisory Committee on Immunization Practices (ACIP). MMWR Recomm Rep 1999;48:1–37.
22. Fiore AE, Wasley A, Bell BP. Prevention of hepatitis A through active or passive immunization: recommendations of the Advisory Committee on Immunization Practices (ACIP). MMWR Recomm Rep 2006;55:1–23.
23. Akriviadis EA, Redeker AG. Fulminant hepatitis A in intravenous drug users with chronic liver disease. Ann Intern Med 1989;110:838–9.
24. Vento S, Garofano T, Renzini C, Cainelli F, Casali F, Ghironzi G, Ferraro T, Concia E. Fulminant hepatitis associated with hepatitis A virus superinfection in patients with chronic hepatitis C. N Engl J Med 1998;338:286–90.
25. Keeffe EB. Is hepatitis A more severe in patients with chronic hepatitis B and other chronic liver diseases? Am J Gastroenterol 1995;90:201–5.
26. Perrillo RP. Current treatment of chronic hepatitis B: benefits and limitations. Semin Liver Dis 2005;25 Suppl 1:20–8.
27. Werle-Lapostolle B, Bowden S, Locarnini S, Wursthorn K, Petersen J, Lau G, Trepo C, Marcellin P, Goodman Z, Delaney WEt, Xiong S, Brosgart CL, Chen SS, Gibbs CS, Zoulim F. Persistence of cccDNA during the natural history of chronic hepatitis B and decline during adefovir dipivoxil therapy. Gastroenterology 2004;126:1750–8.
28. Locarnini S. Molecular virology and the development of resistant mutants: implications for therapy. Semin Liver Dis 2005;25 Suppl 1:9–19.
29. Schaefer S. Hepatitis B virus: significance of genotypes. J Viral Hepat 2005;12:111–24.
30. Chu CJ, Keeffe EB, Han SH, Perrillo RP, Min AD, Soldevila-Pico C, Carey W, Brown RS, Jr., Luketic VA, Terrault N, Lok AS. Hepatitis B virus genotypes in the United States: results of a nationwide study. Gastroenterology 2003;125:444–51.
31. Fung SK, Lok AS. Hepatitis B virus genotypes: do they play a role in the outcome of HBV infection? Hepatology 2004;40:790–2.
32. Garfein RS, Bower WA, Loney CM, Hutin YJ, Xia GL, Jawanda J, Groom AV, Nainan OV, Murphy JS, Bell BP. Factors associated with fulminant liver failure during an outbreak among injection drug users with acute hepatitis B. Hepatology 2004;40:865–73.
33. Wai CT, Fontana RJ, Polson J, Hussain M, Shakil AO, Han SH, Davern TJ, Lee WM, Lok AS. Clinical outcome and virological characteristics of hepatitis B-related acute liver failure in the United States. J Viral Hepat 2005;12:192–8.
34. Lavanchy D. Hepatitis B virus epidemiology, disease burden, treatment, and current and emerging prevention and control measures. J Viral Hepat 2004;11:97–107.
35. Alter MJ. Epidemiology and prevention of hepatitis B. Semin Liver Dis 2003;23:39–46.
36. McQuillan GM, Coleman PJ, Kruszon-Moran D, Moyer LA, Lambert SB, Margolis HS. Prevalence of hepatitis B virus infection in the United States: the National Health and Nutrition Examination Surveys, 1976 through 1994. Am J Public Health 1999;89:14–8.
37. Goldstein ST, Alter MJ, Williams IT, Moyer LA, Judson FN, Mottram K, Fleenor M, Ryder PL, Margolis HS. Incidence and risk factors for acute hepatitis B in the United States, 1982–1998: implications for vaccination programs. J Infect Dis 2002;185:713–9.
38. McMahon BJ. Epidemiology and natural history of hepatitis B. Semin Liver Dis 2005;25 Suppl 1:3–8.

39. Ganem D, Prince AM. Hepatitis B virus infection–natural history and clinical conse-quences. N Engl J Med 2004;350:1118–29.

40. Zuckerman AJ. Prevention of primary liver cancer by immunization. N Engl J Med 1997;336:1906–7.

41. Chang MH, Chen CJ, Lai MS, Hsu HM, Wu TC, Kong MS, Liang DC, Shau WY, Chen DS. Universal hepatitis B vaccination in Taiwan and the incidence of hepatocellular carcinoma in children. Taiwan Childhood Hepatoma Study Group. N Engl J Med 1997;336:1855–9.

42. Mast EE, Margolis HS, Fiore AE, Brink EW, Goldstein ST, Wang SA, Moyer LA, Bell BP, Alter MJ. A comprehensive immunization strategy to eliminate transmission of hepatitis B virus infection in the United States: recommendations of the Advisory Com-mittee on Immunization Practices (ACIP) part 1: immunization of infants, children, and adolescents. MMWR Recomm Rep 2005;54:1–31.

43. Mast EE, Weinbaum CM, Fiore AE, Alter MJ, Bell BP, Finelli L, Rodewald LE, Douglas JM, Jr., Janssen RS, Ward JW. A comprehensive immunization strategy to eliminate transmission of hepatitis B virus infection in the United States: recommendations of the Advisory Committee on Immunization Practices (ACIP) Part II: immunization of adults. MMWR Recomm Rep 2006;55:1–33; quiz CE1–4.

44. Schmilovitz-Weiss H, Ben-Ari Z, Sikuler E, Zuckerman E, Sbeit W, Ackerman Z, Safadi R, Lurie Y, Rosner G, Tur-Kaspa R, Reshef R. Lamivudine treatment for acute severe hepatitis B: a pilot study. Liver Int 2004;24:547–51.

45. Torii N, Hasegawa K, Ogawa M, Hashimo E, Hayashi N. Effectiveness and long-term outcome of lamivudine therapy for acute hepatitis B. Hepatol Res 2002;24:34.

46. Kondili LA, Osman H, Mutimer D. The use of lamivudine for patients with acute hepatitis B (a series of cases). J Viral Hepat 2004;11:427–31.

47. Tillmann HL, Hadem J, Leifeld L, Zachou K, Canbay A, Eisenbach C, Graziadei I, Encke J, Schmidt H, Vogel W, Schneider A, Spengler U, Gerken G, Dalekos GN, Wedemeyer H, Manns MP. Safety and efficacy of lamivudine in patients with severe acute or fulminant hepatitis B, a multicenter experience. J Viral Hepat 2006;13:256–63.

48. Tassopoulos NC, Koutelou MG, Polychronaki H, Paraloglou-Ioannides M, Hadziyan-nis SJ. Recombinant interferon-alpha therapy for acute hepatitis B: a randomized, double-blind, placebo-controlled trial. J Viral Hepat 1997;4:387–94.

49. Davis GL, Albright JE, Cook SF, Rosenberg DM. Projecting future complications of chronic hepatitis C in the United States. Liver Transpl 2003;9:331–8.

50. Lauer GM, Walker BD. Hepatitis C virus infection. N Engl J Med 2001;345:41–52.

51. Thomson BJ, Finch RG. Hepatitis C virus infection. Clin Microbiol Infect 2005;11:86–94.

52. Carey W. Tests and screening strategies for the diagnosis of hepatitis C. Cleve Clin J Med 2003;70 Suppl 4:S7–13.

53. Armstrong GL, Wasley A, Simard EP, McQuillan GM, Kuhnert WL, Alter MJ. The prevalence of hepatitis C virus infection in the United States, 1999 through 2002. Ann Intern Med 2006;144:705–14.

54. Armstrong GL, Alter MJ, McQuillan GM, Margolis HS. The past incidence of hepatitis C virus infection: implications for the future burden of chronic liver disease in the United States. Hepatology 2000;31:777–82.

55. Williams I. Epidemiology of hepatitis C in the United States. Am J Med 1999;107:2S-9S.

56. Alter MJ. Prevention of spread of hepatitis C. Hepatology 2002;36:S93–8.

57. Zein NN. The epidemiology and natural history of hepatitis C virus infection. Cleve Clin J Med 2003;70 Suppl 4:S2–6.

58. Mondelli MU, Cerino A, Cividini A. Acute hepatitis C: diagnosis and management. J Hepatol 2005;42 Suppl:S108–14.

59. Irving WL. Acute hepatitis C virus infection: a neglected disease? Gut 2006;55:1075–7.

60. Pawlotsky JM. Use and interpretation of virological tests for hepatitis C. Hepatology 2002;36:S65–73.

61. Farci P, Alter HJ, Shimoda A, Govindarajan S, Cheung LC, Melpolder JC, Sacher RA, Shih JW, Purcell RH. Hepatitis C virus-associated fulminant hepatic failure. N Engl J Med 1996;335:631–4.

62. Hoofnagle JH. Course and outcome of hepatitis C. Hepatology 2002;36:S21–9.

63. Micallef JM, Kaldor JM, Dore GJ. Spontaneous viral clearance following acute hepatitis C infection: a systematic review of longitudinal studies. J Viral Hepat 2006;13:34–41.

64. Thomas DL, Astemborski J, Rai RM, Anania FA, Schaeffer M, Galai N, Nolt K, Nelson KE, Strathdee SA, Johnson L, Laeyendecker O, Boitnott J, Wilson LE, Vlahov D. The natural history of hepatitis C virus infection: host, viral, and environmental factors. Jama 2000;284:450–6.

65. Farci P, Shimoda A, Coiana A, Diaz G, Peddis G, Melpolder JC, Strazzera A, Chien DY, Munoz SJ, Balestrieri A, Purcell RH, Alter HJ. The outcome of acute hepatitis C predicted by the evolution of the viral quasispecies. Science 2000;288:339–44.

66. Heller T, Rehermann B. Acute hepatitis C: a multifaceted disease. Semin Liver Dis 2005;25:7–17.

67. Updated U.S. Public Health Service Guidelines for the Management of Occupational Exposures to HBV, HCV, and HIV and Recommendations for Postexposure Prophylaxis. MMWR Recomm Rep 2001;50:1–52.

68. National Institutes of Health Consensus Development Conference Statement: Management of hepatitis C: 2002–June 10–12, 2002. Hepatology 2002;36:S3–20.

69. Santantonio T, Sinisi E, Guastadisegni A, Casalino C, Mazzola M, Gentile A, Leandro G, Pastore G. Natural course of acute hepatitis C: a long-term prospective study. Dig Liver Dis 2003;35:104–13.

70. Licata A, Di Bona D, Schepis F, Shahied L, Craxi A, Camma C. When and how to treat acute hepatitis C? J Hepatol 2003;39:1056–62.

71. Kamal SM, Fouly AE, Kamel RR, Hockenjos B, Al Tawil A, Khalifa KE, He Q, Koziel MJ, El Naggar KM, Rasenack J, Afdhal NH. Peginterferon alfa-2b therapy in acute hepatitis C: impact of onset of therapy on sustained virologic response. Gastroenterology 2006;130:632–8.

72. Wiegand J, Buggisch P, Boecher W, Zeuzem S, Gelbmann CM, Berg T, Kauffmann W, Kallinowski B, Cornberg M, Jaeckel E, Wedemeyer H, Manns MP. Early monotherapy with pegylated interferon alpha-2b for acute hepatitis C infection: the HEP-NET acute-HCV-II study. Hepatology 2006;43:250–6.

73. Santantonio T, Fasano M, Sinisi E, Guastadisegni A, Casalino C, Mazzola M, Francavilla R, Pastore G. Efficacy of a 24-week course of PEG-interferon alpha-2b monotherapy in patients with acute hepatitis C after failure of spontaneous clearance. J Hepatol 2005;42:329–33.

74. Kamal SM, Moustafa KN, Chen J, Fehr J, Abdel Moneim A, Khalifa KE, El Gohary LA, Ramy AH, Madwar MA, Rasenack J, Afdhal NH. Duration of peginterferon therapy in acute hepatitis C: a randomized trial. Hepatology 2006;43:923–31.

75. Kamal SM, El Tawil AA, Nakano T, He Q, Rasenack J, Hakam SA, Saleh WA, Ismail A, Aziz AA, Madwar MA. Peginterferon {alpha}-2b and ribavirin therapy in chronic hepatitis C genotype 4: impact of treatment duration and viral kinetics on sustained virological response. Gut 2005;54:858–66.

76. Strader DB, Wright T, Thomas DL, Seeff LB. Diagnosis, management, and treatment of hepatitis C. Hepatology 2004;39:1147–71.

77. Rizzetto M, Canese MG, Arico S, Crivelli O, Trepo C, Bonino F, Verme G. Immunofluorescence detection of new antigen-antibody system (delta/anti-delta) associated to hepatitis B virus in liver and in serum of HBsAg carriers. Gut 1977;18:997–1003.

78. Wang KS, Choo QL, Weiner AJ, Ou JH, Najarian RC, Thayer RM, Mullenbach GT, Denniston KJ, Gerin JL, Houghton M. Structure, sequence and expression of the hepatitis delta (delta) viral genome. Nature 1986;323:508–14.

79. Radjef N, Gordien E, Ivaniushina V, Gault E, Anais P, Drugan T, Trinchet JC, Roulot D, Tamby M, Milinkovitch MC, Deny P. Molecular phylogenetic analyses indicate a wide

and ancient radiation of African hepatitis delta virus, suggesting a deltavirus genus of at least seven major clades. J Virol 2004;78:2537–44.

80. Farci P. Delta hepatitis: an update. J Hepatol 2003;39 Suppl 1:S212–9.

81. Gaeta GB, Stroffolini T, Chiaramonte M, Ascione T, Stornaiuolo G, Lobello S, Sagnelli E, Brunetto MR, Rizzetto M. Chronic hepatitis D: a vanishing Disease? An Italian multicenter study. Hepatology 2000;32:824–7.

82. Sagnelli E, Stroffolini T, Ascione A, Chiaramonte M, Craxi A, Giusti G, Piccinino F. Decrease in HDV endemicity in Italy. J Hepatol 1997;26:20–4.

83. Manock SR, Kelley PM, Hyams KC, Douce R, Smalligan RD, Watts DM, Sharp TW, Casey JL, Gerin JL, Engle R, Alava-Alprecht A, Martinez CM, Bravo NB, Guevara AG, Russell KL, Mendoza W, Vimos C. An outbreak of fulminant hepatitis delta in the Waorani, an indigenous people of the Amazon basin of Ecuador. Am J Trop Med Hyg 2000;63:209–13.

84. Flodgren E, Bengtsson S, Knutsson M, Strebkova EA, Kidd AH, Alexeyev OA, Kidd-Ljunggren K. Recent high incidence of fulminant hepatitis in Samara, Russia: molecular analysis of prevailing hepatitis B and D virus strains. J Clin Microbiol 2000;38:3311–6.

85. Wu JC, Chen CM, Sheen IJ, Lee SD, Tzeng HM, Choo KB. Evidence of transmission of hepatitis D virus to spouses from sequence analysis of the viral genome. Hepatology 1995;22:1656–60.

86. Niro GA, Casey JL, Gravinese E, Garrubba M, Conoscitore P, Sagnelli E, Durazzo M, Caporaso N, Perri F, Leandro G, Facciorusso D, Rizzetto M, Andriulli A. Intrafamilial transmission of hepatitis delta virus: molecular evidence. J Hepatol 1999;30:564–9.

87. Guilhot S, Huang SN, Xia YP, La Monica N, Lai MM, Chisari FV. Expression of the hepatitis delta virus large and small antigens in transgenic mice. J Virol 1994;68:1052–8.

88. Cole SM, Gowans EJ, Macnaughton TB, Hall PD, Burrell CJ. Direct evidence for cytotoxicity associated with expression of hepatitis delta virus antigen. Hepatology 1991;13:845–51.

89. Nisini R, Paroli M, Accapezzato D, Bonino F, Rosina F, Santantonio T, Sallusto F, Amoroso A, Houghton M, Barnaba V. Human CD4+ T-cell response to hepatitis delta virus: identification of multiple epitopes and characterization of T-helper cytokine profiles. J Virol 1997;71:2241–51.

90. Farci P, Mandas A, Coiana A, Lai ME, Desmet V, Van Eyken P, Gibo Y, Caruso L, Scaccabarozzi S, Criscuolo D, et al. Treatment of chronic hepatitis D with interferon alfa-2a. N Engl J Med 1994;330:88–94.

91. Lau DT, Kleiner DE, Park Y, Di Bisceglie AM, Hoofnagle JH. Resolution of chronic delta hepatitis after 12 years of interferon alfa therapy. Gastroenterology 1999;117:1229–33.

92. Lau DT, Doo E, Park Y, Kleiner DE, Schmid P, Kuhns MC, Hoofnagle JH. Lamivudine for chronic delta hepatitis. Hepatology 1999;30:546–9.

93. Wong DC, Purcell RH, Sreenivasan MA, Prasad SR, Pavri KM. Epidemic and endemic hepatitis in India: evidence for a non-A, non-B hepatitis virus aetiology. Lancet 1980;2:876–9.

94. Khuroo MS. Study of an epidemic of non-A, non-B hepatitis. Possibility of another human hepatitis virus distinct from post-transfusion non-A, non-B type. Am J Med 1980;68:818–24.

95. Balayan MS, Andjaparidze AG, Savinskaya SS, Ketiladze ES, Braginsky DM, Savinov AP, Poleschuk VF. Evidence for a virus in non-A, non-B hepatitis transmitted via the fecal-oral route. Intervirology 1983;20:23–31.

96. Tam AW, Smith MM, Guerra ME, Huang CC, Bradley DW, Fry KE, Reyes GR. Hepatitis E virus (HEV): molecular cloning and sequencing of the full-length viral genome. Virology 1991;185:120–31.

97. Reyes GR, Purdy MA, Kim JP, Luk KC, Young LM, Fry KE, Bradley DW. Isolation of a cDNA from the virus responsible for enterically transmitted non-A, non-B hepatitis. Science 1990;247:1335–9.

98. Jameel S. Molecular biology and pathogenesis of hepatitis E virus. Expert Rev Mol Med 1999;1999:1–16.

99. Schlauder GG, Mushahwar IK. Genetic heterogeneity of hepatitis E virus. J Med Virol 2001;65:282–92.

100. Wang L, Zhuang H. Hepatitis E: an overview and recent advances in vaccine research. World J Gastroenterol 2004;10:2157–62.

101. Krawczynski K. Hepatitis E. Hepatology 1993;17:932–41.

102. Krawczynski K, Aggarwal R, Kamili S. Hepatitis E. Infect Dis Clin North Am 2000;14:669–87.

103. Aggarwal R, Naik SR. Hepatitis E: intrafamilial transmission versus waterborne spread. J Hepatol 1994;21:718–23.

104. Khuroo MS, Kamili S, Jameel S. Vertical transmission of hepatitis E virus. Lancet 1995;345:1025–6.

105. Teo CG. Hepatitis E indigenous to economically developed countries: to what extent a zoonosis? Curr Opin Infect Dis 2006;19:460–6.

106. Khuroo MS, Rustgi VK, Dawson GJ, Mushahwar IK, Yattoo GN, Kamili S, Khan BA. Spectrum of hepatitis E virus infection in India. J Med Virol 1994;43:281–6.

107. Khuroo MS, Teli MR, Skidmore S, Sofi MA, Khuroo MI. Incidence and severity of viral hepatitis in pregnancy. Am J Med 1981;70:252–5.

108. Hamid SS, Atiq M, Shehzad F, Yasmeen A, Nissa T, Salam A, Siddiqui A, Jafri W. Hepatitis E virus superinfection in patients with chronic liver disease. Hepatology 2002;36:474–8.

109. Khuroo MS, Kamili S, Dar MY, Moecklii R, Jameel S. Hepatitis E and long-term antibody status. Lancet 1993;341:1355.

110. Arankalle VA, Chadha MS, Dama BM, Tsarev SA, Purcell RH, Banerjee K. Role of immune serum globulins in pregnant women during an epidemic of hepatitis E. J Viral Hepat 1998;5:199–204.

111. Khuroo MS, Dar MY. Hepatitis E: evidence for person-to-person transmission and inability of low dose immune serum globulin from an Indian source to prevent it. Indian J Gastroenterol 1992;11:113–6.

Chronic Hepatitis B and D

Dimitrios Vassilopoulos, MD,[1] and
Stephanos J. Hadziyannis, MD[2]

BACKGROUND

Despite the widespread application of vaccination programs, chronic hepatitis B virus (HBV) infection remains a significant public health problem with 350–400 million people infected worldwide.[1] The prevalence of chronic HBV infection displays a significant geographic variation with areas of high (8–15%), intermediate (1–7%), and low (<1%) endemicity.[1]

Differences in the prevalence and incidence rates of HBV infection are largely linked to different modes and age of HBV transmission as well as with socioeconomic factors. In areas of high HBV endemicity such as the East Asia and sub-Saharan Africa, transmission occurs mainly during the perinatal or during the early childhood period. On the other end, in industrialized countries of North Europe, Australia, and North America where the endemicity is very low (<1%), HBV is transmitted mainly in high-risk adult populations through injection drug use, high-risk sexual behavior, and occupation-related needlesticks (health care workers). However, even in these populations perinatal and early childhood transmission still accounts for the majority of chronic HBV infections.

PATHOGENESIS

The transition of an acute to a chronic HBV infection is mainly influenced by the age of the host at which exposure to the virus occurs.[2] During the perinatal and early childhood period (< 5 years), the majority of infections lead to chronicity. So far, it is unclear what are the exact immune mechanisms that contribute to the inability of the host to eradicate the virus.[3,4] A role of the secreted HBe protein as a potential tolerogen during the neonatal period has been suggested.[5] The absence of an effective host immune response against the replicating virus is obvious in the initial period of chronic HBV infection, widely referred as the "immune tolerant phase" which may last for several years until adolescence or adulthood. During this HBeAg-positive phase of chronic infection, serum HBV DNA levels are very high but alanine aminotransferase (ALT) levels remain persistently normal or nearly normal and liver necroinflammation is minimal.[3,4] Both CD4 and CD8 + T-cells from these patients are hypo-responsive to *in vitro* stimulation, indicative of functional inactivation of the immune system.[6,7] Nevertheless, a number of HBV specific CD8+ T-cells can still be detected in the liver of these patients.[6]

Later on during the adolescent or adulthood years, the tolerance to the HBeAg is gradually lost and immune responses against the replicating virus start to evolve. This leads to increased liver necroinflammation reflected by elevated ALT levels and gradually decreasing levels of viremia.[8] The majority of patients are able to achieve seroconversion from HBeAg to anti-HBe during this unstable phase (HBeAg clearance or immunoactive phase), which is characterized by high levels of intracellular HBcAg in hepatocytes and a vigorous cellular immune response involving CD4 and CD8 lymphocytes. Patients who are unable to clear HBeAg, develop HBeAg positive chronic hepatitis B (CHB), characterized by severe liver necroinflammation, and high HBV DNA levels.

In the majority of individuals with chronic HBV infection, HBeAg clearance is followed by a phase of low viral replication, normal or nearly normal ALT levels and minimal liver necroinflammation.[8] This phase has been termed "HBsAg inactive carrier state" in order to emphasize its overall good prognosis. Although this period was initially considered an immunologically "quiescent" period, a number of recent studies have shown that HBV specific CD8+ cytotoxic T lymphocytes (CTLs) can be detected in the circulation and liver.[9,10] The majority of these CTLs are directed against the core protein and are able to secrete antiviral cytokines and exert cytolytic activities after stimulation.

In about one-third of HBeAg negative patients, viral replication recurs followed by a variable host immune response, leading to chronic liver inflammation referred as HBeAg negative/anti-HBe positive and pre-core mutant CHB.[11] Depending mainly on the infecting HBV genotype, viral strains that replicate during this phase are usually HBV variants with decreased (basic core promoter-BCP mutants) or absent (precore mutants) capability of HBeAg production.[11] Mixed populations of such mutants with wild type (wt) virus may also be detected in such HBeAg negative patients. These mutant strains have been selected under the host immune pressure during the HBeAg clearance phase. In HBeAg-negative patients infected with HBV genotypes B and D and with some genotype C strains, the development of precore HBV variants predominates while in patients with genotype A and in a high percentage of genotype C infection the BCP mutations prevail.

The immunopathogenesis of the HBeAg negative CHB has not been studied in detail. The immune response against the replicating viral strains in the liver appears to be strong enough, similar to that observed during acute hepatitis B.[6,12] Despite this rigorous immune response, the host is unable to clear the virus from the infected hepatocytes, while at the same time, if untreated, it may cause significant chronic liver necroinflammation leading to fibrosis and cirrhosis.

CLINICAL PRESENTATION

The clinical manifestations of CHB are usually mild and most patients remain asymptomatic, until signs of liver decompensation, manifested with ascites,

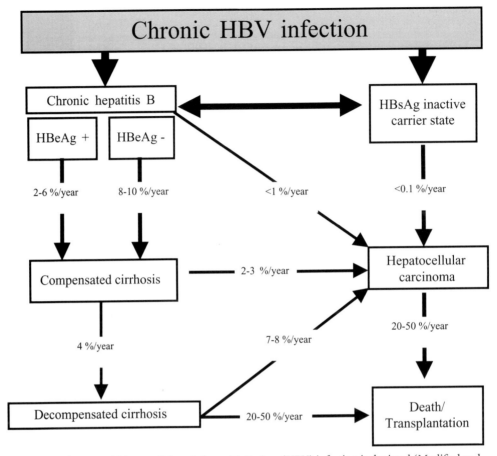

Figure 2.1: The natural history of chronic hepatitis B virus (HBV) infection is depicted (Modified and Reprinted with permission of Wiley-Liss, Inc., a subsidiary of John Wiley & Sons, Inc. from reference. [14])

gastrointestinal bleeding or hepatic encephalopathy, appear. In certain cases, the first clinical manifestations are related to the development of hepatocellular carcinoma (HCC). The natural history of chronic HBV infection[13,14] is depicted in Figure 2.1.

DIAGNOSIS

Chronic HBV infection is diagnosed by a combination of virological, biochemical and serological tests.[15] An infection is considered chronic when HBsAg or HBV DNA is detected in the serum for more than six months. Chronic HBV infection, could be classified as either inactive (HBsAg inactive carrier state) or active (HBeAg negative or positive CHB).[2,16] However, in order to make an accurate diagnosis, monitoring for a period of 12 or more months with frequent measurement of serological markers (HBsAg, HBeAg, anti-HBe, anti-HBs, anti-HBc), ALT, and HBV DNA levels is needed.

The *inactive HBsAg carrier state* is defined by:

- HBsAg (+),
- HBeAg (–)/anti-HBe (±)
- normal or near normal ALT (preferably <0.75x upper limit of normal –ULN, values)
- undetectable or low serum HBV DNA (<10,000 copies/ml or 2,000 IU/ml)

Chronic hepatitis B (HBeAg positive or negative) is defined by:

- HBsAg (+)
- HBeAg (+) or (–)
- persistently or intermittently elevated ALT
- histological evidence of liver necroinflammation and
- increased HBV DNA levels (>2,000–20,000 IU/ml or 10,000–100,000 copies/ml)

Different cut-off HBV DNA values ranging from $0.3–1 \times 10^5$ copies/ml have been proposed in order to differentiate between inactive carriers and patients with HBeAg negative CHB. [17,18] Taking into account the cost of HBV DNA measurement and the absence of a widely accepted cut-off HBV DNA value, frequent monitoring ALT could suffice for the differentiation between the two disease states. However, the most recently proposed cut-off level for ALT is 19 and 30 IU/L for women and men respectively.[19]

There are a number of different HBV DNA assays (quantitative and qualitative) that are currently used in clinical practice with great differences in their sensitivity and linear dynamic range.[15] Newer techniques using the World Health Organization (WHO) international standard for HBV DNA, express HBV DNA levels in international units per milliliter (IU/ml) and allow the comparison between different assays.[15] An IU is equivalent with approximately five copies. Regardless of the exact role of HBV DNA measurement in differentiating inactive carriers from patients with HBeAg negative CHB, its role for the assessment of eligibility, prognosis, and efficacy of antiviral treatment is indispensable.[20]

Based on the genomic variability of HBV, eight different genotypes (designated A to H) and subtypes have been identified.[21] Although it appears that HBV genotypes correlate with the HBeAg seroconversion rate to anti-HBe (spontaneous and after interferon-IFN treatment), severity of liver damage and progression to cirrhosis and HCC[22], there is currently no clear indication for their assessment in clinical practice.

Measurement of IgM anti-HBc levels has been also shown in some studies to correlate with liver inflammation, but its place in the diagnosis and monitoring of CHB has not been definitely established.[16]

Liver biopsy in patients with CHB patients provides significant information regarding the correct diagnosis, severity of liver necroinflammation, stage of fibrosis and the co-existence of unrelated liver diseases.[2] It is also particularly useful in patients with borderline ALT levels ($<2 \times$ ULN) who are considered candidates for antiviral treatment.[23]

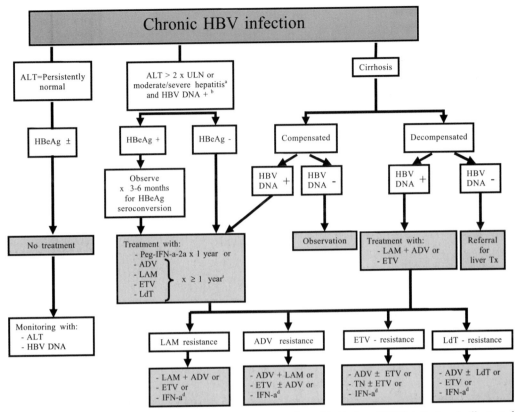

Figure 2.2: A treatment algorithm for patients with chronic hepatitis B virus (HBV) infection is illustrated (Modified and reprinted with permission of Wiley-Liss, Inc., a subsidiary of John Wiley & Sons, Inc. from reference. [2,14,23]) [a]Evaluated by a liver biopsy; [b]For patients with: HBeAg positive chronic hepatitis B (CHB): ≥ 20,000 IU/ml HBeAg negative CHB: ≥ 2,000 IU/ml; [c]In patients with HBeAg positive CHB, therapy with oral nucleos(t)ide agents should be continued for 6 months after HBeAg seroconversion (consolidation period); [d]Not for patients with contraindications to interferon (IFN) or decompensated cirrhosis.
Abbreviations: ALT = alanine aminotransferase, ULN = upper limit of normal, Peg-IFN = Pegylated IFN, ADV = adefovir, LAM = lamivudine, ETV = entecavir, LdT = Telbivudine, TN = Tenofovir, Tx = transplantation.

MANAGEMENT

The decision to treat patients with chronic HBV infection with antiviral treatment should be based on a number of factors including patients' age, ALT values, liver histology, presence of cirrhosis (compensated or decompensated), HBV DNA levels, presence of certain contraindications to antiviral treatment, and patients' preferences.[2,16,20,22] In Figure 2.2, a suggested algorithm for the treatment of patients with chronic HBV infection is depicted.

There are currently five approved drugs for the treatment of chronic HBV infection including two different formulations of IFN, standard IFN-a and pegylated (PEG) IFN-a-2a and 4 oral nucleos(t)ide analogs (lamivudine-LAM, adefovir-ADV, entecavir-ETV, and telbivudine-LdT).[2,20,22]

The treatment strategy for the different groups of patients with chronic HBV infection will be examined separately.

A. Inactive Carrier State

Because the long-term prognosis of these patients is good[24] and in the absence of data indicating that antiviral treatment of any kind has any effect on HBsAg loss, therapy is not recommended.[2,16] Nevertheless, close monitoring of these patients with measurement of ALT values and HBV DNA levels every three to six months is imperative.

B. Chronic Hepatitis B

a. HBeAg POSITIVE

Patients with persistently normal ALT values, independently of HBV DNA levels, should be monitored with ALT measurement without administration of antiviral therapy (Figure 2.1). If ALT and HBV DNA values become elevated there is a high possibility for spontaneous HBeAg seroconversion, so patients should be followed for a period of three to six months, before a decision for initiation of treatment is made.[2,16]

Patients with HBeAg positive CHB, defined by ALT greater than two times the ULN or with moderate/severe hepatitis in liver biopsy and high HBV DNA levels ($>10^5$ copies/ml or $\sim$ 20,000 IU/ml), should be treated.[2] The end-point of treatment in these patients is the sustained loss of HBeAg and development of anti-HBe antibodies (HBeAg seroconversion).

Approved treatments include agents given for a finite period of time (IFN-based regimens) or oral nucleos(t)ide analogues usually given for more than one year.[25] The durability of HBeAg seroconversion differs significantly between these two therapeutic schemes. In 80–90% of patients treated either with standard IFN-a for four to six months or PEG-IFN-a-2a for one year, this response is sustained after treatment discontinuation.[25] On the contrary, patients achieving HBeAg seroconversion, under LAM treatment experience high relapse rates two years after stopping therapy.[25] Based on these results, therapy with oral agents has been proposed to be continued for six months after seroconversion has been achieved.[19] This is referred as period of response consolidation. Longer consolidation periods may be necessary, especially if HBV DNA is detectable at the end of treatment.[25] IFN based regimens given for a definite period of time (4–6 months for standard IFN-a or 1 year for PEG-IFN-a-2a) have the best efficacy for HBeAg seroconversion (28–32%) compared to oral agents given for one year (LAM: 17–22%, ADV: 12%, ETV: 21%, LdT: 22%).[2,20] In the presence of contraindications to IFN, treatment with oral agents is recommendable for more than one year in order to maximize the possibility for HBeAg seroconversion. Long-term data with LAM and ADV have indicated an increasing rate of HBeAg seroconversion when these agents are given for more than one year.[20] This positive effect though is offset by the frequent appearance of LAM-resistant viral strains during long-term treatment ($\sim$70% after 5 years of treatment). The problem of development of HBV resistance to nucleos(t)ide analogs is reversely related to their antiviral potency and their genetic barrier to resistance and is much lower and delayed with ADV and ETV compared to LAM and LdT.[20]

b. HBeAg NEGATIVE PATIENTS

Therapy is indicated when there is clear-cut increase in ALT levels ($>2 \times$ ULN) or moderate/severe hepatitis on liver biopsy and positive HBV DNA.[20]

Since HBV DNA levels are in general lower than in patients with HBeAg positive CHB and they fluctuate significantly, a lower threshold for HBV DNA positivity has been proposed ($\sim$ 2,000 IU or 10,000 copies/ml).[19]

In contrast to HBeAg positive CHB, the goals of antiviral therapy are not clearly defined. A realistic goal for this group of patients is suppression of HBV replication either off-therapy for IFN-based regimens given for a finite period of time or maintained during prolonged therapy with oral nucleos(t)ide analogues.[20]

PEG-IFN-a-2a (180 µg subcutaneously once a week) given for one year achieved virological responses in 43% of patients at the end of therapy and this response was maintained in 30% of them 12 months after stopping therapy.[20] Different oral nucleos(t)ide analogs including LAM, ADV, ETV, and LdT have been tried in patients with HBeAg negative CHB for variable periods of time (>1 year).[20] LAM given for one year achieves virological responses in 65–90% of cases, but this initial response is not maintained due to the accumulating emergence of drug-resistant mutations in the YMDD motif of the HBV polymerase (most common rtM204V/I).[20] Genotypic resistance reaches rates of 65–70% after five years of treatment and is usually followed by increasing HBV DNA (virological breakthrough) and ALT levels (biochemical breakthrough).[20] Nevertheless, 30–35% of patients treated with LAM for five years are able to maintain a virological response on therapy and this has been accompanied by a favorable clinical response.[26] Attempts to discontinue LAM after one to two years of treatment are followed by a high rate of virological relapse,[27,28] signifying the need for long-term therapy.

ADV is a prodrug of an adenosine nucleotide analogue that has been shown to be effective during long-term treatment of HBeAg negative CHB. The virological response was $\sim$51% after one year of therapy[29] further increasing and keeping in $\sim$70% of treated patients after four or five years of therapy.[30] Genotypic resistance to the drug (rtA181V/T and rtN236T) developed in approximately 29% of patients after five years of treatment but only 16% experienced a virologic breakthrough.[30] When ADV was discontinued after one year of treatment, the majority of patients had a virological relapse.[20] These data indicate that, similarly to LAM, treatment for more than one year is needed in order to maintain the virological response. Whether discontinuation of therapy is an achievable option after longer periods of treatment remains to be seen.

ETV is another nucleoside analogue of guanosine with a very high potency compared to ADV and LAM, in terms of virological, biochemical, and histological response. After one year of treatment, the virological response was approximately 95%[31] without evidence of drug-resistance in treatment-naïve patients. The high anti-HBV potency of ETV, its impressive efficacy in terms of rapid HBV suppression to undetectability of HBV DNA by most sensitive PCR assays, combined with its high genetic barrier to HBV resistance, make ETV monotherapy a very attractive option as first line treatment in LAM-naïve CHB patients both HBeAg-positive and HBeAg-negative. However, the hitherto duration of ETV phase III trials is short, their extension design complex and appropriate long-term studies are needed before reaching definite conclusions on its very long-term safety and resistance. Long-term data are also necessary in order to assess its efficacy and durability of response on and off therapy.

Telbivudine (LdT, β-L-2'-deoxythimidine) is an L nucleoside analog of thymidine, approved by FDA on late 2006 for the treatment of chronic hepatitis B at a daily dose of 600 mg. It is a potent anti-HBV agent and has been evaluated in terms of efficacy, safety, side effects, and HBV resistance in comparison to LAM in a very large cohort of 1,367 HBeAg-positive and HBeAg-negative CHB patients (GLOBE trial).[32] The year 1 and 2 results showed that LdT is equally safe but more effective than LAM in terms of absolute HBV DNA reduction from baseline and time of undetectability and in treatment failures and HBV resistance are less frequent with LdT compared to LAM. However, there is no significant difference from LAM in HBeAg loss and seroconversion to anti-HBe.[32,34] Moreover, it has been well documented both in LdT and LAM treated patients, that the rates of HBeAg seroconversion are significantly increased if a profound and rapid HBV suppression to undetectability of serum HBV DNA at week 24 is achieved, this effect being also associated with enhanced T-cell reactivity to the HBc protein.[35]

C. Cirrhosis

a. COMPENSATED

Patients with compensated cirrhosis (HBeAg positive or negative) without evidence of active viral replication, should be observed closely[2] and referred for liver transplantation when liver decompensation develops.

If viral replication is documented, then therapy with IFN-based regimens or oral nucleos(t)ide analogs can be given. The response rate in patients treated with IFN-based regimens, LAM and ADV do not seem to differ from patients without underlying cirrhosis.[36] Cirrhotics patients treated with LAM, exhibited a reduced risk for development of hepatic decompensation and HCC, but during treatment ($\sim$32 months), half of these patients developed LAM-resistance with adverse clinical sequelae (decompensation, HCC, death).[37] So far, there have not been adequate long-term data available for ADV and ETV, but their overall low rate of resistance makes them good candidates for first line treatment in these patients.

b. DECOMPENSATED

For patients without active viral replication, referral to a liver transplant center is obligatory.[2] For patients with decompensated cirrhosis and active viral replication, antiviral treatment with oral agents is indicated, because IFN-based regimens are contraindicated in this setting.[2,16] The majority of data regarding nucleos(t)ide analog therapy in patients with decompensated cirrhosis are available for LAM[36], indicating a favorable virological response and clinical improvement (decrease $\geq$ 2 of Child-Pugh score) in about half of the cases. As already noted, drug-resistance is a major issue leading to adverse outcomes. Although, very long-term data are not available for ADV and ETV, these agents should be considered as initial therapy for cirrhotic patients. Close monitoring for adverse events, particularly renal impairment, is extremely important in cirrhotics on oral agents especially ADV.

On the other hand, the combination of two potent antivirals without cross-resistance preferably with high genetic barrier to HBV resistance has actually entered clinical practice and is emerging as the best long-term treatment paradigm of patients with decompensated cirrhosis.[38]

D. Patients with LAM-Resistance

The rate of drug-resistant mutations reaches ~70 % after five years of LAM treatment and is associated with ALT elevation, hepatic flares and, especially in patients with advanced liver disease, hepatic decompensation and even death.[39] LAM-resistance has been treated with different nucleoside analogues (such as ADV or ETV) or IFN-a.[22] Recent data though suggest that the rate of drug-resistance when switching to ADV monotherapy in LAM-resistant cases is higher compared to LAM-naïve patients.[40] Thus, it is possibly more appropriate adding-on rather than switching to ADV, in LAM-resistant cases.[41,42] This is particularly relevant in patients with liver decompensation or in the transplant setting.

E. Patients with ADV-Resistance

In patients who had not been treated previously with nucleoside analogs, LAM or ETV can be added while for patients with previous LAM-resistance, adding LAM may not be the appropriate option because re-emerging LAM-resistant strains have been reported.[2]

F. Patients with ETV Resistance

Approximately 30% of LAM-resistant patients treated with ETV for three years, developed genotypic HBV-resistance to ETV.[43] Whether or not a combination strategy similar to ADV, should be employed here, remains unknown. Based on *in vitro* data, switching or adding ADV or tenofovir can be tried.[2]

G. Patients with LdT Resistance

The treatment strategy should be similar to that followed in patients with LAM-resistance.

Combination Antiviral Therapies

A number of combination approaches have been tried in chronic hepatitis B with the goals to achieve higher viral suppression and less viral resistance. Despite the theoretical advantages of such approach, especially if we consider the established experience from other chronic viral infections such as HIV, the data on combination therapies in chronic hepatitis B have been rather disappointing so far.

The better-studied combination schemes included either IFN-a (standard or PEG-IFN-a) and LAM or the combination of nucleos(t)ide analogs (LAM +ADV or LAM+LdT).[2] Adding LAM to IFN-a in five clinical trials, did not result in a greater sustained virological response after discontinuing IFN-a. LAM-resistant strains were still encountered in the combination arm despite the fact that their frequency was lower compared to LAM monotherapy.[2]

Similar results in terms of virological response were obtained in studies comparing LAM+ADV to LAM in nucleoside naïve patients, where still LAM-resistance was detected.[2] In patients with LAM-resistance, adding ADV is probably the best approach compared to switching to ADV, as outlined above.[41,42] In a small study, LdT + LAM was not betted that LdT monotherapy.[33]

In patients with decompensated liver disease either treatment naïve or LAM-resistant, combination therapy with two potent nucleoside analogs lacking cross resistance, is gaining increasing clinical acceptability in terms of efficacy, tolerability, safety, and negligible HBV resistance.[38,44]

CHRONIC HEPATITIS D

Background

Chronic hepatitis D is due to hepatitis D virus (HDV) infection occurring exclusively in HBV infected individuals.[45] The virus enters the host either simultaneously with HBV (co-infection) or during the course of chronic HBV infection (super-infection). Approximately 5% of HBV infected patients worldwide are infected with HDV.[45] Although its prevalence has declined over the last three decades, still it represents a serious health problem in different areas of the world.[45,46,47]

Pathogenesis

HDV is a single-stranded RNA virus that needs HBV for its assembly and transmission.[48] HDV particles are spherical particles containing an outer envelope comprised of the HBV surface proteins (HBsAg, Pre-S1, pre-S2), the circular HDV RNA and the hepatitis delta antigen. HDV after entering the hepatocytes, possibly through the same receptor as HBV, replicates in the nucleus of the infected cells, leading through immune-mediated cell destruction to chronic inflammation and liver fibrosis. Although the pathogenetic mechanisms leading to liver inflammation have not been elucidated, similar pathogenetic mechanisms to chronic HBV infection probably operate.[49]

Three different HDV genotypes have been reported until today with different geographic distribution. Genotype I is the most prevalent genotype in North America and Europe and has been associated with a more severe clinical course in recent studies.[50] A new classification scheme of HDV into 8 clades has been recently proposed.[51]

Clinical Presentation

The clinical course of chronic HDV infection has been traditionally viewed as more severe leading earlier to cirrhosis and HCC, compared to chronic HBV infection. Although, this is true for certain patient populations, a significant proportion of HDV infected individuals demonstrate a more benign course of infection. Nevertheless, chronic HDV infection still accounts for approximately 40% of cirrhosis in HBsAg positive children and in endemic areas of HDV infection, is one of the major causes leading to liver transplantation.

Diagnosis

The diagnosis of chronic HDV infection is made by the detection of IgG anti-HDV antibodies in the serum of chronically infected HBV patients. In certain, cases, IgM anti-HDV antibodies can also be detected. The diagnosis is established by the detection of HDV RNA in the serum using a sensitive reverse transcription PCR (RT-PCR). Non-detectability of HDV RNA in the serum is indicative of HDV clearance either after therapy or spontaneously.

Management

Despite the significance progress that has been made in the therapy of chronic hepatitis B, the treatment of chronic hepatitis D remains challenging.[44] The difficulty in achieving HDV clearance lies on the absence of a specific inhibitor of HDV replication. Therefore, most efforts have been concentrated in the goal of achieving long-lasting suppression of HBV replication and diminution of circulating levels of HBsAg. The clinical studies that have been reported so far included a small number of patients with rather disappointing results. The best results have been achieved with IFNa either in its standard form (9 million units TIW) or as PEG-IFN-a-2b (1.5 μg/Kg weekly) given for at least one year.[46] In two recent studies, the rate of sustained virological response after treatment with PEG-IFN-a-2b, ranged between 25 and 43%[52,53] Trials with PEG-IFN-a-2a are also underway and their results are expected soon.

In conclusion, PEG-IFNa administered for at least 12 months is the current treatment of choice for patients with chronic hepatitis D. The duration of therapy in patients who do not clear HDV after one year of treatment remains unclear. For patients who achieve a significant reduction of HDV RNA after one year of treatment continuation of therapy is recommended.[46]

REFERENCES

1. M. J. Alter. Epidemiology of hepatitis B in Europe and worldwide. J Hepatol, 2003; 39 Suppl 1:S64–9.
2. A. S. Lok and B. J. McMahon. Chronic hepatitis B. Hepatology, 2007;45:507–39.
3. F. V. Chisari and C. Ferrari. Hepatitis B virus immunopathogenesis. Annu Rev Immunol, 1995;13:29–60.
4. B. Rehermann and M. Nascimbeni. Immunology of hepatitis B virus and hepatitis C virus infection. Nat Rev Immunol, 2005;5:215–29.
5. D. Milich and T. J. Liang. Exploring the biological basis of hepatitis B e antigen in hepatitis B virus infection. Hepatology, 2003;38:1075–86.
6. C. Ferrari, G. Missale, C. Boni et al. Immunopathogenesis of hepatitis B. J Hepatol, 2003;39 Suppl 1:S36–42.
7. K. Visvanathan and S. R. Lewin. Immunopathogenesis: role of innate and adaptive immune responses. Semin Liver Dis, 2006;26:104–15.
8. S. J. Hadziyannis. Hepatitis B e antigen negative chronic hepatitis B: from clinical recognition to pathogenesis and treatment. Viral Hepat Rev, 1995;1:7–36.
9. M. K. Maini, C. Boni, C. K. Lee et al. The role of virus-specific CD8+; cells in liver damage and viral control during persistent hepatitis B virus infection. J Exp Med, 2000;191:1269–80.

10. G. J. Webster, S. Reignat, D. Brown et al. Longitudinal analysis of CD8+ T cells specific for structural and nonstructural hepatitis B virus proteins in patients with chronic hepatitis B: implications for immunotherapy. J Virol, 2004;78:5707–19.

11. S. J. Hadziyannis and D. Vassilopoulos. Hepatitis B e antigen-negative chronic hepatitis B. Hepatology, 2001;34:617–24.

12. S. J. Hadziyannis and D. Vassilopoulos. Immunopathogenesis of hepatitis B e antigen negative chronic hepatitis B infection. Antiviral Res, 2001;52:91–8.

13. G. Fattovich. Natural history and prognosis of hepatitis B. Semin Liver Dis, 2003;23: 47–58.

14. H. J. Yim and A.S. Lok. Natural history of chronic hepatitis B virus infection: what we knew in 1981 and what we know in 2005. Hepatology, 2006;43:S173–81.

15. S. Bowden. Serological and molecular diagnosis. Semin Liver Dis, 2006;26:97–103.

16. R. de Franchis, A. Hadengue, G. Lau et al. EASL International Consensus Conference on Hepatitis B. 13–14 September, 2002 Geneva, Switzerland. Consensus statement long version; J Hepatol, 2003;39 Suppl 1:S3–25.

17. C. J. Chu, M. Hussainand and A. S. Lok. Quantitative serum HBV DNA levels during different stages of chronic hepatitis B infection. Hepatology, 2002;36:1408–15.

18. E. K. Manesis, G.V. Papatheodoridis and S. J. Hadziyannis. Serum HBV-DNA levels in inactive hepatitis B virus carriers. Gastroenterology, 2002;122:2092–3.

19. E. B. Keeffe, D.T. Dieterich, S. H. Han et al. A treatment algorithm for the management of chronic hepatitis B virus infection in the United States: an update. Clin Gastroenterol Hepatol, 2006;4:936–62.

20. S. J. Hadziyannis. New developments in the treatment of chronic hepatitis B. Expert Opin Biol Ther, 2006;6:913–21.

21. S. Locarnini. Molecular virology of hepatitis B virus. Semin Liver Dis, 2004; 24 Suppl 1:3–10.

22. R. P. Perrillo. Therapy of hepatitis B – viral suppression or eradication? Hepatology, 2006;43:S182–93.

23. M. K. Osborn and A. S. Lok. Antiviral options for the treatment of chronic hepatitis B. J, Antimicrob Chemother, 2006;57:1030–4.

24. M. Manno, C. Camma, F. Schepis et al. Natural history of chronic HBV carriers in northern Italy: morbidity and mortality after 30 years. Gastroenterology, 2004;127:756–63.

25. J. J. Feld and E. J. Heathcote. Hepatitis B e antigen-positive chronic hepatitis B: natural history and treatment. Semin Liver Dis, 2006; 26:116–29.

26. G. V. Papatheodoridis, E. Dimou, K. Dimakopoulos et al. Outcome of hepatitis B e antigen-negative chronic hepatitis B on long-term nucleoside analog therapy starting with lamivudine. Hepatology, 2005;42:121–9.

27. S. K. Fung, F. Wong, M. Hussain et al. Sustained response after a 2-year course of lamivudine treatment of hepatitis B e antigen-negative chronic hepatitis B. J Viral Hepat, 2004;11:432–8.

28. T. Santantonio, M. Mazzola, T. Iacovazzi et al. Long-term follow-up of patients with anti-HBe/HBV DNA-positive chronic hepatitis B treated for 12 months with lamivudine. J Hepatol, 2000;32:300–6.

29. S. J. Hadziyannis, N. C. Tassopoulos, E. J. Heathcote et al. Adefovir dipivoxil for the treatment of hepatitis B e antigen-negative chronic hepatitis B. N Engl J Med, 2003;348: 800–7.

30. S. J. Hadziyannis, N. C. Tassopoulos, E. J. Heathcote et al. Long-term Therapy With Adefovir Dipivoxil for HBeAg-Negative Chronic Hepatitis B for up to 5 Years. Gastroenterology, 2006;131:1743–51.

31. C. L. Lai, D. Shouval, A.S. Lok et al. Entecavir versus lamivudine for patients with HBeAg-negative chronic hepatitis B. N Engl J Med,2006;354:1011–20.

32. S. Thongsawat, C. L. Lai, E. Gane et al. Telbivudine displays consistent antiviral efficacy across patient subgroups for the treatment of chronic hepatitis B: Results from the GLOBE study. J Hepatol 2006;44 Suppl 2:S49.

33. C. L. Lai, N. Leung, E. K. Teo et al. A 1-year trial of telbivudine, lamivudine, and the combination in patients with hepatitis B e antigen-positive chronic hepatitis B. Gastroenterology, 2005;129:528–36.

34. C. L. Lai, E. Gane, Y. F. Liaw et al. Telbivudine LdT; vs. lamivudine for chronic hepatitis B: First-year results from the international phase III globe trial. Hepatology, 2005;42 Suppl 1:748A.

35. H. Cooksley, J. Hou, L. Vitek et al. Impact Of Nucleoside Treatment On Antiviral T-Cell Reactivity In Chronic Hepatitis B: Major Differences Depending On Early Viral Suppression, HBeAg Status And HBV Genotype. Hepatology, 2006;44 Suppl 1:547–8A.

36. C. M. Chu and Y. F. Liaw. Hepatitis B virus-related cirrhosis: natural history and treatment. Semin Liver Dis, 2006;26:142–52.

37. Y. F. Liaw, J. J. Sung, W. C. Chow et al. Lamivudine for patients with chronic hepatitis B and advanced liver disease. N Engl J Med, 2004;351;1521–31.

38. S. J. Hadziyannis. Treatment paradigms on hepatitis B e antigen-negative chronic hepatitis B patients. Expert Opin Investig Drugs, 2007;16:777–86.

39. A. Bartholomeusz and S. A. Locarnini. Antiviral drug resistance: clinical consequences and molecular aspects. Semin Liver Dis, 2006;26:162–70.

40. S. K. Fung, H. B. Chae, R. J. Fontana et al. Virologic response and resistance to adefovir in patients with chronic hepatitis B. J Hepatol, 2006;44:283–90.

41. I. Rapti, E. Dimou, P. Mitsoula et al. Adding-on versus switching-to adefovir therapy in lamivudine-resistant HBeAg-negative chronic hepatitis B. Hepatology, 2007;45:307–13.

42. Y. F. Liaw. Rescue therapy for lamivudine-resistant chronic hepatitis B: When and how? Hepatology, 2007;45:266–68.

43. R. J. Colonno, R. E. Rose, K. Pokomowski et al. Assessment At Three Years Shows High Barrier To Resistance Is Maintained In Entecavir-Treated Nucleoside Naive Patients While Resistance Emergence Increases Over Time In Lamivudine Refractory Patients. Hepatology, 2006; 44, Suppl 1:229A–30A

44. E. B. Keeffe, S. Zeuzem, R. S. Koff et al. Report of an international workshop: roadmap for management of patients receiving oral therapy for chronic hepatitis B. Clin Gastroenterol Hepatol, 2007;5:890–7.

45. S. J. Hadziyannis. Hepatitis D. Clin Liver Dis, 1999;3:309–25.

46. P. Farci. Treatment of chronic hepatitis D: New advances, old challenges. Hepatology, 2006;44:536–9.

47. H. Wedemeyer, B. Heidrichand, M. P. Manns. Hepatitis D virus infection – not a vanishing disease in Europe! Hepatology, 2007;45:1331–2.

48. J. M. Taylor. Hepatitis delta virus. Virology, 2006;344:71–6.

49. M. Fiedler and M. Roggendorf. Immunology of HDV infection. Curr Top Microbiol Immunol, 2006;307:187–209.

50. C. W. Su, Y. H. Huang, T. I. Huo et al. Genotypes and viremia of hepatitis B and D viruses are associated with outcomes of chronic hepatitis D patients. Gastroenterology, 2006;130:1625–35.

51. P. Deny. Hepatitis delta virus genetic variability: from genotypes I, II, III to eight major clades? Curr Top Microbiol Immunol, 2006;307:151–171.

52. C. Castelnau, F. Le Gal, M. P. Ripault et al. Efficacy of peginterferon alpha-2b in chronic hepatitis delta: relevance of quantitative RT-PCR for follow-up. Hepatology, 2006;44:728–35.

53. G. A. Niro, A. Ciancio, G. B. Gaeta et al. Pegylated interferon alpha-2b as monotherapy or in combination with ribavirin in chronic hepatitis delta. Hepatology, 2006;44:713–20.

Chronic Hepatitis C

Sam Galhenage, MD,
and John G. McHutchison, MD

BACKGROUND

The hepatitis C virus (HCV) is a small, single-stranded, blood-borne RNA virus of the family *Flaviviridae*. It was first identified in 1989 as a major cause of parenterally transmitted non-A non-B hepatitis. Infection with HCV is a leading cause of chronic liver disease worldwide. A proportion of patients with chronic infection develop progressive liver damage with cirrhosis and complications of end-stage liver disease over 20–40 years. The mortality from chronic hepatitis C (CHC) is also rising and is expected to double or triple over the next two decades.[1,2] HCV is now the leading indication for liver transplantation in developed countries and will continue to pose an important health and economic burden for at least the next 10–20 years.

EPIDEMIOLOGY AND TRANSMISSION

There are an estimated 180 million people with CHC infection worldwide, with 3–4 million new infections per year. Overall, the estimated global prevalence of infection is 1–3%.[3] In Western countries the true prevalence of HCV is likely to be significantly underestimated. In the United States for example, an estimated 4 million people have been infected;[4] however, important epidemiological surveys have excluded particular groups traditionally at high risk for infection, such as prisoners, the institutionalized, and the homeless.[5–7]

Following a peak incidence in the 1980s, a sharp decline in the number of new cases of CHC infection has been subsequently observed.[8] Consequently, the majority of patients seen with CHC infection today largely represent individuals first infected with the virus over a period extending from the 1960s to the 1980s. Several factors have been responsible for the declining incidence of this infection. First, the introduction of screening anti-HCV blood tests in Western countries from 1992 has reduced the number of new cases of transfusion-associated HCV to almost zero.[9] Second, high-risk injection drug use is less common today compared with the pre-human immunodeficiency virus era of the 1960s and

1970s.[4] In particular, anti-HIV educational programs promoting safer injection practices such as needle exchange, and reduced needle sharing, appear to have had a beneficial effect in reducing HCV incidence.[1,9]

Parenteral exposure through either injecting drug use or transfusion of blood products remains the most efficient means of HCV transmission. Injecting drug use (IDU) is the major risk factor for acquiring infection in the developed world. IDU accounts for an estimated 60% of all newly acquired HCV infections.[8] Seroprevalence among individual drug users is at least 50%, with rates of 60–70% reported in some series.[10,11] As previously described, transfusion-associated HCV infection has become rare in the developed world since routine testing for HCV began in 1992. Prior to this, patients receiving multiple transfusions were at particularly high risk of acquiring infection, such as patients with thalassemia or hemophiliacs treated with clotting factor concentrates before 1987. The risk of infection is now less than 1/1,000,000 per unit transfused.[12] The subsequent implementation of nucleic acid testing for HCV in donated blood, rather than detectable HCV specific antibodies, has further decreased the risk of transfusion-associated HCV. However, transfusion-associated HCV remains a problem in many developing countries which do not have adequate screening procedures and where only around 40% of donated blood is tested for HCV.[13]

Health care workers who acquire HCV infection account for approximately 4% of all newly diagnosed infections. However the 1.5% prevalence of HCV among health care workers is lower or not substantially different from that observed in the general population.[4] The average risk of infection from percutaneous exposure to blood has been reported as 1.8%.[8] No infections have been reported in association with mucous membrane or non-intact skin exposures. Thus, given the extremely low risk of transmission, there are currently no recommendations regarding the restriction of health care workers with HCV infection.

Transplant recipients who receive organs from HCV-infected donors have a high risk of acquiring infection and developing chronic liver disease. Some studies report near universal transmission of the virus.[14] However, most transplant centers have developed effective screening programs, and only selectively utilize anti-HCV positive donors for HCV-infected patients.

Sexual transmission of HCV can also occur, and may account for up to 15–20% of HCV infections in the United States.[8,15] However, transmission by this means is inefficient. This is particularly the case among stable heterosexual partners, with a reported 0.1% annual risk of infection.[16] Seroprevalence of HCV is increased among promiscuous heterosexuals and possibly male homosexuals. In addition, the risk of transmission is likely to be higher if the index case is coinfected with HIV.[17] Other factors associated with higher anti-HCV positivity include younger age at intercourse, a history of sexually transmitted disease, and non-use of condoms.[4]

The risk of transmission from an infected mother to a newborn ranges from 2–6%, and is not associated with delivery method or breastfeeding.[18,19] Transmission occurs almost exclusively in HCV RNA positive mothers and is more likely to occur with higher levels of viremia at the time of birth. Higher HCV RNA levels are also likely to account for the approximately 2–5 fold higher risk of transmission in mothers coinfected with HCV and HIV.[20,21]

Table 3.1. Screening Recommendations for Hepatitis C Infection

History of illicit injecting drug use
Recipients of blood products or solid organs before 1992
Patients receiving hemodialysis
Unexplained elevation in aminotransferase levels or chronic liver disease
Patients with human immunodeficiency virus (HIV) infection
Current sexual partners of people infected with HCV
Children born to HCV positive mothers
Healthcare workers after needle stick injury or mucosal exposure to HCV

Routine screening is not recommended in: asymptomatic adults, healthcare workers, pregnant women, household (nonsexual) contacts of HCV-infected persons, unless a specific risk factor for HCV infection exists. However, testing is often performed to provide reassurance.
Need for testing is uncertain in transplant recipients, intranasal cocaine users, or individuals with tattoos, body piercings, and history of sexually transmitted diseases or multiple sexual partners.

Adapted from recommendations from Centers for Disease Control and Prevention (CDC).

Rarer causes of HCV infection include healthcare-related transmission, including chronic hemodialysis and the use of unsterile needles (e.g., for immunization). The incidence and prevalence of transmission by this route has steadily declined in Western countries with the use of adequate sterilization procedures. In approximately 9% of cases, the route of transmission is unknown.[8,15] Potential risks of unclear importance include so-called household transmission (for example, sharing of razors or toothbrushes), tattooing, body piercing, intranasal cocaine use, dental procedures, and acupuncture. Transmission via these routes is frequently difficult to prove. Failure to remember or disclose relevant or seemingly obscure medical history (for example, childhood vaccination practices) may also account for a significant percentage of "unknown" causes. Screening recommendations for HCV infection are outlined in Table 3.1.

PATHOGENESIS OF CHRONIC INFECTION

Prospective studies have indicated that approximately 75–85% of HCV-infected individuals go on to develop chronic infection,[22–24] which is defined as the persistence of HCV RNA in the blood for greater than six months. The rate of spontaneous clearance of the virus after this period is low. In 15% of individuals, the natural immune system is able to clear the acute infection spontaneously. This is more likely to occur in women and younger patients. Conversely, African American men and patients with asymptomatic acute infection are more prone to developing chronic infection.[24–26]

The precise reasons why HCV infection persists in some patients but spontaneously resolves in others is not understood. The availability of informative data has been limited by the lack of robust cell culture systems and small animal models of infection as well as the difficulty in identifying patients immediately after inoculation with HCV. As such, a great deal remains to be discovered regarding several key areas in CHC pathogenesis. These include the interaction of HCV with host cells, the role of host antiviral cellular immune response and the mechanisms of HCV persistence.

Several theories regarding the ability of HCV to persist and lead to chronic infection have been proposed. The virus has a rapid turnover (serum half-life of a few hours, replication rate of 10^{10} to 10^{12} virions per day) and frequently mutates due to the lack of an error proof reading by HCV RNA dependent RNA polymerase.[27] This results in large concentrations of the virus circulating in the serum as a population of several different variants known collectively as quasispecies. This may help the virus to avoid early recognition and evade host immune mechanisms.

Defective early host immune responses have also been noted in association with persistent HCV infection.[27] The appearance of anti-HCV antibodies is typically delayed for 7–8 weeks, and is not associated with clinical outcome, reflecting ongoing viral infection rather than protective immunity.[28] The failure to generate a vigorous T cell response in response to the virus has been noted in those with persistent infection. The predominant type of T cell response is also important. For example, a persistent CD4+ type 1 (Th1) proinflammatory cytokine response producing interleukin-2, interferon-gamma, and tumor necrosis factor favors self-limiting acute HCV infection, as opposed to the CD4+ type 2 or Th2 anti-inflammatory response (interleukins 4, 5, and 6; B cell activation) apparent in those with chronic infection.[29,30] Host genetic factors that may be associated with increased viral clearance include the presence of specific major histocompatibility complex class II alleles HLA-DRB1 and DQB1.[31,32] However, the mechanisms that determine these immune response profiles await further investigation.

PROGRESSION OF CHRONIC LIVER DISEASE

The natural history of HCV disease involves progression from acute to chronic infection, and from chronic infection to cirrhosis, and finally, from cirrhosis to decompensated liver disease or hepatocellular carcinoma (Figure 3.1). The

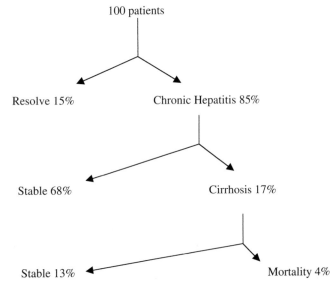

Figure 3.1. Natural History of Hepatitis C infection. *Source:* Reference 33.

chronic phase of HCV infection is often asymptomatic for decades, and may remain so. Approximately 10–20% of patients will develop cirrhosis over two decades or longer. For those with compensated cirrhosis, the risk of decompensation is approximately 3–4% per year and the five-year survival is 90%.[34,35] Once decompensated disease occurs, the prognosis declines sharply, and five-year survival decreases to 50%. Up to 3–4% of patients with established cirrhosis develop liver cancer annually.[22,34]

There is a wide variation in HCV disease progression among infected populations due to the presence of multiple host and perhaps viral contributors. Host factors that increase the risk of progressive liver disease include infection in males, older age at infection, Caucasian race (relative to African American race), HIV coinfection, concurrent HBV or schistosomal infection, higher levels of alcohol use, iron overload, obesity, insulin resistance or diabetes mellitus, and concurrent hepatic steatosis. Alcohol accelerates liver injury even among those with low or moderate levels of intake.[36–38] Of potential importance are genetic predispositions associated with the immune response and hepatic fibrogenesis which may theoretically also affect disease progression. The contribution of viral factors in determining disease progression is less certain; HCV RNA levels do not appear to correlate with disease severity.[13] There is no convincing data on the role of HCV genotype and quasispecies in disease progression.

CLINICAL MANIFESTATIONS

Acute HCV infection is subclinical in approximately two-thirds of cases. In the remainder, the predominant symptoms are malaise and weakness with a minority developing jaundice. Acute liver failure is extremely uncommon. Most patients with chronic infection are asymptomatic or experience mild nonspecific symptoms. Fatigue is most commonly reported, as are psychological disorders including depression, reduced vitality and diminished social functioning.[4] Other symptoms of variable frequency include anorexia, nausea, right-upper-quadrant abdominal discomfort, myalgia, and arthralgia. These symptoms do not accurately reflect disease activity but appear to occur more commonly with advancing liver disease and may significantly affect quality of life. Signs of advanced liver disease include muscle weakness, weight loss, pruritus, dark urine, fluid retention, and abdominal swelling. Physical examination may reveal an enlarged liver and spleen, jaundice, ascites, and ankle edema. Ascites is the most common form of decompensation,[35] followed by bleeding from esophageal varices, encephalopathy, and jaundice. Survival is not impaired until cirrhosis has developed. Some of the less common extrahepatic manifestations of chronic HCV infection are listed in Table 3.2.

LABORATORY TESTS AND CLINICAL EVALUATION

Diagnostic tests for HCV consist of serological tests that detect antibodies to HCV and molecular assays that detect and/or quantify HCV RNA concentrations. HCV genotype testing and liver biopsy provide additional information regarding risk assessment and prognosis as well as treatment duration and responses.

Table 3.2. Extrahepatic Manifestations of Chronic Hepatitis C Infection

Essential mixed cryoglobulinemia
Cryoglobulins are found in over 50% of patients.[39] They result in formation and deposition of circulating immune complexes in small to medium blood vessels which may result in a vasculitis involving skin (palpable purpura), joints (arthralgias), kidneys, peripheral nerves, and brain.
Monoclonal gammopathies
Lymphoma
Typically B cell Non-Hodgkin's lymphoma
Diabetes mellitus
Linked to HCV in several epidemiologic studies[40–42]
Thyroiditis
Antithyroid antibodies are present in 10–20% with chronic HCV,[43,44] particularly females, and mostly result in hypothyroidism
Seronegative arthritis
Keratoconjunctivitis sicca
Glomerulonephritis
Sialadenitis
Lichen planus
Neuropathies
Cognitive dysfunction
Porphyria cutanea tarda

An array of serum tests, including hematologic, biochemical, metabolic, and immune markers are employed for diagnosis and monitoring before and after treatment, as well as for screening for other types of liver disease and complications of HCV infection.

Diagnostic Tests

Both serologic and molecular tests are used to diagnose HCV infection. Serologic testing, of which the most commonly employed is the enzyme immunoassay (EIA), is highly sensitive for detecting antibodies to HCV.[45] EIA is a relatively inexpensive and semi-automated test that is useful for screening purposes, indicating exposure to HCV but not reflective of active viral replication. False negative results may occur in acute HCV, HCV associated cryoglobulinemia, renal failure, and in the immunocompromised.[13]

Subsequent generation EIAs (EIA-2 and EIA-3) are now the most commonly employed screening assay and have higher levels of sensitivity and specificity, detecting anti-HCV antibodies earlier during seroconversion (7–10 weeks post-inoculation compared with 16 weeks for the first-generation assay).[45,46] EIA-3 is approved for screening blood products in the United States.

Following the detection of anti-HCV antibodies by EIA, confirmatory testing for HCV should be performed either with recombinant immunoblot assay (RIBA) or more accurately with molecular testing for HCV RNA in the serum. RIBA uses recombinant HCV-encoded antigens to detect antibodies in patient serum. RIBA may be helpful in interpreting positive anti-HCV results, especially in low prevalence situations where risk factors for HCV are not evident or the clinical suspicion of HCV is low.[47] RIBA does not appear to have a meaningful role in diagnosis of HCV and is now rarely performed with the advent of more reliable third-generation antibody and HCV RNA testing.

The detection of HCV RNA in the serum using the reverse transcriptase polymerase chain reaction (RTPCR) is a highly sensitive assay that is able to detect extremely small concentrations of virus. It is now considered the gold standard test for diagnosis of HCV. Due to its high cost it is usually not employed as a screening test except in newborns (who may harbor maternal HCV antibodies), seronegative chronic hepatitis, or immunocompromised individuals who may lack serologic evidence of HCV infection. Serum levels of HCV RNA are also routinely performed as a means of predicting and monitoring the response to antiviral treatment. Both qualitative and quantitative assays are available for this purpose.

Following a diagnosis of HCV infection, genotype testing should be performed, as this determines both the duration and likelihood of response to interferon-based treatment. Genotype 1 accounts for 60–70% of infections in the United States and Europe. Genotypes 2 and 3 represent 19–22% of infections, with genotype 3 more common in India, the Far East, and Australia.[4] The remaining genotypes (4, 5, and 6) account for less than 5% of infections. Genotype 4 is seen more commonly in Africa and Egypt, the Middle East, and several Mediterranean countries; genotype 5 is seen in South Africa and genotype 6 in South China and Southeast Asia.[48]

Liver Biopsy

Liver biopsy remains an important test in the diagnostic evaluation for HCV infection, and is the most accurate way of assessing the severity of liver damage caused by the virus. A biopsy provides direct evidence of necroinflammatory activity and liver fibrosis, the presence of which provides useful information in determining prognosis and potential for disease progression. Liver biopsy can also establish the presence of concomitant liver diseases, for example steatosis and alcoholic injury, and assist in treatment decisions and modifications. In particular, the amount of inflammation and fibrosis on liver biopsy has been shown to be the best clinical predictor of disease progression. In one study of 70 HCV positive patients, patients with only mild hepatic inflammation and no fibrosis had only a 1.2% annual risk of progressing to cirrhosis. This compared with a 4.6% annual risk in patients with moderately severe inflammation, and nearly all patients with severe inflammation or bridging fibrosis developing cirrhosis within 10 years.[40] If cirrhosis is present on biopsy, then screening these patients for complications of CHC is indicated, such as 6–12 monthly abdominal ultrasound and 6-monthly serum alpha-fetoprotein for hepatocellular carcinoma, and upper gastrointestinal endoscopy for detection of esophageal varices. Histological features consistent with CHC infection are summarized in Table 3.3.

The Metavir score has been specifically designed and validated for patients with CHC infection. It is now the most commonly used method of grading and staging the severity of liver disease, and consists of both an activity and fibrosis score. The activity score is graded according to the intensity of necroinflammation (A0 = no activity, A1 = mild activity, A2 = moderate activity, A3 = severe activity). The fibrosis score is assessed on a 5 point scale (0 = no fibrosis,

---

Table 3.3. Histologic Features of Chronic Hepatitis C Infection

Infiltration of portal tracts with lymphocytes and macrophages
Inflammation at the interface between the portal tract and liver parenchyma (interface hepatitis). Portal tract infiltrates may coalesce to form lymphoid aggregates
Foci of necrosis within liver parenchyma (piecemeal necrosis)
Fibrosis which commonly begins around portal tracts
Steatosis is frequent, though usually mild and appears to be virally mediated and more common in genotype 3 infected patients, as opposed to host metabolic factors in genotype 1 patients.[50]

---

1 = portal fibrosis without septa, 2 = portal fibrosis with few septa, 3 = numerous septa without cirrhosis, 4 = cirrhosis).

Despite frequent use, liver biopsy has inherent limitations. Complications include significant pain in approximately 20%[51] of patients and rarely bleeding, and patients are often hesitant to undergo the procedure. Furthermore, sampling variability may lead to incorrect staging of the severity of liver disease in as many as 15–30% of patients.[52,53] Thus, it is important that specimens are of a length that enables more accurate assessment of fibrosis and activity scores. A biopsy length of at least 10–15 mm is considered adequate although this may not be achieved in a significant number of patients.[54] The Metavir score is also subject to discordant interpretation, even among experienced pathologists.[53] Finally, because fibrosis progression may not be linear over time, measuring fibrosis at a single point in time may not accurately predict disease progression. Noninvasive measures of hepatic fibrosis, such as use of transient elastography (Fibroscan) or serodiagnostic markers, such as Fibrotest or Fibrospect may be a reasonable alternative to biopsy in selected patients, and are in widespread clinical use in some countries.

Serum Tests

Among patients with CHC infection, a wide variation in serum aminotransaminase values is noted. In up to 30% of patients, alanine aminotransferase (ALT) values are persistently normal.[22] In the remainder, mild elevations are usually present, with the majority having an ALT of less than twice normal. Generally there is no definitive correlation between aminotransferase levels and liver histology or disease progression.[55] Therefore, transaminase levels do not allow the discernment of different stages of liver disease. Nonetheless, there is a general tendency for patients with substantially elevated ALT levels (especially if over 5 times normal) to have higher levels of necroinflammation and progress more rapidly than patients with persistently normal ALT.[55] Patients with normal ALT almost always show evidence of chronic inflammation, although liver injury is usually minimal or mild. The presence of a raised aspartate aminotransferase (AST) to ALT ratio and a low platelet count may be a 'clue' to the presence of advanced fibrosis or cirrhosis.[56]

Other serum tests that form part of the diagnostic work up for CHC infection should include evaluation for other types of liver disease (e.g., hepatitis B serological assays, iron studies, copper, and ceruloplasmin) as well as markers of autoimmune liver disease (e.g., anti-nuclear antibody, anti-smooth muscle, and anti-mitochondrial antibodies). The results of these investigations are also useful in shaping HCV treatment decisions.

TREATMENT OF CHRONIC HEPATITIS C INFECTION

The overall aim of treating patients with CHC infection is to prevent progressive hepatic fibrosis and its clinical consequences by permanently eradicating viral RNA. The eradication of HCV, defined as a sustained virological response (SVR), is defined as the absence of HCV RNA by a sensitive PCR assay 24 weeks after the end of treatment. The potential long-term benefits of viral clearance include the normalization of serum aminotransferase levels, a reduction in hepatic necroinflammation and fibrosis, an improvement or return to normal in health-related quality of life measures, improved survival, and a reduction in the risk of hepatocellular carcinoma.[57]

Treatment Decisions

A decision to treat CHC infection is a complex and individualized one, and thus referral to a hepatologist is recommended once a diagnosis of HCV is made. When considering a patient for treatment of CHC infection, the clinician must weigh the potential benefits of a permanent cure and/or suppression of liver inflammation and disease progression against the risks and potential side effects and costs of treatment. The presence or absence of symptoms alone is not an indication for treatment. Instead, many factors are involved that shape this decision. These include the extent of liver damage or fibrosis on biopsy and the risk of progression; as well as the presence of comorbidities and contraindications to treatment. Potential host factors of importance include age and occupation, the patient's psychological profile or 'mindset', treatment preferences, the likelihood of adherence to treatment, social situation and support, and the ongoing presence of risk factors for HCV or chronic liver disease (e.g., alcohol consumption and injecting drug use). Due to all these considerations, only around 50–60% of HCV patients seem to be candidates for therapy and a smaller number of patients actually receive treatment.[58] Thus, to maximize the potential benefits of antiviral treatment, adequate counseling and education of the patient is essential and requires a multidisciplinary team of experienced staff who can provide and prompt and accurate information in a supportive manner.

Treatment is generally recommended for those patients with an increased risk of developing cirrhosis. Current National Institutes of Health (NIH) guidelines define these higher risk patients as those with detectable HCV RNA levels and a liver biopsy with portal and bridging fibrosis (Metavir F2 or greater) and at least moderate inflammation and necrosis.[22] The majority of patients fulfilling these criteria will have persistently elevated ALT levels. Those with milder forms of liver disease and normal transaminases should be given the option of deferring therapy depending on their preferences and motivation. A plan of watchful waiting and monitoring is commonly employed in these patients.

Because patients with genotypes 2 or 3 have a SVR rate of approximately 80%, a liver biopsy is not mandatory to make an initial treatment decision. However, many clinicians still favor biopsy in order to facilitate screening for

HCC in the event of cirrhosis. The seriousness of the histological findings may also help to decide the aggressiveness of continued antiviral therapy in the event that it is poorly tolerated, or to help determine the urgency for newer treatment regimes in the event of non-response to previous therapies.

Treatment Options

The current standard of care for treatment-naive CHC patients is a combination of pegylated interferon-α administered once weekly by subcutaneous injection and oral ribavirin given twice daily. The interferons are a group of naturally occurring cytokines that exhibit immunomodulatory, antiproliferative, and antiviral effects. Interferon administration for CHC infection began initially as standard interferon, which has a short half-life of 6–8 hours and was administered thrice weekly. Pegylation of interferon (PEG-IFN) refers to the covalent attachment of an inert water-soluble polymer of ethylene glycol to the interferon molecule, available in 2 preparations, either a linear chain (α-2b) or branched chain (α-2a). Pegylation improves the pharmacokinetic profile of interferon through a combination of mechanisms, including reduced rates of absorption and renal clearance.[59] The resultant increase in half-life and steady state concentrations of the drug lead to a more favorable therapeutic effect in achieving viral eradication.[60] PEG–IFN α-2a is administered as a fixed dose of 180 µg weekly (Pegasys, Hoffman-La Roche), whereas PEG-IFN α-2b is available as a weight based dose of 1.5 μg/kg/week. (Pegintron, Schering Plough). It is not yet clear whether differences in these two forms of interferon have significant clinical differences, and head-to-head studies are currently in progress. Currently, either preparation in combination with interferon is considered appropriate for clinical use.

Ribavirin is a purine nucleoside analogue with antiviral effects against HCV when combined with IFN-α. Its mode of action is not fully understood. Several mechanisms have been postulated, including: (1) depletion of intracellular guanosine triphosphate (important for viral RNA synthesis), (2) inhibition of the 5 prime cap structure of viral mRNA, (3) mutagenic and inhibitory effects on HCV RNA dependent RNA polymerases, and (4) altering the balance towards a favorable proinflammatory cytokine response.[61–63]

The safety and efficacy of pegylated interferon and ribavirin therapy has been confirmed in several large randomized controlled trials.[64–66] In these studies, combination therapy has been shown to achieve an overall SVR rate of 54–61%. The success of this treatment varies according to HCV genotype. In patients infected with genotypes 2 and 3, SVR rates are approximately 80%. Therapy is less successful in genotype 1 infected patients, with SVR ranging from 42–46%. The optimum duration of treatment determined by these trials is 24 weeks for genotypes 2 and 3 and 48 weeks for genotype 1. Evidence also supports improved SVR with the use of higher doses of ribavirin in genotype 1 patients.[66] Thus, recommended ribavirin doses are 800 mg/day for genotypes 2 and 3, increasing to 1000 mg/day for genotype 1 patients weighing below 75 kg and 1200 mg/day for genotype 1 patients above 75 kg in weight. Data on the efficacy of treatment for genotypes 4, 5, and 6 are limited; therefore recommended treatment dosing and schedules follow those for genotype 1 infection. Patient factors predictive of a favorable response to combination therapy are listed in Table 3.4.

> **Table 3.4. Favorable Predictors of Response to Combination Therapy for Chronic Hepatitis C Infection**
>
> Virus-specific
> - HCV genotype 2 or 3
> - Low HCV RNA concentrations
>
> Demographic
> - Female
> - Younger age
> - Lower body mass index
>
> Histologic
> - Absence of fibrosis
> - Absence of steatosis

During successful antiviral treatment, HCV RNA concentrations in the serum promptly fall to undetectable levels and remain negative throughout therapy and thereafter. More than 98% of patients who achieve an SVR remain HCV RNA negative and are considered to have had a durable response when followed for an additional five years.[57] Reversal of hepatic fibrosis occurs in many patients (including those with Metavir F4 fibrosis) based on available follow-up data. Available information on longer-term outcomes following successful treatment is lacking. Properly conducted randomized controlled trials are needed to verify the assumption that the achievement of an SVR reduces morbidity and mortality from chronic liver disease. Currently, most clinicians agree that the development of cirrhosis and HCC are reduced in most, but not all, of these patients.

Pretreatment Assessment and Evaluation

Successful treatment of CHC infection relies on careful patient selection and detailed assessment of comorbidities, including psychiatric history. Contraindications to pegylated interferon and ribavirin therapy are listed in Table 3.5. A summary of tests that are required prior to initiating treatment is provided in Table 3.6. Treatment has a greater chance of success if patients have adequate social support and are well informed and compliant about treatment dosing and follow-up schedules. Thus, adequate education about the disease, treatment, and recognition of its side effects are of paramount importance. An appropriately staffed multidisciplinary team involving doctors, nurses, allied health care professionals, and support groups is therefore necessary. In particular, a good patient-doctor-nurse relationship is vital to a successful outcome.

Assessing Early Treatment Response

Early response to treatment is best determined by the levels of HCV RNA in the serum at 12 weeks of therapy. A $\geq 2 \log_{10}$ reduction or undetectable HCV RNA concentrations at week 12 is defined as an early virological response (EVR). Overall, 75–85% of HCV patients receiving combination therapy experience an EVR.[67] The failure to achieve this reduction at week 12 is a predictor of nonresponse to continued treatment. Studies have shown that only 1–2% of

---

Table 3.5. Contraindications to Combination Therapy for Chronic Hepatitis C Infection

Absolute Contraindications
Uncontrolled malignancy
Symptomatic coronary artery disease
Uncontrolled diabetes mellitus
Severe pulmonary disease
End-stage renal failure
Decompensated liver disease (total serum bilirubin > 25 μmol/l; prothrombin time international
normalised ratio > 1.5; albumin > 34 g/l; platelet count > 75000 × 10^9/l; presence of hepatic
encephalopathy, bleeding gastroesophageal varices, orascites)
Haemoglobinopathies (ribavirin)
Uncontrolled depression or other significant psychiatric illness
Pregnancy (ribavirin – embryocidal/teratogenic effects, IFN – abortifacient properties)
Unwilling to use 2 forms of contraception during treatment and for 6 months post-treatment
Uncontrolled autoimmune disorders or autoimmune hepatitis exacerbated by interferon
Non-liver solid organ transplantation (renal, cardiac)

Relative Contraindications
Active intravenous drug use
Alcohol abuse
Non compliance with medical, psychiatric or addiction therapies, HCV treatment instructions etc.
Underlying cytopenia, e.g., baseline neutrophil count < 1.5 × 10^9/L, Hb < 13 g/dL formen, < 12 g/dL
for women
Chronic renal insufficiency: cautious use of IFN if creatinine clearance < 50 ml/min; ribavirin
contraindicated

Table 3.6. Recommended Pretreatment Investigations for Patients With Chronic Hepatitis C Infection

HCV genotype

HCV RNA level

Biochemical investigations
*Liver tests (30% have persistently normal serum ALT; elevated serum bilirubin and low serum albumin
levels may reflect cirrhosis); urea and electrolytes, thyroid function tests, serum fasting glucose.*

Pregnancy test

Hematological investigations
Complete blood count and coagulation testing

Autoantibody tests
*Screening for autoimmune hepatitis (e.g., antinuclear and smooth muscle antibodies) and CHC-related
autoimmune diseases (e.g., antithyroid antibodies)*

Screening for other liver diseases
*HBV serology, α-FP (HCC), iron studies (haemochromatosis), serum copper and caeruloplasmin
(Wilson's disease)*

Liver ultrasound +/− CT scan
Detection of HCC (in patients with cirrhosis)

Liver biopsy

ECG in older patients or with a history of cardiac disease
Underlying cardiac disease as this may be exacerbated by treatment-relatedanemia

these patients achieve an SVR with continued treatment.[64,65,67,68] In view of this, it is recommended that genotype 1 patients without an EVR cease combination therapy at 12 weeks. Treatment should also be discontinued if HCV RNA remains detectable at 24 weeks in those patients who were HCV RNA positive at 12 weeks but had a $\geq 2 \log_{10}$ reduction in viral load. Assessment of EVR is not necessary in genotypes 2 and 3, as over 90% of these patients are HCV RNA negative at week 12, and rates of SVR are high. These early stopping rules reduce treatment costs, encourage patient compliance, and help early nonresponders avoid prolonged exposure to drugs with potentially harmful side effects that will have minimal benefits on virologic response.

Conversely, the presence of an EVR is not necessarily an accurate predictor of SVR, as only 65–75% of patients with EVR actually go on to achieve a SVR.[64,67] Instead, it has recently been shown that the rapidity of an EVR and the rate at which HCV RNA declines early in treatment is a better predictor of SVR, especially in genotype 1 infected patients.[68] Available data suggest that patients who have become HCV RNA negative by four weeks (rapid viral responders, RVR) represent a highly responsive treatment group. These patients, if they remain HCV RNA negative at weeks 12 and 24, have a greater than 90% chance of SVR.[68]

Management of Side Effects of Antiviral Therapy and the Effect of Dose Reduction

Side effects of pegylated IFN and ribavirin therapy are observed in approximately 80% of treated individuals.[69] Common adverse effects of treatment are listed in Table 3.7. Adverse events range from relatively common flu-like and psychological symptoms associated with IFN, to dermatologic reactions, hematologic, and thyroid abnormalities, to less common but more serious effects including major psychiatric illnesses. Due to the more severe adverse effects of combination therapy, at least 10–15% of patients withdraw from treatment prematurely.[64–66,69] Thus, early recognition and management of symptoms and frequent follow-up are vital in maintaining adherence and enhancing response rates. Many of these disturbances can be managed effectively with adjunctive pharmacotherapies such as antipyretics and antidepressants, rather than dose reductions. The latter tends to be reserved for treatment-related anemia, thrombocytopenia, and neutropenia, although the use of growth factors in these settings to combat anemia and neutropenia is commonplace, albeit with little evidence to support this concept.[70] Special consideration should be given to avoiding dose reductions of IFN or ribavirin for treatment effects during the first 12 weeks of therapy. The actual "amount" of dose reduction that impairs response has not been clearly defined, but it is clear that dose reduction has less of an impact in reducing EVR and SVR rates than complete discontinuation of these drugs.[57]

Treatment of Specific Patient Populations

Our current understanding of outcomes to antiviral therapy is based largely on clinical data from highly selected patient groups. In day-to-day practice however, distinct populations emerge in which the clinical course of HCV infection differs, or for which treatment decisions are difficult or controversial. In these patients, the clinician should consider antiviral treatment on an individual patient basis.

Table 3.7. Side Effects of Pegylated Interferon Plus Ribavirin for Chronic Hepatitis C Infection

'Flu-like' symptoms (IFN)
Fatigue
Headache
Anorexia
Nausea
Myalgia
Arthralgia
Fever
Rigors

Hair and skin conditions (IFN and ribavirin)
Injection site reactions (IFN)
Localized inflammatory lesions
Generalized skin reactions e.g. photosensitivity reactions (ribavirin);
hypersensitivity and allergic reactions e.g. pruritus, urticarial lesions
Exacerbation of immune-mediated skin disease e.g. psoriasis, lichen planus
Cellulitis
Vasculitis
Alopecia (IFN)

Neuropsychiatric disturbances (IFN)
Insomnia
Irritability
Impaired concentration
Depression (up to a third of patients with PEG-IFN therapy)

Hematological abnormalities (IFN and ribavirin)
Anemia (ribavirin – dose dependent reversible intravascular hemolytic anemia;
IFN – bone marrow suppression)
Thrombocytopenia (IFN)
Neutropenia (IFN) - severe ($< 0.5 \times 10^9$) occurs in $< 5\%$ patients

Thyroid dysfunction (IFN)
Frequently subclinical
Hypo- or hyperthyroidism (can be irreversible)

Rare
Pneumonitis
Cardiac arrhythmias (IFN)
Seizures (IFN)
Ophthalmologic disorders
Autoimmune disorders
Pancreatitis

Normal Serum ALT Levels and/or Minimal Liver Disease on Biopsy

These patients are likely to have slower rates of progression to cirrhosis, particularly if a prolonged duration of infection has been established. Thus, most do not require treatment and can be reassured with periodic follow-up every 6–12 months. Liver biopsy should be repeated after 3–5 years to ensure that those who develop significant fibrosis do receive appropriate antiviral treatment. In approximately one-third of patients, progression of fibrosis will occur.[71] Considerations that may favor treatment even in patients with mild liver disease include the following: (1) future childbearing plans; (2) specific concerns related to infectivity e.g. health care workers; (3) the presence of significant symptoms which may be associated with viremia e.g. fatigue; (4) patient mindset strongly favoring treatment; (5) extrahepatic manifestations of CHC infection (e.g., cryoglobulinaemia with systemic involvement); and (6) the presence of cofactors that increase the risk of progressive liver damage, such as HIV or significant steatosis on biopsy.

Patients with Cirrhosis

Patients with stable or compensated cirrhosis can be treated effectively but should be closely monitored, due to the greater likelihood of complications occurring during therapy. The efficacy of long-term interferon monotherapy to reverse fibrosis in these patients is being evaluated in clinical trials, and is discussed later. Interferon is inappropriate and potentially dangerous for patients with decompensated cirrhosis, and these patients should be referred to dedicated liver units with experience in liver transplantation prior to any consideration regarding antiviral therapy.

Recurrent Liver Disease Post-Transplant

Recurrence of HCV infection is universal following transplant.[72,73] Histological evidence of recurrence is apparent in approximately 50% of HCV-infected recipients in the first post-operative year.[74] Due to various reasons, the progression of liver disease and development of cirrhosis-related complications is accelerated in the post-transplant setting, and a sizeable proportion of patients are candidates for retransplantation. In the absence of large studies of patients in the post-transplant setting, the decision to proceed with antiviral treatment should be individualized. Successful treatment can be undertaken, although therapy is poorly tolerated overall and dose reduction frequencies of PEG-IFN and/or ribavirin of greater than 80% have been consistently reported.[75–77] IFN also carries a potential increased risk of allograft rejection, although there is no compelling evidence to support this association thus far.

Patients with Comorbid Liver Disease due to Other Causes

In patients with liver disease due to iron overload and hepatitis C, adjuvant treatment with venesection is often performed; however, there is no convincing evidence that this approach improves viral eradication. Interferon is contraindicated in patients with autoimmune hepatitis due to the potential for disease exacerbation. Treatment of patients with a history of excessive alcohol consumption is discussed below. For most other chronic liver diseases, such as hepatitis B infection, concurrent HCV infection is uncommon and when present can be treated on its own merits.

Children

HCV infection in children is usually due to perinatal transmission.[27] Newborns and younger children have a higher likelihood of spontaneous viral clearance.[18] Chronic viral infection is usually asymptomatic. With increasing age and duration of infection, the risk of fibrosis increases, although full progression to cirrhosis is an uncommon occurrence.[78] Multi-centered trials of combination therapy are in progress. Available data suggest that children respond at least as well as adults and they generally tolerate treatment well.[79] However, treatment should be avoided in children less than three years of age due to the increased potential for neurological side effects.[27]

Alcohol and Injecting Drug Use

Epidemiological studies have shown that approximately 30% of patients with alcoholic liver disease are infected with HCV.[80] There is good evidence from retrospective trial data that individuals with a history of moderate to heavy alcohol consumption ($\geq$ 30–50 g/day) in the setting of CHC infection are more likely to develop advanced fibrosis, cirrhosis, and HCC.[36–38] The effect of continued alcohol use during treatment has not been clearly defined, due to the fact that most large clinical trials have required a prolonged period of abstinence prior to enrollment. However, it should be noted that tolerance and compliance with antiviral therapy is traditionally poorer in these patients, and the psychological effects of interferon can potentially increase rates of recidivism. Patients are currently advised to refrain from alcohol before and during treatment, and this recommendation should be more strictly applied to individuals with more advanced liver disease.

The decision to treat actively injecting drug users is also controversial, due to a widespread belief that many of these individuals are noncompliant with treatment schedules and that continued high-risk behavior may result in reinfection. Again, all registration trials have excluded active drug users and thus available data on treatment success is limited. In general, a six-month period of abstinence is recommended prior to the initiation of antiviral therapy, aided by registration in a substance abuse program. There is emerging evidence that these patients are able to achieve rates of viral eradication comparable to others if they are managed jointly by specialists in hepatology and addiction medicine.[81,82]

Relapsers and Nonresponders to Previous Treatment

Patients not responsive to prior short-acting interferon therapy, either alone or in combination with ribavirin, can be retreated with pegylated interferon and ribavirin with an incremental gain in SVR of 10–20%.[83–85] In general, retreatment should be considered for patients with more advanced liver fibrosis or cirrhosis. Specific factors associated with a greater chance of retreatment response include previous interferon monotherapy (vs. prior interferon and ribavirin), adequate adherence to previous therapy, and prior relapse response (as opposed to nonresponse). The use of prophylactic therapies (e.g., antidepressants, hematopoietic growth factors) should be utilized to minimize adverse effects and dose reductions that may have occurred with previous antiviral treatment. Retreatment with combination therapy for longer durations (e.g., 48 weeks with genotypes 2 and 3) and with maximal doses of ribavirin of 1,000–1,200 mg/day is also practiced by some clinicians to maximize chances of success.

Therapeutic options are limited in patients who have not responded to pegylated interferon and ribavirin therapy. For patients with milder forms of liver disease, regular clinical observation and monitoring of liver biochemistry is appropriate until more effective therapies are available. Appropriate lifestyle measures should also be employed to minimize the effects of risk factors such as alcohol and steatosis, if present, on disease progression. For nonresponders with more advanced liver fibrosis, the option of enrollment in a clinical trial should be considered. Several large clinical trials are evaluating the utility of long-term maintenance therapy with low-dose pegylated interferon in preventing disease progression and complications of end-stage liver disease.[86] Interim results have been promising; however routine clinical use should be avoided until benefits in long-term outcomes have been clearly demonstrated.

Future Treatment Options

New therapeutic strategies currently in clinical trials include shortening or lengthening the duration of existing antiviral therapy depending on early viral responses, novel interferon preparations such as albumin-bound and omega interferon, alternatives to ribavirin, direct viral enzyme inhibitors targeted against the HCV protease or polymerase, and agents involved in modulating host immune responses and hepatic fibrogenesis. In the near future, increasing treatment success is likely to rest on continued use of interferon as a platform for synergistic combinations of these new agents.[87] Continuing challenges faced by newer therapeutic approaches will include the development of viral resistance and concerns regarding tolerability of multiple drug regimens. Effective vaccines for HCV remain elusive, with clinical trials still in the early phases of development.

SUMMARY

Despite a declining incidence in Western countries, the global prevalence of long-term CHC infection will remain relatively constant in the foreseeable future. Thus, morbidity and mortality from complications of cirrhosis are expected to remain a serious and significant problem over the next two decades. Many of these patients will be referred for liver transplantation, adding to the considerable health and economic burden of the disease. Much remains to be understood regarding the precise host and viral mechanisms that allow chronic infection and progression of liver disease in some affected individuals. It is hoped that the recent development of an efficient infectious HCV culture system will be helpful in expanding our knowledge in these areas. Although therapy for chronic HCV has improved dramatically in recent years, current interferon based therapy is effective in only half of all treated patients and is associated with significant adverse effects. Future therapies will likely entail combinations of existing therapies with novel, more targeted agents that specifically disrupt viral replication and/or modulate the host immune response.

REFERENCES

1. Armstrong GL, Alter MJ, McQuillan GM, Margolis HS. The past incidence of hepatitis C virus infection: implications for the future burden of chronic liver disease in the United States. Hepatology 2000 Mar;31(3):777–82
2. Kim WR. The burden of hepatitis C in the United States. Hepatology 2002 Nov;36(5 Suppl 1):S30–4.

3. Initiative for Vaccine Research, Viral Cancers, Hepatitis C. World health Organization, 2006. Accessed 1st November, 2006, at http://www.who.int/vaccine_research/diseases/viral_cancers/en/index2.html

4. McHutchison JG. Understanding hepatitis C. Am J Manag Care 2004 Mar;10(2 Suppl):S21–9.

5. Alter MJ, Kruszon-Moran D, Nainan OV, McQuillan GM, Gao F, Moyer LA, Kaslow RA, Margolis HS. The prevalence of hepatitis C virus infection in the United States, 1988 through 1994. N Engl J Med 1999 Aug 19;341(8):556–62.

6. Cheung RC, Hanson AK, Maganti K, Keeffe EB, Matsui SM. Viral hepatitis and other infectious diseases in a homeless population. J Clin Gastroenterol 2002 Apr;34(4):476–80.

7. Ruiz JD, Molitor F, Sun RK, Mikanda J, Facer M, Colford JM Jr, Rutherford GW, Ascher MS. Prevalence and correlates of hepatitis C virus infection among inmates entering the California correctional system. West J Med 1999 Mar;170(3):156–60.

8. Centers for Disease Control. Hepatitis C Slide Kit. Division of Viral Hepatitis, CDC. Accessed November 2006. http://www.cdc.gov/ncidod/diseases/hepatitis/slideset/hep_c/hcv_epi_for_distrib_000925.pdf

9. Alter MJ. Epidemiology of hepatitis C. Hepatology 1997 Sep;26(3 Suppl 1):62S–65S.

10. Garfein RS, Vlahov D, Galai N, Doherty MC, Nelson KE. Viral infections in short-term injection drug users: the prevalence of the hepatitis C, hepatitis B, human immunodeficiency, and human T-lymphotropic viruses. Am J Public Health 1996 May;86(5):655–61.

11. Rhodes T, Platt L, Maximova S, Koshkina E, Latishevskaya N, Hickman M, Renton A, Bobrova N, McDonald T, Parry JV. Prevalence of HIV, hepatitis C and syphilis among injecting drug users in Russia: a multi-city study. Addiction 2006 Feb;101(2):252–66.

12. Pomper GJ, Wu Y, Snyder EL. Risks of transfusion-transmitted infections: 2003. Curr Opin Hematol 2003 Nov;10(6):412–8.

13. Patel K, Muir AJ, McHutchison JG. Diagnosis and treatment of chronic hepatitis C infection. BMJ 2006 Apr 29;332(7548):1013–7.

14. Pereira BJ, Milford EL, Kirkman RL, Levey AS. Transmission of hepatitis C virus by organ transplantation. N Engl J Med 1991 Aug 15;325(7):454–60.

15. Alter MJ. Prevention of spread of hepatitis C. Hepatology 2002 Nov;36(5 Suppl 1):S93–8.

16. Dienstag JL. Sexual and perinatal transmission of hepatitis C. Hepatology 1997 Sep;26(3 Suppl 1):66S–70S.

17. Lissen E, Alter HJ, Abad MA, Torres Y, Perez-Romero M, Leal M, Pineda JA, Torronteras R, Sanchez-Quijano A. Hepatitis C virus infection among sexually promiscuous groups and the heterosexual partners of hepatitis C virus infected index cases. Eur J Clin Microbiol Infect Dis 1993 Nov;12(11):827–31.

18. Mast EE, Hwang LY, Seto DS, Nolte FS, Nainan OV, Wurtzel H, Alter MJ. Risk factors for perinatal transmission of hepatitis C virus (HCV) and the natural history of HCV infection acquired in infancy. J Infect Dis 2005 Dec 1;192(11):1880–9. Epub 2005 Oct 28.

19. Ohto H, Terazawa S, Sasaki N, Sasaki N, Hino K, Ishiwata C, Kako M, Ujiie N, Endo C, Matsui A, et al. Transmission of hepatitis C virus from mothers to infants. The Vertical Transmission of Hepatitis C Virus Collaborative Study Group. N Engl J Med 1994 Mar 17;330(11):744–50.

20. Zanetti AR, Tanzi E, Paccagnini S, Principi N, Pizzocolo G, Caccamo ML, D'Amico E, Cambie G, Vecchi L. Mother-to-infant transmission of hepatitis C virus. Lombardy Study Group on Vertical HCV Transmission. Lancet 1995 Feb 4;345(8945):289–91.

21. Roberts EA, Yeung L. Maternal-infant transmission of hepatitis C virus infection. Hepatology 2002 Nov;36(5 Suppl 1):S106–13.

22. National Institutes of Health. Consensus Statement Publication: Management of Hepatitis C. Hepatology 2002;36:S3–S20.

23. Centers for Disease Control and Prevention. Recommendations for prevention and control of hepatitis C virus (HCV) infection and HCV-related chronic disease. MMWR Recomm Rep 1998;47(RR-19):1–39.

24. Seeff LB. Natural history of chronic hepatitis C. Hepatology 2002 Nov;36(5 Suppl 1):S35–46.

25. Hoofnagle JH. Course and outcome of hepatitis C. Hepatology 2002 Nov;36(5 Suppl 1):S21–9.

26. Vogt M, Lang T, Frosner G, Klingler C, Sendl AF, Zeller A, Wiebecke B, Langer B, Meisner H, Hess J.Prevalence and clinical outcome of hepatitis C infection in children who underwent cardiac surgery before the implementation of blood-donor screening. N Engl J Med 1999 Sep 16;341(12):866–70.

27. McHutchison JG et al. Management Issues in hepatitis C Infection. Handbook. Science Press Ltd, Lonndon, UK. 2004.

28. Chang KM. Immunopathogenesis of hepatitis C virus infection. Clin Liver Dis 2003 Feb;7(1):89–105.

29. Lauer GM, Walker BD. Hepatitis C virus infection. N Engl J Med 2001 Jul 5;345(1): 41–52.

30. Mizukoshi E, Rehermann B. Immune responses and immunity in hepatitis C virus infection. J Gastroenterol 2001 Dec;36(12):799–808.

31. Alric L, Fort M, Izopet J, Vinel JP, Duffaut M, Abbal M. Association between genes of the major histocompatibility complex class II and the outcome of hepatitis C virus infection. J Infect Dis 1999 May;179(5):1309–10.

32. Thursz M, Yallop R, Goldin R, Trepo C, Thomas HC. Influence of MHC class II geno-type on outcome of infection with hepatitis C virus. The HENCORE group. Hepatitis C European Network for Cooperative Research. Lancet 1999 Dec 18–25;354(9196): 2119–24.

33. Alter MJ, Kruszon-Moran D, Nainan OV, McQuillan GM, Gao F, Moyer LA, Kaslow RA, Margolis HS. The prevalence of hepatitis C virus infection in the United States, 1988 through 1994. N Engl J Med 1999 Aug 19;341(8):556–62.

34. Di Bisceglie AM. Natural history of hepatitis C: its impact on clinical management. Hepatology 2000 Apr;31(4):1014–8.

35. Fattovich G, Giustina G, Degos F, Tremolada F, Diodati G, Almasio P, Nevens F, Solinas A, Mura D, Brouwer JT, Thomas H, Njapoum C, Casarin C, Bonetti P, Fuschi P, Basho J, Tocco A, Bhalla A, Galassini R, Noventa F, Schalm SW, Realdi G. Morbidity and mortality in compensated cirrhosis type C: a retrospective follow-up study of 384 patients. Gastroenterology 1997 Feb;112(2):463–72.

36. Hutchinson SJ, Bird SM, Goldberg DJ. Influence of alcohol on the progression of hepatitis C virus infection: a meta-analysis. Clin Gastroenterol Hepatol 2005 Nov;3(11): 1150–9.

37. Poynard T, Bedossa P, Opolon P. Natural history of liver fibrosis progression in patients with chronic hepatitis C. The OBSVIRC, METAVIR, CLINIVIR, and DOSVIRC groups. Lancet 1997 Mar 22;349(9055):825–32.

38. Westin J, Lagging LM, Spak F, Aires N, Svensson E, Lindh M, Dhillon AP, Norkrans G, Wejstal R. Moderate alcohol intake increases fibrosis progression in untreated patients with hepatitis C virus infection. J Viral Hepat 2002 May;9(3): 235–41.

39. Lunel F, Musset L, Cacoub P, Frangeul L, Cresta P, Perrin M, Grippon P, Hoang C, Valla D, Piette JC, et al. Cryoglobulinemia in chronic liver diseases: role of hepatitis C virus and liver damage. Gastroenterology 1994 May;106(5):1291–300. Erratum in: Gastroenterology 1995 Feb;108(2):620.

40. Mason AL, Lau JY, Hoang N, Qian K, Alexander GJ, Xu L, Guo L, Jacob S, Regenstein FG, Zimmerman R, Everhart JE, Wasserfall C, Maclaren NK, Perrillo RP. Association of diabetes mellitus and chronic hepatitis C virus infection. Hepatology 1999 Feb;29(2):328–33.

41. Mehta SH, Brancati FL, Strathdee SA, Pankow JS, Netski D, Coresh J, Szklo M, Thomas DL. Hepatitis C virus infection and incident type 2 diabetes. Hepatology 2003 Jul;38(1):50–6.

42. Zein CO, Levy C, Basu A, Zein N. Chronic hepatitis C and type II diabetes mellitus: a prospective cross-sectional study. Am J Gastroenterol 2005 Jan;100(1):48–55.

43. Antonelli A, Ferri C, Fallahi P, Ferrari SM, Ghinoi A, Rotondi M, Ferrannini E. Thyroid disorders in chronic hepatitis C virus infection. Thyroid 2006 Jun;16(6):563–72.

44. Huang MJ, Tsai SL, Huang BY, Sheen IS, Yeh CT, Liaw YF. Prevalence and signifi- cance of thyroid autoantibodies in patients with chronic hepatitis C virus infection: a prospective controlled study. Clin Endocrinol (Oxf.) 1999 Apr;50(4):503–9.

45. Ferreira-Gonzalez A, Shiffman ML. Use of diagnostic testing for managing hepatitis C virus infection. Semin Liver Dis 2004;24 Suppl 2:9–18.

46. Gretch DR. Use and interpretation of HCV diagnostic tests in the clinical setting. Clin Liver Dis 1997 Nov;1(3):543–57, vi.

47. Rios M, Diago M, Rivera P, Tuset C, Cors R, Garcia V, Carbonel P, Gonzalez C. Epidemiological, biological and histological characterization of patients with indeter- minate third-generation recombinant immunoblot assay antibody results for hepatitis C virus. J Viral Hepat 2006 Mar;13(3):177–81.

48. Dusheiko G, Schmilovitz-Weiss H, Brown D, McOmish F, Yap PL, Sherlock S, McIn- tyre N, Simmonds P. Hepatitis C virus genotypes: an investigation of type-specific differences in geographic origin and disease. Hepatology 1994 Jan;19(1):13–8.

49. Yano M, Kumada H, Kage M, Ikeda K, Shimamatsu K, Inoue O, Hashimoto E, Lefkow- itch JH, Ludwig J, Okuda K. The long-term pathological evolution of chronic hepatitis C. Hepatology 1996 Jun;23(6):1334–40.

50. Powell EE, Jonsson JR, Clouston AD. Steatosis: co-factor in other liver diseases. Hepa- tology 2005 Jul;42(1):5–13.

51. Castera L, Negre I, Samii K, Buffet C. Pain experienced during percutaneous liver biopsy. Hepatology 1999 Dec;30(6):1529–30.

52. Regev A, Berho M, Jeffers LJ, Milikowski C, Molina EG, Pyrsopoulos NT, Feng ZZ, Reddy KR, Schiff ER. Sampling error and intraobserver variation in liver biopsy in patients with chronic HCV infection. Am J Gastroenterol 2002 Oct;97(10):2614–8.

53. Bedossa P, Dargere D, Paradis V. Sampling variability of liver fibrosis in chronic hepatitis C. Hepatology 2003 Dec;38(6):1449–57.

54. Schiano TD, Azeem S, Bodian CA, Bodenheimer HC Jr, Merati S, Thung SN, Hytiroglou P. Importance of specimen size in accurate needle liver biopsy evalua- tion of patients with chronic hepatitis C. Clin Gastroenterol Hepatol 2005 Sep;3(9): 930–5.

55. Haber MM, West AB, Haber AD, Reuben A. Relationship of aminotransferases to liver histological status in chronic hepatitis C. Am J Gastroenterol 1995 Aug;90(8):1250–7.

56. Pohl A, Behling C, Oliver D, Kilani M, Monson P, Hassanein T. Serum aminotransferase levels and platelet counts as predictors of degree of fibrosis in chronic hepatitis C virus infection. Am J Gastroenterol 2001 Nov;96(11):3142–6.

57. Bacon BR. Managing hepatitis C. Am J Manag Care 2004 Mar;10(2 Suppl):S30–40.

58. Shad J, Person J, Brann O, Moon S, Pockros PJ, Nyberg L, Pianco S, et al. How often are referred chronic hepatitis C patients candidates for antiviral therapy [Abstract]. Hepatology 2000;32(Suppl): 283A.

59. Shiffman ML. Pegylated interferons: what role will they play in the treatment of chronic hepatitis C? Curr Gastroenterol Rep 2001 Feb;3(1):30–7.

60. Zeuzem S, Feinman SV, Rasenack J, Heathcote EJ, Lai MY, Gane E, O'Grady J, Reichen J, Diago M, Lin A, Hoffman J, Brunda MJ. Peginterferon alfa-2a in patients with chronic hepatitis C. N Engl J Med 2000 Dec 7;343(23):1666–72.

61. Hoofnagle JH, Seeff LB. Peginterferon and ribavirin for chronic hepatitis C. N Engl J Med 2006 Dec 7;355(23):2444–51.

62. Vo NV, Young KC, Lai MM. Mutagenic and inhibitory effects of ribavirin on hepatitis C virus RNA polymerase. Biochemistry 2003 Sep 9;42(35):10462–71.

63. Ning Q, Brown D, Parodo J, Cattral M, Gorczynski R, Cole E, Fung L, Ding JW, Liu MF, Rotstein O, Phillips MJ, Levy G. Ribavirin inhibits viral-induced macrophage production of TNF, IL-1, the procoagulant fgl2 prothrombinase and preserves Th1 cytokine production but inhibits Th2 cytokine response. J Immunol 1998 Apr 1;160(7):3487–93.

64. Manns MP, McHutchison JG, Gordon SC, Rustgi VK, Shiffman M, Reindollar R, Goodman ZD, Koury K, Ling M, Albrecht JK. Peginterferon alfa-2b plus ribavirin compared with interferon alfa-2b plus ribavirin for initial treatment of chronic hepatitis C: a randomised trial. Lancet 2001 Sep 22;358(9286):958–65.

65. Fried MW, Shiffman ML, Reddy KR, Smith C, Marinos G, Goncales FL Jr, Haussinger D, Diago M, Carosi G, Dhumeaux D, Craxi A, Lin A, Hoffman J, Yu J. Peginterferon alfa-2a plus ribavirin for chronic hepatitis C virus infection. N Engl J Med 2002 Sep 26;347(13):975–82.

66. Hadziyannis SJ, Sette H Jr, Morgan TR, Balan V, Diago M, Marcellin P, Ramadori G, Bodenheimer H Jr, Bernstein D, Rizzetto M, Zeuzem S, Pockros PJ, Lin A, Ackrill AM;PEGASYS International Study Group. Peginterferon-alpha2a and ribavirin combination therapy in chronic hepatitis C: a randomized study of treatment duration and ribavirin dose. Ann Intern Med 2004 Mar 2;140(5):346–55.

67. Davis GL, Wong JB, McHutchison JG, Manns MP, Harvey J, Albrecht J. Early virologic response to treatment with peginterferon alfa-2b plus ribavirin in patients with chronic hepatitis C. Hepatology 2003 Sep;38(3):645–52.

68. Ferenci P, Fried MW, Shiffman ML, Smith CI, Marinos G, Goncales FL Jr, Haussinger D, Diago M, Carosi G, Dhumeaux D, Craxi A, Chaneac M, Reddy KR. Predicting sustained virological responses in chronic hepatitis C patients treated with peginterferon alfa-2a (40 KD)/ribavirin. J Hepatol 2005 Sep;43(3):425–33.

69. Fried MW. Side effects of therapy of hepatitis C and their management. Hepatology 2002 Nov;36(5 Suppl 1):S237–44.

70. Curry MP, Afdhal NH. Use of growth factors with antiviral therapy for chronic hepatitis C. Clin Liver Dis 2005 Aug;9(3):439–51, vii.

71. Ghany MG, Kleiner DE, Alter H, Doo E, Khokar F, Promrat K, Herion D, Park Y, Liang TJ, Hoofnagle JH. Progression of fibrosis in chronic hepatitis C. Gastroenterology 2003 Jan;124(1):97–104.

72. Everhart JE, Wei Y, Eng H, Charlton MR, Persing DH, Wiesner RH, Germer JJ, Lake JR, Zetterman RK, Hoofnagle JH. Recurrent and new hepatitis C virus infection after liver transplantation. Hepatology 1999 Apr;29(4):1220–6. Erratum in: Hepatology 1999 Oct;30(4):1110.

73. Barcena R, Del Campo S, Sanroman AL, Nuno J, Zelaya R, Honrubia A, Vicente E, Monge G. Prospective study of hepatitis C virus infection after orthotopic liver transplantation. Transplant Proc 1997 Feb-Mar;29(1–2):515–6.

74. Sreekumar R, Gonzalez-Koch A, Maor-Kendler Y, Batts K, Moreno-Luna L, Poterucha J, Burgart L, Wiesner R, Kremers W, Rosen C, Charlton MR. Early identification of recipients with progressive histologic recurrence of hepatitis C after liver transplantation. Hepatology 2000 Nov;32(5):1125–30.

75. Samuel D, Bizollon T, Feray C, Roche B, Ahmed SN, Lemonnier C, Cohard M, Reynes M, Chevallier M, Ducerf C, Baulieux J, Geffner M, Albrecht JK, Bismuth H, Trepo C. Interferon-alpha 2b plus ribavirin in patients with chronic hepatitis C after liver transplantation: a randomized study. Gastroenterology 2003 Mar;124(3):642–50.

76. Chalasani N, Manzarbeitia C, Ferenci P, Vogel W, Fontana RJ, Voigt M, Riely C, Martin P, Teperman L, Jiao J, Lopez-Talavera JC;Pegasys Transplant Study Group. Peginterferon alfa-2a for hepatitis C after liver transplantation: two randomized, controlled trials. Hepatology. 2005 Feb;41(2):289–98. Erratum in: Hepatology 2005 Aug;42(2):506.

77. Charlton M. The Dilemma of Recurrent HCV Infection Following Liver Transplantation. AASLD Postgraduate Course Book, 2006, pp. 55–62.

78. Badizadegan K, Jonas MM, Ott MJ, Nelson SP, Perez-Atayde AR. Histopathology of the liver in children with chronic hepatitis C viral infection. Hepatology 1998 Nov;28(5):1416–23.

79. Gonzalez-Peralta RP, Kelly DA, Haber B, Molleston J, Murray KF, Jonas MM, Shelton M, Mieli-Vergani G, Lurie Y, Martin S, Lang T, Baczkowski A, Geffner M, Gupta S, Laughlin M;International Pediatric Hepatitis C Therapy Group. Interferon alfa-2b in combination with ribavirin for the treatment of chronic hepatitis C in children: efficacy, safety, and pharmacokinetics. Hepatology 2005 Nov;42(5):1010–8.

80. Rosman AS, Waraich A, Galvin K, Casiano J, Paronetto F, Lieber CS. Alcoholism is associated with hepatitis C but not hepatitis B in an urban population. Am J Gastroenterol 1996 Mar;91(3):498–505.

81. Backmund M, Reimer J, Meyer K, Gerlach JT, Zachoval R. Hepatitis C virus infection and injection drug users: prevention, risk factors, and treatment. Clin Infect Dis 2005 Apr 15;40 Suppl 5:S330–5.

82. Jeffrey GP, Macquillan G, Chua F, Galhenage S, Bull J, Young E, Hulse G, O'neil G. Hepatitis C virus eradication in intravenous drug users maintained with subcutaneous naltrexone implants. Hepatology 2007 Jan;45(1):111–7.

83. Krawitt EL, Ashikaga T, Gordon SR, Ferrentino N, Ray MA, Lidofsky SD; New York New England Study Team. Peginterferon alfa-2b and ribavirin for treatment-refractory chronic hepatitis C. J Hepatol 2005 Aug;43(2):243–9.

84. Taliani G, Gemignani G, Ferrari C, Aceti A, Bartolozzi D, Blanc PL, Capanni M, Esperti F, Forte P, Guadagnino V, Mari T, Marino N, Milani S, Pasquazzi C, Rosina F, Tacconi D, Toti M, Zignego AL, Messerini L, Stroffolini T;Nonresponder Retreatment Group. Pegylated interferon alfa-2b plus ribavirin in the retreatment of interferon-ribavirin nonresponder patients. Gastroenterology 2006 Apr;130(4):1098–106.

85. Jacobson IM, Gonzalez SA, Ahmed F, Lebovics E, Min AD, Bodenheimer HC Jr, Esposito SP, Brown RS Jr, Brau N, Klion FM, Tobias H, Bini EJ, Brodsky N, Cerulli MA, Aytaman A, Gardner PW, Geders A randomized trial of pegylated interferon alpha-2b plus ribavirin in the retreatment of chronic hepatitis C. Am J Gastroenterol. 2005 Nov;100(11):2453–62.

86. Shiffman ML, Di Bisceglie AM, Lindsay KL, Morishima C, Wright EC, Everson GT, Lok AS, Morgan TR, Bonkovsky HL, Lee WM, Dienstag JL, Ghany MG, Goodman ZD, Everhart JE;Hepatitis C Antiviral Long-Term Treatment Against Cirrhosis Trial Group. Peginterferon alfa-2a and ribavirin in patients with chronic hepatitis C who have failed prior treatment. Gastroenterology 2004 Apr;126(4):1015–23;discussion 947.

87. McHutchison JG, Bartenschlager R, Patel K, Pawlotsky JM. The face of future hepatitis C antiviral drug development: recent biological and virologic advances and their translation to drug development and clinical practice. J Hepatol 2006 Feb;44(2):411–21. Epub 2005 Dec 7.

HIV and Viral Hepatitis

Mark S. Sulkowski, MD

BACKGROUND

Communities and populations at high risk for HIV infection are also likely to be at risk for coinfection with hepatitis B virus (HBV) or hepatitis C virus (HCV). HIV, HBV, and HCV are bloodborne pathogens transmitted through similar routes, for example, via injection drug use (IDU), sexual contact, or from mother to child during pregnancy or birth.[1] A substantial proportion of HIV-infected individuals are coinfected with HBV, HCV, or both viruses, and in the context of effective HIV therapy, liver-related morbidity and mortality among HIV patients is a significant challenge. Current approaches to management of HIV/HBV and HIV/HCV coinfection are detailed in this course.

HEPATITIS C IN THE HIV-INFECTED PATIENT

Epidemiology

HCV and HIV have similar modes of transmission, but the transmission efficiency of each virus differs substantially. HCV is primarily transmitted by percutaneous exposure to blood – namely, via IDU. Coinfection with HCV and HIV is relatively common given the shared routes of transmission, and about 30% of all HIV-infected persons in the United States are also infected with HCV.[3] The prevalence of HIV/HCV coinfection varies depending on the route of HIV transmission, ranging from 10–14% among persons reporting high-risk sexual exposure to approximately 85–90% among those reporting IDU.[3] Despite the lower prevalence of chronic HCV infection among persons not engaged in IDU, recent outbreaks of acute HCV infection have been reported among HIV-infected men who have sex with other men, particularly those who engage in unprotected, traumatic sexual practices.[4] Accordingly, clinicians should counsel such patients to avoid high-risk sexual practices and should consider the possibility of acute HCV infection when treating patients with unexplained elevations in liver enzyme levels.

Natural History

Infection with HIV clearly exacerbates the natural history of HCV infection. HIV-infected patients are less likely to clear hepatitis C viremia, have higher HCV RNA loads, and experience more rapid progression of HCV-related liver disease than those without HIV infection.[5] As early as 1993, Eyster and colleagues reported that HCV RNA levels were higher in people with hemophilia who became HIV infected than in those who remained HIV negative, and liver failure occurred exclusively in HIV/HCV-coinfected patients.[6] More recently, among 1,816 HCV-positive patients with hemophilia who were prospectively monitored, Goedert and colleagues estimated the 16-year cumulative incidence of end-stage liver disease (ESLD) among men with and without HIV to be 14.0% and 2.6%, respectively.[7] Furthermore, among those men with HIV/HCV coinfection, the ESLD risk increased 8.1 fold with HBV surface antigenemia, 2.1 fold with CD4+ cell counts below 200 cells/mm^3, and 1.04 fold per additional year of age. Finally, the effect of HIV on HCV was summarized in a meta-analysis of studies by Graham and coworkers that assessed the correlation between HIV coinfection and the progression of HCV-related liver disease.[8] HIV coinfection was associated with a relative risk of ESLD of 6.14 and a relative risk of cirrhosis of 2.07 when compared with HCV monoinfection.

Given these data, and as survival among patients with HIV increases because of the use of potent antiretroviral therapies and prevention of traditional opportunistic pathogens, HCV-related morbidity and mortality among HIV-infected individuals can be expected to increase. Gebo and coworkers evaluated rates of admission at the Johns Hopkins University Hospital, Baltimore, Maryland, from 1995–2000 among HIV-infected patients and found that admissions for liver-related complications among HCV-positive patients increased nearly five-fold from 5.4 to 26.7 admissions per 100 person-years during that time.[9] Similarly, among 23,441 HIV-infected North American and European patients followed in the Data Collection on Adverse Events of Anti-HIV Drugs (D:A:D) study, liver disease was the second leading cause of death, with an incidence of 0.23 cases per 100 person-years follow-up behind HIV/AIDS (0.59 cases per 100 person-years) and ahead of cardiovascular disease (0.14 cases per 100 person-years).[10] Accordingly, in the era of potent antiretroviral therapy, HCV-related liver disease is currently and will continue to be a major cause of hospital admissions and deaths among HIV-infected persons. As such, effective HCV treatment strategies are needed.

Treatment of HCV-HIV Co-Infected Patients

Current guidelines endorsed by the National Institutes of Health, the U.S. Public Health Service, the American Association for the Study of Liver Diseases, the Infectious Diseases Society of America, and the European Consensus Conference Panel state that HCV should be treated in the HIV/HCV-coinfected person.[11–14] Current HCV therapies are associated with significant toxicity and have limited efficacy, however, and should therefore be provided to patients whose risk of serious liver disease is judged to outweigh the risk of morbidity due to the adverse effects of therapy, and who are most likely to respond to treatment (Table 4.1).

Table 4.1. Recommendations for the Management of HCV in HIV-Infected Patients(11)

Recommendation

- Anti-HCV testing should be performed in all HIV-infected patients
- HCV RNA testing should be performed to confirm HCV infection in HIV-infected patients who are seropositive for anti-HCV, as well as in those who are seronegative and have evidence of unexplained liver disease
- HCV should be treated in the HIV/HCV-coinfected patient in whom the likelihood of serious liver disease and a treatment response are judged to outweigh the risk of morbidity from the adverse effects of therapy
- Initial treatment of HCV in most HIV-infected patients consists of peginterferon alfa plus ribavirin for 48 weeks
- Given the high likelihood of adverse events, HIV/HCV-coinfected patients on HCV treatment should be monitored closely
- Ribavirin should be used with caution in patients with limited myeloid reserves and in those taking ZDV or d4T. When possible, patients receiving ddI should be switched to an equivalent antiretroviral before beginning ribavirin
- HIV-infected patients with decompensated liver disease may be candidates for orthotopic liver transplantation

---

The goal of HCV therapy is to achieve a sustained virologic response (SVR), defined as undetectable HCV RNA six months after HCV treatment is completed. Based on data from four randomized controlled trials, first-line HCV treatment in most HIV-infected persons consists of peginterferon alfa plus ribavirin for 48 weeks (Table 4.2).[15–18] Overall, these studies indicate that treatment may eradicate HCV infection in 14–29% of HIV-infected patients coinfected with HCV genotype 1 and in 43–62% of those coinfected with HCV genotype 2 or 3. Treatment efficacy was low (18%), however, in genotype 1 patients with high levels of HCV viremia ($> 800,000$ IU/mL), representing a substantial proportion of coinfected patients in the United States.

Lack of early virologic response at Week 12 of therapy is highly predictive of virologic failure among HIV/HCV-coinfected patients. In the APRICOT study, SVR was observed in less than 2% of patients who did not achieve at least a 2-$\log_{10}$ IU/mL reduction in HCV RNA from baseline or undetectable HCV RNA levels after 12 weeks of treatment (negative predictive value: 98–100%). Accordingly, current guidelines indicate that HCV treatment should be discontinued among HIV-infected patients who fail to achieve an early virologic response at 12 weeks of treatment to avoid exposing patients to the risks of treatment when they are very unlikely to achieve SVR. Recently, Payan and colleagues reported that the failure to suppress serum HCV RNA levels below 460,000 IU/ml after four weeks of therapy was associated with a negative predictive value of 100% among subjects enrolled in the RIBAVIC.[19] These data suggest that clinical decisions regarding the continuation of therapy may be made earlier in some person with HCV/HIV coinfection, particularly those experiencing significant toxicity.

Adverse events are common among HCV/HIV-coinfected patients receiving peginterferon alfa plus ribavirin. Approximately 12–25% of coinfected patients in clinical trials discontinued therapy early because of an adverse event, and serious adverse events occurred in 17–29%. The most common adverse effects of

Table 4.2. Comparison of 4 Randomized Controlled Trials of Peginterferon Plus Ribavirin in HIV/HCV-Coinfected Patients

Parameter	APRICOT (15)	ACTG A5071 (16)	ANRS HC02 RIBAVIC (17)	Laguno et al. (18)
Number of subjects	868	133	412	95
Country Regimen	Multinational	United States	France	Spain
■ Peginterferon	Peginterferon alfa-2a 180 µg/wk	Peginterferon alfa-2a 180 µg/wk	Peginterferon alfa-2b 1.5 µg/kg/wk	Peginterferon alfa-2b 100–150 µg/wk (weight-based)
■ Ribavirin	800 mg/day	Dose escalated from 600 to 800 to 1000 mg/day at 4-week intervals	800 mg/day	600–1200 mg/day (weight-based)
■ Duration	48 wks	48 wks	48 wks	48 wks*
Baseline characteristics				
■ White, %	79	33	93	100
■ Mean CD4+ cell count, cells/mm³	530	474	482	570
■ Undetectable HIV-1 RNA, %	60	60	67	70
■ On ART, %	84	86	83	88
■ Bridging fibrosis or cirrhosis, %	16	11[†]	39	33
■ Genotype 1, %	61	77	59	55
■ HCV RNA > 800,000 IU/mL, %	72	83[‡]	–	47
SVR by genotype, %				
■ 1	29	14		
■ 1 & 4	–	–	17	38
■ 2 & 3	62	73	44	53

ACTG, AIDS Clinical Trials Group; ANRS; National AIDS Research Agency (France); ART, antiretroviral therapy.

*24 wks for HCV genotype 2 or 3 *and* HCV RNA < 800,000 IU/mL.

[†] Patients with cirrhosis.

[‡] HCV RNA > 1 million IU/mL.

HCV therapy include fatigue, depression, irritability, insomnia, and weight loss. Didanosine and zidovudine have been found to have important interactions with peginterferon and ribavirin. Didanosine has been associated with severe mitochondrial toxicity leading to pancreatitis, hepatic failure, and death, particularly among patients taking ribavirin.[20] As such, didanosine is contraindicated in patients receiving HCV treatment. Concomitant use of zidovudine and HCV therapy has been associated with higher rates of anemia, ribavirin dose reductions, and use of epoetin alfa compared with rates seen in patients not taking zidovudine.[21,22]

Not unexpectedly, in light of the relatively low HCV eradication rates and high rates of toxicity observed in carefully selected clinical trial subjects, the effectiveness of HCV therapy has been even more modest in clinical practice. In

1 urban setting with a high prevalence of HCV genotype 1 coinfection, African American ethnicity, and polysubstance abuse, the rate of referral for hepatitis C care and initiation of HCV treatment was relatively low.[23] More importantly, although the SVR rate among those initiating HCV treatment with standard interferon or peginterferon plus ribavirin was comparable (21%) to that observed in controlled trials, the overall effectiveness in this population was negligible, as less than 1% of the full cohort of HIV/HCV-coinfected patients receiving HIV care were treated and achieved an SVR. These and similar data from other settings suggest that new paradigms for HCV care are urgently needed in the United States and beyond – paradigms that incorporate patient and provider education, as well as case management to address competing patient needs, such as substance abuse, psychiatric illness, and HIV infection. These data also highlight the need for novel HCV therapies with improved efficacy and safety for coinfected patients.

Summary

HCV coinfection is common in HIV-positive patients in the United States and Europe. Because HIV infection can accelerate the progression of HCV-related liver disease, consideration of HCV treatment is generally recommended for all HIV/HCV-coinfected patients. However, the effectiveness of current HCV treatment regimens (i.e., peginterferon plus ribavirin) may be limited in some settings, e.g., in individuals with HCV genotype 1 and a high HCV load, in African American patients, in individuals with active drug and alcohol abuse, and in patients with uncontrolled mental illness or HIV disease. Current strategies must focus the delivery of HCV treatment to those with the greatest medical need. New and investigational agents have the potential to improve outcomes and should be studied early and aggressively in HIV/HCV-coinfected patients.

HEPATITIS B IN THE HIV-INFECTED PERSON

Epidemiology

HBV can be transmitted by sexual intercourse, percutaneous exposure, or from mother to infant. Among persons coinfected with HIV in the United States, HBV is most often transmitted by sexual intercourse (both heterosexual and between men), followed by IDU.[24,25] In Asia and sub-Saharan Africa, HBV is principally transmitted from mother to infant or during early childhood. Because the routes of transmission of HIV and HBV are similar, there is evidence of prior HBV infection in approximately 90% of HIV-infected persons whereas chronic HBV infection, indicated by reactive hepatitis B surface antigen (HBsAg) is detected in 5–15% of HIV-infected persons globally.

Natural History

The outcome of HBV infection varies according to age at acquisition and the immune status of the host. HBV infection persists in 50–90% of persons infected at birth or early childhood. In contrast, among adults, fewer than 5% of HBV infections become chronic. Recovery from HBV infection is characterized by clearance of HBsAg and HBeAg from blood in association with the formation of antibodies to both antigens. Viral recovery is most likely to occur during the first year after infection, but spontaneous clearance of HBsAg and HBeAg can occur indefinitely. HIV infection has been associated with the failure to seroconvert following acute infection and a greater risk of developing chronic hepatitis B infection compared to HIV seronegative persons.[26] It is now appreciated that HBV DNA can be detected in some persons with serologic evidence of recovery, indicating that there is ongoing replication that is contained by a vigorous immune response. Several studies have demonstrated relatively high rates of "occult" hepatitis B infection in persons with HIV infection.[27] This incomplete clearance probably explains relapses that have been reported in immunosupressed persons, such as those who develop AIDS, which illustrates the dynamic nature of hepatitis B infection, particularly in persons with HIV disease.

Among those in whom HBsAg is persistently detected, some never develop substantial liver enzyme elevation or significant histologic disease. Typically, the serum of such persons contains HBsAg but no or very low levels of HBV DNA, and HBeAg is usually not detected. Others with persistent HBsAg develop significant liver disease that can progress to cirrhosis or hepatocellular carcinoma. Persons at risk for cirrhosis and hepatocellular carcinoma usually have HBsAg and HBV DNA in their serum; furthermore, the presence of HBeAg is associated with an additional increased risk of these outcomes. Emerging data suggest that HBV DNA levels may be best predictor of clinical progression of HBV infection to cirrhosis and hepatocellular carcinoma. In a prospective cohort study of 3,653 Taiwanese patients aged 30–65 years who were HBsAg-positive (and HIV-negative), an elevated serum HBV DNA level ($>$ 10,000 copies/mL) was the strongest predictor for the development of cirrhosis and hepatocellular carcinoma independent of HBeAg status or serum ALT levels.[28,29] Thus, the level of HBV replication appears to be closely linked to the development of liver disease. In general, persons with HIV coinfection have higher levels of hepatitis B viremia compared to those with HBV infection alone.[30] This may explain the increase risk of HBV-related liver disease in person with HBV and HIV coinfection.

The stage of hepatitis B infection in persons with concurrent HIV disease is typically assessed by HBV serologic testing (HBsAg, HBeAg), serum ALT level and magnitude of hepatitis B viremia (i.e., HBV viral load). Some experts recommend liver biopsy to assess histologic activity and fibrosis in HIV/HBV coinfected persons with normal or minimally elevated serum ALT levels and low levels of HBV DNA ($<$10,000 IU/mL).[31] However, other experts suggest that because of the negative impact of HIV on the risk of HBV-related disease (see below) that all HIV/HBV coinfected persons should be considered to be at risk for the development of cirrhosis and/or hepatocellular carcinoma.

The natural history of HBV infection is modified by HIV infection, which can result in higher rates of HBV persistence (HBsAg, HBeAg, HBV DNA detection) and relapse (reemergence of HBsAg, HBeAg, or HBV DNA) (Figure 4.2). Among those with persistent HBV infection, the severity of liver disease is substantially increased in the setting of HIV coinfection with markedly increased risk of liver-related mortality. Among subjects followed a long-term cohort study, Thio and coworkers reported that the liver-related mortality rate was higher in men with HIV-1 and HBsAg (14.2/1000) than in those with only HIV-1 infection (1.7/1000,

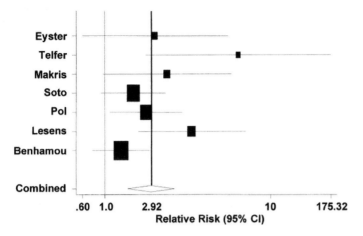

Figure 4.1. Adjusted relative risk of decompensated liver disease or histological cirrhosis in patients with HIV/HCV coinfection compared with patients who have HCV infection alone (adapted from meta-analysis published by Graham and colleagues)[8]

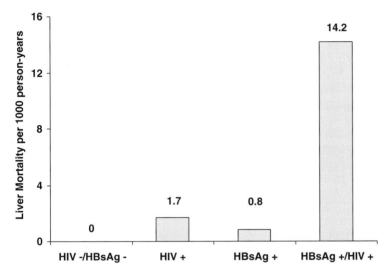

Figure 4.2. Comparison of liver-related mortality by HIV and HBsAg status among 5,293 men followed in the Multicenter AIDS Cohort Study (MACS)[32]

p < 0.001) or only HBsAg (0.8/1000, p < 0.001)(Figure 4.1).[32] In coinfected individuals, the liver-related mortality rate was highest with lower nadir CD4+ cell counts and was twice as high after 1996, when highly active antiretroviral therapy was introduced. The effect of antiretroviral-related immune restoration has been associated with spontaneous recovery from chronic HBV infection but, in other studies, with flares of hepatitis B. The effects of HBV infection on HIV natural history are less apparent but may include a higher incidence of liver enzyme elevations associated with antiretroviral therapy.[33]

Diagnosis

Ongoing HBV infection is diagnosed by the detection of viral antigens (HBsAg or HBeAg) and HBV DNA in blood. When infection is acute, IgM antibodies to the core protein are also detected, generally together with HBV antigens and HBV DNA. When the infection has been established for more than 12 months, IgG (but not IgM) antibodies to the core protein are detectable along with viral antigens and HBV DNA. Chronic hepatitis B infection is characterized by the presence of HBsAg with or without HBeAg. During the course of an infection, the loss of HBeAg and development of anti-HBe, is usually associated with a decrease in serum HBV viral load, and is associated with a favorable prognosis. However, the loss of HBeAg may also reflect the emergence of HBeAg-negative HBV with precore and core promoter mutations that alter the normal HBeAg synthesis. In this situation, HBV replication remains active as indicated by detectable HBV DNA. Thus, persons with detectable HBsAg and anti-HBe should be assessed for evidence of active HBV replication by HBV DNA assays. All persons with detectable HbsAg should undergo screening for hepatocellular carcinoma with serum AFP and liver ultrasound at regular intervals (6–12 months).

When individuals recover from acute hepatitis B, HBeAg and HBsAg are no longer detectable in the blood, although low levels of HBV DNA may be detected with sensitive assays. With recovery, antibodies to the HBV surface, E, and core antigens become detectable. Because recombinant and serum-derived HBV vaccines include HBsAg determinants, prior vaccination, and immunity are reflected by the presence of anti-HBs in serum.

Antibodies to the HBV core can be detected in some persons without HBsAg, HBeAg, or antibodies to these antigens. Isolated HBV core antibody serology occurs frequently in persons engaging in IDU (who are generally also HCV infected) and among both HIV-infected and HIV-uninfected persons.[34] The probability that isolated antibody to the HBV core represents HBV infection (versus a false-positive reaction) is related to the prevalence of HBV infection and the anticore antibody titer. For example, in low-prevalence settings, such as among volunteer blood donors, persons with low titers of antibody to the HBV core without other HBV markers rarely have anamnestic responses to HBV vaccination (detection of antibody to the surface antigen) after a single dose, thus suggesting that these may be false-positive anticore reactions.[35] However, individuals with isolated hepatitis B core antibodies who are at high risk for HBV infection and those with high-titer core antibodies are more likely to have evidence of prior HBV infection, as indicated by anamnestic responses to vaccination or by the detection of HBV DNA by PCR. Given the high risk for HBV infection, it is reasonable to assume that the finding of isolated HBV core antibody in HIV-infected persons represent evidence of past infection. However, controversy exists as to the need to assess HIV-infected persons with isolated antiHBc for active HBV replication with assays to detect HBV DNA. In addition, the need for HBV vaccine in such persons is also unclear and some experts recommend the provision of HBV vaccine to all HIV-infected persons who are HBsAb negative independent of anti-HBc status.

OF HBV-HIV CO-INFECTED PATIENTS

Several medications are approved by the United States Food and Drug Administration (FDA) for the treatment of chronic HBV: interferon alfa, peginterferon alfa-2a, adefovir, lamivudine, telbivudine, and entecavir. In addition, tenofovir and emtricitabine are approved for the treatment of HIV infection and are dually active against HBV (Tables 4.3 and 4.4).

Standard or Pegylated Interferon Alfa

Few studies have addressed the efficacy of interferon alfa treatment in patients with HIV/HBV coinfection. The pegylated form of interferon appears to be more

Table 4.3. Medications Approved by the FDA for the Treatment of Chronic HBV Infection

Drug	Dose and Duration	Indicated for Chronic HBV in HIV-Infected Patients*	Active Against HIV and HBV
Interferon alfa	▪ 5 MU daily or 10 MU 3 times per week by injection ▪ Duration 16–48 weeks	No	No
Peginterferon alfa-2a	▪ 180 μg weekly by injection ▪ Duration 6–12 months	No	Yes
Lamivudine	▪ 300 mg/day in HIV-positive individuals ▪ Minimum treatment 12 months	No	Yes
Emtricitabine	▪ 200 mg/day ▪ Optimal duration unknown	No	Yes
Adefovir	▪ 10 mg/day ▪ Optimal duration unknown	No	No[†]
Tenofovir	▪ 300 mg/day ▪ Optimal duration unknown	No	Yes
Entecavir	▪ 0.5 mg/day in lamivudine-naive patients ▪ mg/day in lamivudine-experienced patients ▪ Optimal duration unknown	Yes	Yes
Telbivudine	▪ 600 mg/day lamivudine naïve patients	No	No

MU, million units.

* Indicated by FDA for treatment of chronic HBV in HIV-infected persons.

[†] Not considered active against HIV at doses used in HBV therapy.

Table 4.4. Tenofovir versus adefovir for treatment of HBV in individuals coinfected with HIV[45]

Study Group	n	HBV DNA DAVG$_{48}$, log$_{10}$ copies/mL		
		Adefovir Arm	Tenofovir Arm	Difference
Intent-to-treat population	52	−3.12	−4.03	0.91
Modified intent-to-treat population	47	−3.35	−4.46	1.11
As-treated population	41	−3.48	−4.76	1.28

HBV DNA DAVG$_{48}$, time-weighted mean change in HBV DNA at week 48.

effective than standard interferon alfa for the treatment of chronic hepatitis B in HIV-uninfected persons but there are no published data on peginterferon efficacy in HIV/HBV-coinfected patients. However, limited data suggests that interferon therapy will be relatively ineffective for the treatment of HBV in HIV-infected persons.[36]

Lamivudine

Lamivudine is a nucleoside analogue that, in its active triphosphate form, inhibits HBV DNA polymerase and HIV reverse transcriptase. Although HBV DNA levels decrease by an average of 2.7 $\log_{10}$ copies/mL in HIV/HBV-coinfected persons taking lamivudine for 1 year, the incidence of lamivudine-resistant HBV is approximately 20% per year in HIV-infected persons.[37, 38] When lamivudine-resistant variants emerge, HBV DNA levels increase, liver enzyme levels may rise, and the resulting hepatitis can be fatal in a minority of patients. In addition, the bulk of available data suggest that the benefit in preventing progression of liver disease is substantially diminished with the presence of lamivudine-resistant HBV. Thus, the clinical effectiveness of lamivudine monotherapy is limited by the frequent emergence of resistant HBV variants.

Entecavir

Entecavir is a nucleoside analogue and is licensed for the treatment of chronic HBV infection in both HIV-infected and -uninfected persons. Entecavir inhibits all three functions of the HBV polymerase, including base priming, reverse transcription of the negative strand, and synthesis of the positive strand of HBV DNA. The presence of lamivudine-resistant variants causes decreased susceptibility to entecavir; thus, the recommended doses are 1 mg in lamivudine-experienced patients and 0.5 mg in lamivudine-naive patients.[39] In a randomized controlled trial of 68 HIV/HBV-coinfected persons with lamivudine-resistant HBV, 24 weeks of entecavir resulted in a 3.66 $\log_{10}$ copies/mL reduction in HBV DNA, which is similar to reductions observed in HBV monoinfection.[40] However, after 48 weeks of entecavir treatment, only 9% of patients achieved suppression of HBV replication below 300 copies/mL. To date, resistance to entecavir has rarely been reported among patients with wild-type HBV infection. However, entecavir resistance occurred in 7% of HBV-monoinfected patients with lamivudine-resistant HBV who received entecavir for 48 weeks and 39% of those treated for four years. Thus, while active against lamivudine resistant variants, entecavir should not be used as monotherapy to treat such patients. Finally, although initial reports indicated that entecavir was not active against HIV, clinical observations of significant reduction of HIV RNA level in three coinfected patients receiving entecavir for the treatment of HBV in the absence of treatment for HIV infection led to additional *in vitro* experiments confirming anti-HIV activity of entecavir and the potent for the selection of drug resistant HIV variants(41). Accordingly, entecavir should only be used for the management of HBV in HIV-infected persons receiving effective antiretroviral therapy.

Adefovir

Adefovir dipivoxil is a nucleotide analogue that, in its active diphosphate form, inhibits DNA polymerase and reduces HBV DNA levels by an average of 3.5 $\log_{10}$ copies/mL at 48 weeks.[27] Adefovir is licensed for the treatment of chronic hepatitis B in patients with HBV monoinfection and is active against lamivudine-resistant HBV. In one study, a total of 35 HIV/HBV-coinfected persons were treated with adefovir for 192 weeks and achieved a substantial reduction in HBV DNA (>4 $\log_{10}$).[42] It is clear from this study and from data in HBV-monoinfected patients that the incidence of clinically evident HBV resistance to adefovir is substantially lower than that to lamivudine. However, prolong use (~5 years) of adefovir in HIV seronegative persons with HBeAg negative HBV infection the cumulative probabilities of resistance was 0%, 3%, 11%, 18%, and 29% at 1, 2, 3, 4, and 5 years, respectively. Furthermore, the use of adefovir in HIV/HBV-coinfected patients may theoretically involve a risk of selecting HIV cross-resistance to tenofovir, because adefovir is active against HIV at higher doses than those used in HBV management. Nonetheless, HIV resistance following adefovir treatment has not been reported to date.[43]

Tenofovir

Tenofovir is a nucleotide analogue approved by the FDA for the treatment of HIV. This agent is structurally related to adefovir, differing by one methyl group. In vitro, tenofovir's activity against HBV is at least equivalent to that of adefovir, with a similar IC_{50}. In a prospective, nonrandomized study involving 53 patients with lamivudine-resistant HBV and high HBV viral load, all 35 patients treated with tenofovir had HBV DNA $< 10^5$ copies/mL at 48 weeks, compared with 44% of 18 patients treated with adefovir ($P = .001$).[44] In the setting of HIV/HBV coinfection, where lamivudine-resistant HBV is commonplace, tenofovir's activity against HBV has been demonstrated to be noninferior to that of adefovir. ACTG A5127 was a randomized, placebo-controlled trial in which 52 HIV-HBV-coinfected patients, most (74–80%) of whom had previously used lamivudine, received either tenofovir or adefovir.[45] The time-weighted mean change in HBV DNA did not differ significantly between treatment arms at Week 48 by any analysis method used, and tenofovir reached the protocol-defined criteria for noninferiority to adefovir (Table 4.5).

Emtricitabine

Emtricitabine is a nucleoside analogue that, following intracellular phosphorylation, exerts potent inhibition of both HIV and HBV replication. FTCB-301 was an international, randomized study in which 248 HBV-infected patients who were naive to HBV nucleoside/nucleotide analogue therapy received either emtricitabine or placebo.[46] At Week 48, 54% of patients in the emtricitabine group had HBV DNA < 400 copies/mL compared with 2% in the placebo group ($P < .001$). Resistance mutations emerged in 13% of those treated with emtricitabine. HBV variants resistant to emtricitabine also display decreased sensitivity to lamivudine and entecavir.

Telbivudine

Telbivudine is thymidine nucleoside analogue approved for chronic hepatitis B patients which has no activity against HIV. After 52 weeks of therapy, HBeAg positive and negative patients, telbivudine 600 mg/day was associated with a HBV DNA decrease of 6.45 log10 in HBeAg positive and 4.45 log10 in HBeAg negative patients. Viral suppression to undetectable levels was achieved in 60% of HBeAg positive patients randomized to telbivudine compared to only 40% of those receiving lamivudine. Resistant variants emerged in 8.1% (HBeAg-negative) and 21% (HBeAg-positive) of patients taking telbivudine for 52 weeks. HBV variants resistant to telbivudine are also resistant to emtricitabine and lamivudine. Among HIV-infected persons, telbivudine may have a unique role in that it can be safely used in persons not taking fully suppressive antiretroviral drugs.

Combination Therapy versus Monotherapy

Data that support the use of combination HBV therapy in preference to the use of single agents in HIV/HBV-coinfected patients are limited. GS 903 was a randomized trial designed to compare the efficacy of two first-line antiretroviral regimens in HIV-infected patients.[47] All participants received efavirenz and lamivudine, plus either tenofovir or stavudine. The inclusion of a small number of individuals with HBV coinfection allowed the investigators to compare the efficacy of lamivudine monotherapy versus lamivudine plus tenofovir dual therapy for treatment of HBV. At Week 48, the mean reduction in HBV DNA among six patients treated with lamivudine alone was 3.0 $\log_{10}$ copies/mL compared with 4.7 $\log_{10}$ copies/mL in five patients who received dual therapy ($P = .055$).

Nelson and colleagues from the United Kingdom have reported results from an open-label, randomized trial comparing lamivudine versus tenofovir versus lamivudine plus tenofovir for treatment of HBV in HIV/HBV-coinfected individuals.[48] Treatment was administered as part of a HAART regimen. Among 27 patients who were naive to lamivudine at entry, the median reduction in HBV DNA at Week 24 was significantly greater with use of the combination regimen (5.03 $\log_{10}$ copies/mL versus 3.31 $\log_{10}$ copies/mL in the lamivudine monotherapy arm and 4.66 $\log_{10}$ copies/mL in the tenofovir monotherapy arm; $P = .045$ dual therapy arm versus lamivudine arm). In 32 lamivudine-experienced patients, switching to or adding tenofovir resulted in superior antiviral activity at Week 24 compared with remaining on lamivudine alone ($P < .001$).

Treatment Approach

Because HIV infection can accelerate progression of HBV-related liver disease, treatment of chronic hepatitis B is generally recommended for all HIV/HBV-coinfected patients. However, the best strategy for management of HBV infection has not been fully defined. Among patients with chronic HBV infection with no current indication for antiretroviral therapy (e.g., CD4+ cell count > 350 cells/mm^3), some experts recommend avoiding drugs active against HIV (e.g., emtricitabine, lamivudine, entecavir, and tenofovir) and suggest using adefovir, telbivudine, or peginterferon. However, other experts recommend the institution of a fully suppressive antiretroviral regimen that includes the use of two agents active against HBV. This recommendation is based on the rationale that control of HIV infection may represent an important step in preventing HBV-related liver disease. Use of HBV therapy among HIV/HBV-coinfected patients for whom HIV treatment is indicted is less controversial: Most experts recommend the use of an antiretroviral regimen that includes the use of two agents that are active against HBV (e.g., tenofovir plus emtricitabine or lamivudine). No consensus has been reached on the management of coinfected patients with lamivudine-resistant HBV. However, most experts recommend the use of tenofovir plus continuation emtricitabine or lamivudine (despite HBV resistance to these agents) whereas other experts recommend the use of two drugs active against lamivudine resistant HBV: tenofovir and entecavir.

Prevention

Vaccination and the observance of universal precautions are the chief public health measures for preventing HBV infection. HBV vaccination is indicated for all children and adults who are at increased risk of HBV infection, including virtually all HIV-infected patients, people with multiple sexual partners, men who have sex with men, and people engaging in IDU. The vaccine used in most well-resourced nations is a recombinant surface antigen expressed in yeast. When used as licensed (3 doses administered to the intradeltoid muscle), more than 95% of adults develop antibody responses that are considered protective. Postvaccination antibody testing is recommended one to two months after the third vaccine dose for people with an increased risk of exposure.

In HIV-infected patients, HBV vaccination appears to be safe, as measured by the change in HIV viral load or the subsequent progression of HIV infection. HBV vaccine immunogenicity is reduced in HIV-infected patients, especially those with low CD4+ cell counts.[49] Improved HBV vaccine responses have been described in HIV-infected patients given three additional vaccine injections or the use of higher doses of vaccine. It should be noted, however, that neither of these measures is currently routinely recommended to prevent hepatitis B infection in people with HIV infection.

Summary

Due to shared modes of transmission, HBV coinfection is common in HIV-positive patients in the United States, Europe, Africa, India, and China. HIV modifies the natural history of HBV infection, leading to increased rates of chronic infection following acquisition of disease and greater likelihood of HBV-liver morbidity and mortality. Accordingly, all HIV-infected persons should be screened for hepatitis B with HBsAb and HBsAg testing. Persons found to be HBsAb negative should be vaccinated against HBV, preferably at relatively high CD4 cell counts. Persons found to HBsAg positive must undergo further diagnostic evaluation including testing for HBeAg, HBV DNA, serum ALT, AFP, and liver imaging (e.g., ultrasound). Because HIV infection can accelerate progression of HBV-related liver disease, treatment of chronic hepatitis B is generally recommended for all HIV/HBV-coinfected patients. However, the best strategy for management of HBV infection has not been fully defined. Most experts recommend the use of combination therapy for HBV with tenofovir plus emtricitabine or lamivudine in the setting of a fully suppressive antiretroviral drug regimen. In persons seeking to avoid an antiretroviral therapy, adefovir and/or telbivudine are options for therapy.

REFERENCES

1. Koziel MJ, Peters MG. Viral hepatitis in HIV infection. N Engl J Med 2007; 356(14):1445–54.
2. Sherman KE, Rouster SD, Chung R, Rajicic N. Hepatitis C prevalence in HIV-infected patients: a cross-secctional analysis of the US adult clinical trials group. Antiviral Therapy 2000 (suppl 1) 2000;5:64.
3. Sulkowski MS, Thomas DL. Hepatitis C in the HIV-Infected Person. Ann Intern Med 2003;138(3):197–207.
4. Danta M, Brown D, Bhagani S, Pybus OG, Sabin CA, Nelson M, et al. Recent epidemic of acute hepatitis C virus in HIV-positive men who have sex with men linked to high-risk sexual behaviours. AIDS 2007;21(8):983–91.
5. Thomas DL, Astemborski J, Rai RM, Anania FA, Schaeffer M, Galai N, et al. The natural history of hepatitis C virus infection: host, viral, and environmental factors. JAMA 2000;284(4):450–6.
6. Eyster ME, Diamondstone LS, Lien JM, Ehmann WC, Quan S, Goedert JJ. Natural history of hepatitis C virus infection in multitransfused hemophiliacs: effect of coin-fection with human immunodeficiency virus. The Multicenter Hemophilia Cohort Study. J Acquir Immune Defic Syndr 1993;6:602–10.
7. Goedert JJ, Eyster ME, Lederman MM, Mandalaki T, De Moerloose P, White GC, et al. End-stage liver disease in persons with hemophilia and transfusion- associated infections. Blood 2002;100(5):1584–9.
8. Graham CS, Baden LR, Yu E, Mrus JM, Carnie J, Heeren T, et al. Influence of human immunodeficiency virus infection on the course of hepatitis c virus infection: a meta-analysis. Clin Infect Dis 2001;33(4):562–9.
9. Gebo KA, Diener-West M, Moore RD. Hospitalization rates differ by hepatitis C satus in an urban HIV cohort. J Acquir Immune Defic Syndr 2003;34(2):165–73.
10. Weber R, Sabin CA, Friis-Moller N, Reiss P, El Sadr WM, Kirk O, et al. Liver-related deaths in persons infected with the human immunodeficiency virus: the D:A:D study. Arch Intern Med 2006;166(15):1632–41.
11. Strader DB, Wright T, Thomas DL, Seeff LB. Diagnosis, management, and treatment of hepatitis C. Hepatology 2004;39(4):1147–71.
12. Alberti A, Clumeck N, Collins S, Gerlich W, Lundgren JD, Palu G, et al. Short statement of the first european consensus conference on the treatment of chronic hepatitis B and C in HIV-coinfected patients. J Hepatol 2005;42(5):615–24.
13. Benson CA, Kaplan JE, Masur H, Pau A, Holmes KK. Treating Opportunistic Infections Among HIV-Infected Adults and Adolescents. MMWR 2004;53(RR15):1–112.
14. Soriano V, Puoti M, Sulkowski M, Cargnel A, Benhamou Y, Peters M, et al. Care of patients coinfected with HIV and hepatitis C virus: 2007 updated recommendations from the HCV-HIV International Panel. AIDS 2007;21(9):1073–89.
15. Torriani FJ, Rodriguez-Torres M, Rockstroh JK, Lissen E, Gonzalez-Garcia J, Lazzarin A, et al. Peginterferon Alfa-2a plus ribavirin for chronic hepatitis C virus infection in HIV-infected patients. N Engl J Med 2004;351(5):438–50.
16. Chung RT, Andersen J, Volberding P, Robbins GK, Liu T, Sherman KE, et al. Peginterferon Alfa-2a plus ribavirin versus interferon alfa-2a plus ribavirin for chronic hepatitis C in HIV-coinfected persons. N Engl J Med 2004;351(5):451–9.
17. Carrat F, Bani-Sadr F, Pol S, Rosenthal E, Lunel-Fabiani F, Benzekri A, et al. Pegylated interferon alfa-2b vs standard interferon alfa-2b, plus ribavirin, for chronic hepatitis C in HIV-infected patients: a randomized controlled trial. JAMA 2004;292(23):2839–48.
18. Laguno M, Murillas J, Blanco JL, Martinez E, Miquel R, Sanchez-Tapias JM, et al. Peginterferon alfa-2b plus ribavirin compared with interferon alfa-2b plus ribavirin for treatment of HIV/HCV co-infected patients. AIDS 2004;18(13):F27–36.
19. Payan C, Pivert A, Morand P, Fafi-Kremer S, Carrat F, Pol S, et al. Rapid and early virological response to chronic Hepatitis C treatment with IFN alpha-2b or PEG- IFN alpha-2b plus ribavirin in HIV/HCV co-infected patients. Gut 2007.

20. Fleischer R, Boxwell D, Sherman KE. Nucleoside analogues and mitochondrial toxicity. Clin Infect Dis 2004;38(8):e79–e80.

21. Alvarez D, Dieterich DT, Brau N, Moorehead L, Ball L, Sulkowski MS. Zidovudine use but not weight-based ribavirin dosing impacts anaemia during HCV treatment in HIV-infected persons. J Viral Hepat 2006;13(10):683–9.

22. Sulkowski MS, Dieterich DT, Bini EJ, Brau N, Alvarez D, DeJesus E, et al. Epoetin Alfa Once Weekly Improves Anemia in HIV/Hepatitis C Virus-Coinfected Patients Treated With Interferon/Ribavirin: A Randomized Controlled Trial. J Acquir Immune Defic Syndr 2005;39(4):504–6.

23. Mehta SH, Lucas GM, Mirel LB, Torbenson M, Higgins Y, Moore RD, et al. Limited effectiveness of antiviral treatment for hepatitis C in an urban HIV clinic. AIDS 2006;20(18):2361–9.

24. Thomas DL, Cannon RO, Shapiro CN, Hook EW, Alter MJ, Quinn TC. Hepatitis C, hepatitis B, and human immunodeficiency virus infections among non-intravenous drug-using patients attending clinics for sexually transmitted diseases. J Infect Dis 1994;169(5):990–5.

25. Gilson RJC, Hawkins AE, Beecham MR, Ross E, Waite J, Briggs M, et al. Interactions between HIV and hepatitis B virus in homosexual men: Effects on the natural history of infection. AIDS 1997;11(5):597–606.

26. Kellerman SE, Hanson DL, McNaghten AD, Fleming PL. Prevalence of chronic hepatitis B and incidence of acute hepatitis B infection in human immunodeficiency virus-infected subjects. J Infect Dis 2003;188(4):571–7.

27. Shire NJ, Rouster SD, Rajicic N, Sherman KE. Occult Hepatitis B in HIV-Infected Patients. J Acquir Immune Defic Syndr 2004;36(3):869–75.

28. Iloeje UH, Yang HI, Su J, Jen CL, You SL, Chen CJ. Predicting cirrhosis risk based on the level of circulating hepatitis B viral load. Gastroenterology 2006;130(3): 678–86.

29. Chen CJ, Yang HI, Su J, Jen CL, You SL, Lu SN, et al. Risk of hepatocellular carcinoma across a biological gradient of serum hepatitis B virus DNA level. JAMA 2006;295(1):65–73.

30. Thio CL, Netski DM, Myung J, Seaberg EC, Thomas DL. Changes in hepatitis B virus DNA levels with acute HIV infection. Clin Infect Dis 2004;38(7):1024–9.

31. Soriano V, Puoti M, Bonacini M, Brook G, Cargnel A, Rockstroh J, et al. Care of patients with chronic hepatitis B and HIV co-infection: recommendations from an HIV-HBV International Panel. AIDS 2005;19(3):221–40.

32. Thio CL, Seaberg EC, Skolasky RL, Phair J, Visscher B, Munoz A, et al. HIV-1, hepatitis B virus, and risk of liver-related mortality in the Multicenter AIDS Cohort Study (MACS). Lancet 2002;360:1921–6.

33. Sulkowski MS, Thomas DL, Mehta SH, Chaisson RE, Moore RD. Hepatotoxicity associated with nevirapine or efavirenz-containing antiretroviral therapy: role of hepatitis C and B infections. Hepatology 2002;35(1):182–9.

34. Gandhi RT, Wurcel A, Lee H, McGovern B, Boczanowski M, Gerwin R, et al. Isolated antibody to hepatitis B core antigen in human immunodeficiency virus type-1-infected individuals. Clin Infect Dis 2003;36(12):1602–5.

35. Gandhi RT, Wurcel A, Lee H, McGovern B, Shopis J, Geary M, et al. Response to hepatitis B vaccine in HIV-1-positive subjects who test positive for isolated antibody to hepatitis B core antigen: implications for hepatitis B vaccine strategies. J Infect Dis 2005;191(9):1435–41.

36. Di M, V, Thevenot T, Colin JF, Boyer N, Martinot M, Degos F, et al. Influence of HIV infection on the response to interferon therapy and the long-term outcome of chronic hepatitis B. Gastroenterology 2002;123(6):1812–22.

37. Dore GJ, Cooper DA, Barrett C, Goh LE, Thakrar B, Atkins M. Dual efficacy of lamivudine treatment in human immunodeficiency virus/hepatitis B virus-coinfected persons in a randomized, controlled study (CAESAR). The CAESAR Coordinating Committee. J Infect Dis 1999;180(3):607–13.

38. Benhamou Y, Bochet M, Thibault V, Di M, V, Caumes E, Bricaire F, et al. Long-term incidence of hepatitis B virus resistance to lamivudine in human immunodeficiency virus-infected patients. Hepatology 1999;30(5):1302–6.

39. Tenney DJ, Levine SM, Rose RE, Walsh AW, Weinheimer SP, Discotto L, et al. Clinical emergence of entecavir-resistant hepatitis B virus requires additional substitutions in virus already resistant to Lamivudine. Antimicrob Agents Chemother 2004;48(9):3498–507.

40. Pessoa W, Gazzard B, Huang A, Brandao-Mello C, Cassetti L, Correa M, et al. Entecavir in HIV/HBV co-infected patients:safety and efficacy in a phase II study (ETV-038). 12th Conference on Retroviruses and Opportunistic Infections 2005;Abstract 123.

41. McMahon MA, Jilek BL, Brennan TP, Shen L, Zhou Y, Wind-Rotolo M, et al. The HBV drug entecavir – effects on HIV-1 replication and resistance. N Engl J Med 2007;356(25):2614–21.

42. Benhamou Y, Thibault V, Calvez V, Vig P, Valantin MA, Guyon P, et al. Three-year treatment with adefovir dipivoxil in chronic hepatitis B patients with lamivudine-resistant HBV and HIV co-infection results in significant and sustained clinical improvement. 11th Conference on Retroviruses and Opportunistic Infections Abstract 835. 2004.

43. Thio CL. Treatment of lamivudine-resistant hepatitis B in HIV-infected persons: is adefovir dipivoxil the answer? J Hepatol 2005.

44. Van Bommel F, Wunsche T, Mauss S, Reinke P, Bergk A, Schurmann D, et al. Comparison of adefovir and tenofovir in the treatment of lamivudine-resistant hepatitis B virus infection. Hepatology 2004;40(6):1421–5.

45. Peters MG, Anderson J, Lynch P, Jacobson J, Sherman K, Alston-Smith B, et al. Tenofovir Disoproxil Fumarate is not inferior to adefovir dipivoxil for the treatment of hepatitis B virus in subjects who are co-infected with HIV: results of ACTG A5127. 12th Conference on Retroviruses and Opportunistic Infections 2005;Abstract 124.

46. Lim SG, Ng TM, Kung N, Krastev Z, Volfova M, Husa P, et al. A double-blind placebo-controlled study of emtricitabine in chronic hepatitis B. Arch Intern Med 2006;166(1):49–56.

47. Dore GJ, Cooper DA, Pozniak AL, DeJesus E, Zhong L, Miller MD, et al. Efficacy of Tenofovir Disoproxil Fumarate in Antiretroviral Therapy-Naive and -Experienced Patients Coinfected with HIV-1 and Hepatitis B Virus. J Infect Dis 2004;189(7): 1185–92.

48. Nelson M, Portsmouth S, Stebbing J, Atkins M, Barr A, Matthews G, et al. An open-label study of tenofovir in HIV-1 and Hepatitis B virus co- infected individuals. AIDS 2003;17(1):F7–F10.

49. Fonseca MO, Pang LW, de Paula CN, Barone AA, Heloisa LM. Randomized trial of recombinant hepatitis B vaccine in HIV-infected adult patients comparing a standard dose to a double dose. Vaccine 2005;23(22):2902–8.

Nonalcoholic Fatty Liver Disease

Poonam Mishra, MD, Nila Rafiq, MD,
and Zobair M. Younossi, MD, MPH, FACG, FACP

INTRODUCTION

Nonalcoholic fatty liver disease (NAFLD) resembles alcoholic liver disease but it occurs in individuals who do not have a history of significant alcohol consumption. The term nonalcoholic steatohepatitis (NASH) was coined by Ludwig and colleagues in 1980 to describe the biopsy findings of steatohepatitis occurring in obese, diabetic, women who did not consume excessive amounts of alcohol.[1]

NAFLD is now recognized as one of the most common causes of chronic liver disease in the United States and many other parts of the world.[2,3] It is recognized as the hepatic manifestation of metabolic syndrome, a cluster of metabolic abnormalities that include central obesity, hypertriglyceridemia, hypertension, and type II diabetes mellitus.[4,5]

NAFLD is an umbrella term that encompasses a wide spectrum of clinical and pathologic entities ranging from simple steatosis, which typically follows a benign course, to NASH, which can potentially progress to cirrhosis, liver failure, and hepatocellular carcinoma.[6,7] "Burned-out NASH" is a leading cause of cryptogenic cirrhosis.[8,9] In the United States, cryptogenic cirrhosis accounts for about 10% of all liver transplants and can recur after transplantation.[10] A population-based study showed that subjects with NAFLD have a higher risk for all cause mortality than the general population.[11] Needless to say, NAFLD has major health and health care utilization implications worldwide.

NAFLD Epidemiology

Investigations of the epidemiology of NAFLD and NASH are hampered by the lack of accurate, sensitive, and noninvasive disease markers. However, we know that the increasing prevalence of NAFLD and NASH parallels the increased prevalence of obesity and metabolic syndrome. Increases in the prevalence of overweight and obesity among U.S. adults between 1976 and 2002 are depicted in Figure 5.1,[12] and the increasing prevalence of diabetes and NAFLD between 1980 and 2005 are shown in Figure 5.2.[13,14] However, the reported prevalence of

Figure 5.1. Prevalence of
Overweight and Obesity Among
U.S. adults. *Age-adjusted by the
direct method to the year 2000 U.S.
Bureau of the Census estimates
using the age groups 20–39, 40–59,
and 60–74 years. National Center
for Health Statistics Web site:
http://www.cdc.gov/nchs/products/
pubs/pubd/hestats/obese/obse99.htm.

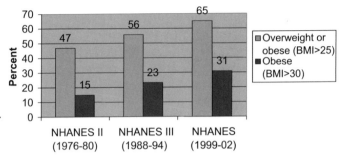

Figure 5.2. Prevalence of Diabetes
and NAFLD. *Approximately 50% of
patients with DM have NAFLD.
NAFLD values have been
extrapolated. Center for Disease
Control and Prevention Web site
http://www.cdc.gov/diabetes/statistics/
prev/national/figpersons.htm.

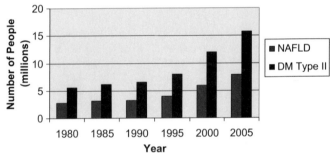

NAFLD varies depending on the study population and the screening modality
(i.e., liver enzymes, imaging studies, liver histology).

The estimated prevalence rate for NAFLD in the U.S. general population
ranges from 3% to 36.9%. The Dallas Heart Study (2,200 adults) assessed NAFLD
with liver imaging (Proton-nuclear magnetic resonance spectroscopy) and found
a prevalence rate of 34%.[15]

The National Health and Nutrition Examination Survey (NHANES III)
estimated the prevalence of NAFLD at 23% on the basis of unexplained elevations
of aminotransferases.[16,17] Another recent study showed that the prevalence of
unexplained elevations in liver enzymes nearly doubled between NHANES 1999–
2002 and NHANES III (1988–1994).[18] Recent findings indicate the rates for
NAFLD in the United States now range between 17% and 33%[15,19] and between
5.7% and 17% for NASH.[19]

Despite the limitations in the published data, certain facts are consistent.
NAFLD and NASH occur among both genders and all ethnicities, and in all age
groups, including children. Among adults, the prevalence of NAFLD increases
with age. NHANES III showed that the peak prevalence of NAFLD is earlier in
men (4th decade) than women (6th decade). Racial and ethnic differences have
been reported in some recent studies.[16,19,20,21] Compared with non-Hispanic
whites, NAFLD is more prevalent among Hispanics and less prevalent among
non-Hispanic blacks.[16,19,20,21] These racial and ethnic differences in NAFLD are
independent of various demographic and metabolic factors.[17]

NASH in Children

NASH was first reported in children in 1980s. The rates of childhood obesity have increased worldwide.[22,23] Simultaneously, NAFLD has been recognized as an important cause of chronic liver disease in children, and may occur in very young children. A Japanese group reported the first description of childhood NAFLD in a 15-year-old obese girl with "maturity-onset" diabetes mellitus who had cirrhosis resulting from NASH.[24] A large clinical series from San Diego included 43 children with histological data; 30 were male and more than half were Hispanic. Nearly 50% of these patients had acanthosis nigricans. Seventy-five percent had fasting hyperinsulinemia and insulin resistance as determined by homeostasis model of insulin resistance (HOMA-IR).[25]

NAFLD is more prevalent in children with metabolic syndrome, which can be secondary to childhood cancer, hypothalamic or pituitary dysfunction, or altered growth hormone secretion.[26,27,28] NAFLD is also associated with Prader-Willi syndrome and polycystic ovary syndrome.[29,30] Furthermore, NAFLD occurs in patients with congenital forms of lipodystrophy.[31,32] Finally, NAFLD shows familial clustering and a child with NAFLD often has a family history significant for obesity and/or fatty liver disease in the parents or grandparents.[33]

Natural History

Substantial evidence suggests that patients with NASH are more likely to progress to cirrhosis than those with simple steatosis or with steatosis and nonspecific inflammation. However, cirrhosis has been reported in 3% of patients with simple steatosis, and 15–20% of NASH patients may progress to cirrhosis.[34,35,36,37] The prognosis of NASH-related cirrhosis is similar to cirrhosis from other causes of liver disease.[38,39] Hepatocellular carcinoma is part of the spectrum of NAFLD, and screening should be considered in patients with NASH-related cirrhosis.[40,41,42,43]

Despite the risk of progression to end-stage liver disease in patients with NASH, we still lack accurate and noninvasive methods to monitor or predict this progression. At this point, liver biopsy may be still necessary to determine disease progression or regression. Some clinical variables have been associated with increased risk for progression to fibrosis, including age over 45 years, obesity, type II diabetes mellitus, and AST/ALT ratio over 1.[44] A study in overweight patients showed that body mass index (BMI) ≥ 28 kg/m^2, ALT ≥ 2 upper limits of normal (ULN), age ≥ 50 years, and serum triglycerides ≥ 1.7 mmol/L were independently associated with advanced fibrosis.[45]

Substantial evidence suggests that fatty liver disease can aggravate parenchymal injury in other chronic liver diseases and may alter their natural history. Steatosis can be caused by both viral and metabolic factors in patients with chronic hepatitis C, and is being reported as a cofactor in promoting fibrosis, impairing the efficacy of antiviral drug therapy and possibly enhancing carcinogenesis.[46,47,48,49,50,51,52] A retrospective study by Sharma et al. showed that patients with HCV genotype 3 were younger, had lower serum cholesterol levels, and a higher prevalence of moderate to severe steatosis compared to non-genotype 3 patients. The study showed a strong association between HCV genotype 3 infection and steatosis. Moreover, this steatosis is etiologically distinct and unrelated to the usual factors predisposing NAFLD. Increasing evidence indicates that steatosis and its associated metabolic abnormalities can also exacerbate other diseases such as alcoholic liver disease, hepatitis B, genetic hemochromatosis, and possibly drug-induced liver disease.[52,53] The underlying pathology appears to be related to increased susceptibility of the hepatocytes to apoptosis adipocytokines produced by white adipose tissue and enhanced oxidative injury in the presence of fatty liver.[52] These findings suggest that fatty liver has significant medical implications even when it is not the primary diagnosis for the liver disease.

Clinical Presentation

NAFLD and NASH are usually clinically silent. Most patients with NAFLD are asymptomatic and elevated liver enzymes are incidentally discovered during routine laboratory examination or a workup for other medical conditions.[1,34,37,54,55,56] NAFLD and NASH must be considered in all individuals with elevated liver enzymes (See Figure 5.3) and components of metabolic syndrome.[5] A recent Japanese study reported that weight gain and the presence of the metabolic syndrome at baseline are independent predictors of the development of NAFLD.[57] Two studies so far suggest that weight gain precedes the development of NAFLD.[57,58]

Conditions associated with NAFLD are metabolic risk factors such as obesity (truncal or central obesity), Type II diabetes mellitus, hypertriglyceridemia, low HDL, hyperinsulinemia, hypertension, polycystic ovary syndrome, and lipodystrophy.[30,59]

Secondary causes of NAFLD include early types of jejunoileal bypass surgery,[54] medications such as methotrexate, amiodarone, tamoxifen, glucocorticoids, and estrogens.[59] Additionally, total parenteral nutrition and severe malnutrition may also lead to fatty liver.[54,59,60]

It is important to remember that NAFLD is a diagnosis of exclusion, so other causes of chronic liver disease must be ruled out, especially alcoholic liver disease, HCV, and Wilson's disease (in young patients). It is important to remember that histologically, alcoholic steatohepatitis (ASH) and NASH cannot be distinguished. Therefore, an accurate history of alcohol intake including the quantity of alcohol consumption is imperative. To make the diagnosis of "nonalcoholic" liver disease, the cut-off for female patients is no more than 10 grams of alcohol per day and for male patients no more than 20 grams per day.[54,61] However, consumption of even lesser amounts of alcohol may be deleterious in patients with other risk factors such as obesity, metabolic syndrome, viral hepatitis and other chronic liver diseases. Nevertheless, obtaining an accurate alcohol intake history may pose its own challenges as patients often underestimate their alcohol consumption.

As noted previously, NAFLD patients are generally asymptomatic with mild elevation of liver enzymes. Nevertheless, a few patients may present with malaise, fatigue, right upper quadrant discomfort, and mild abdominal pain.[62] Physical examination may reveal mild hepatomegaly in some patients.[1,34,42,56,63] The most common laboratory abnormality is mild to moderate elevations in aminotransferases – two to five times the upper limits of normal.[1,34,64] On the other hand, many patients with NAFLD, especially those with morbid obesity who

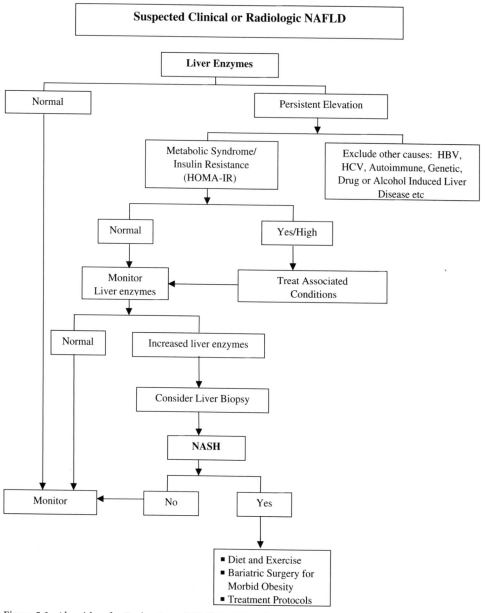

Figure 5.3. Algorithm for Evaluation of NAFLD. Abbreviations: HBV, hepatitis B virus, HCV, hepatitis C virus, HOMA-IR, homeostasis model of insulin resistance.

are undergoing bariatric surgery, may have normal liver enzymes.[65,66] Liver enzymes in patients with NAFLD can fluctuate and do not correlate with the degree of steatosis or fibrosis. Significant liver disease has been described in NAFLD patients with normal liver enzymes.[65,66] No consensus among experts point to a standard cut-off for liver enzymes because population studies have revised the normal limits of ALT downward based on gender and individuals with obesity or metabolic syndrome.[67] Alkaline phosphatase elevations are rare and quite mild in some NAFLD patients.[1,34,42,62,68,69] Serum albumin and bilirubin levels remain normal unless cirrhosis has developed.[1,68]

Radiologic modalities such as ultrasound and CT scans can detect steatosis but are not able to differentiate simple steatosis from NASH.[70] Ultrasound is a sensitive screening tool when more than 33% of liver parenchyma is involved with steatosis.[70,71] However, ultrasound is not quantitative and cannot stage hepatic fibrosis. Saadeh and coworkers have shown the role of different radiologic modalities in distinguishing between NASH and less- aggressive forms of NAFLD.[70] Twenty-five patients with NAFLD (8 with steatosis and 17 with NASH) underwent simultaneous radiological assessments with ultrasonography, CT, and MRI within three months after liver biopsy. None of the radiological features included in the CT, ultrasonography, or MRI protocols could distinguish patients with the pathologic diagnosis of NASH. Ultrasonography and CT were 100% and 93% sensitive in detecting >33% fat, with positive predictive values of 62% and 72% respectively. Data from this study showed that despite excellent sensitivity in detecting significant steatosis, these modalities are unable to distinguish between NASH and other forms of NAFLD.[70]

Magnetic resonance spectroscopy is a non-invasive method to measure hepatic triglyceride content and this novel technique holds promise for the future.[72] Other radiologic modalities that show promise include contrast-enhanced ultrasound and fast MRI.[73]

Transient elastography (Fibroscan) is a relatively novel method for evaluating liver fibrosis by measuring liver stiffness.[74] Investigators showed that liver stiffness significantly correlates with fibrosis stage regardless of the cause of liver disease. However, it may be difficult to obtain reliable measurements in subjects with NAFLD with central obesity [74,75]

Dual energy X-ray absorptiometry (DEXA) is used to assess body fat distribution. A pilot study investigating pioglitazone for treatment of NASH showed that the main side effect was weight gain, which correlated with increase in total body adiposity by DEXA.[76] This modality may be used in the future to monitor therapeutic interventions for NAFLD on adipose tissue.

Histologic Diagnosis

Because clinical, laboratory, and radiologic tests for the diagnosis of NASH have significant limitations, liver biopsy remains the gold standard for the definitive diagnosis of NASH. Histologically, NAFLD is indicated by the presence of fatty infiltration of the liver defined as fat in >5% of hepatocytes.[77,78] On the other hand, the minimum histological criteria for NASH include hepatic steatosis, mixed lobular inflammation, and hepatocellular ballooning.[32] Other pathologic findings such as Mallory bodies or perisinusoidal fibrosis can make the diagnosis even stronger.

The progression of NASH to cirrhosis may be accompanied by a loss of the typical histologic features of NASH, resulting in cryptogenic cirrhosis.[37,79] Recently, the NASH Clinical Research Network has developed a histological scoring system to provide a single pathologic scoring system for NAFLD. This scoring system requires further external validation but will be very helpful in clinical trials of patients with NASH.[80]

Some experts have classified NAFLD as primary NAFLD associated with the metabolic syndrome and insulin resistance. Fatty liver disease occurring secondary to medication, surgical procedures, and TPN has been classified as secondary causes of NAFLD. Some NAFLD patients may not meet the criteria for metabolic syndrome but may have one or more components of metabolic syndrome, namely obesity, diabetes mellitus, or hypertriglyceridemia. Additionally, some NAFLD patients may not have any of these risk factors in the presence of insulin resistance.[81]

Pathogenesis

Our understanding of the pathophysiology of NAFLD and NASH is still evolving (Figure 5.4). It is of utmost importance to fully understand these pathogenic mechanisms if we are to develop novel therapeutic modalities that specifically target this disease. NASH pathogenesis appears to result from a "multiple-hit" process as described in the following section.

The initial insult is the development of macrovesicular steatosis with the accumulation of hepatic fat as the result of increased lipolysis and increased delivery of free fatty acids (FFA) to the liver.[54,61] Hepatic steatosis is the result of three different metabolic pathways; decreased hepatic FFA oxidation, increased hepatic de novo lipogenesis, or decreased lipid export from the liver. This is secondary to fatty acid dysregulation associated with elevated serum insulin levels related to insulin resistance.[82] An animal model created to study NASH placed rats and mice on methionine and choline deficient diets (MCD). Results showed that these two components are vital for hepatic beta oxidation and VLDL production. Tsuguhito's new model placed rats and mice on a MCD diet plus high fat, exhibiting a greater degree of insulin resistance.[83] This model demonstrates that a high fat diet further enhances insulin resistance and accelerates the development of steatosis, inflammation, and ultimately fibrosis.[83] In addition, hepatic steatosis in itself causes hepatic insulin resistance contributing to this vicious cycle.[84]

The second hit includes oxidative stress from reactive oxygen species produced in mitochondria and by cytochrome P-450 enzymes, leading to inflammation and necrosis.[85,86] Oxidative stress is caused by endotoxins, cytokines, and environmental toxins. Oxidative stress, in turn, promotes lipid peroxidation in the hepatocyte membrane and its by products, which can lead to the secretion of pro-inflammatory cytokines and activate stellate cells, resulting in fibrosis.[87]

Additionally, central obesity seems to play a major role in the pathogenesis of NAFLD. The increased omental fat mass is an important endocrine and paracrine organ. White adipose tissue is now recognized as an endocrine organ that secretes several adipokines and cytokines including adiponectin, leptin, resistin, visfatin, TNF-α, angiotensinogen, and free fatty acids.[88] Adiponectin is an adipokine that is decreased in obesity. Furthermore, plasma adiponectin levels are decreased in NAFLD and exogenous adiponectin improves hepatic steatosis in animal models of non-alcoholic fatty liver.[89] The pro-inflammatory cytokine, TNF-alfa, is increased in NAFLD patients and therapy directed against it can be beneficial.[90,91,92,93] Serum leptin levels are increased in NAFLD. Theoretically, leptin may enhance fibrogenesis in NASH through its direct effect on hepatic stellate cells or its indirect effects on production of TGF-β in sinusoidal and Kupffer cells.[94,95,96,97] In summary, there is increasing evidence that these adipokines as well as factors involved in apoptotic pathway can act as "second hits" in the pathogenesis of NASH and its progression.

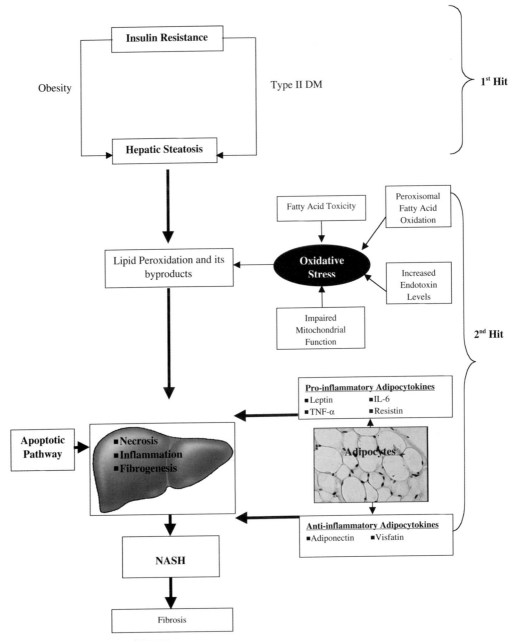

Figure 5.4. Pathogenesis of NASH.

Predictors of NASH, Advanced fibrosis, and Mortality

Researchers have attempted to define a panel of clinical criteria that can predict which NAFLD patients will have aggressive disease or advanced fibrosis. A panel of this kind would help predict prognosis and ameliorate the need for liver biopsy, which carries its own morbidity and mortality.[98]

A study by Angulo and coworkers evaluated 144 patients with NASH and showed that ages greater than 45 years, AST/ALT > 1, obesity, and the presence

---

Table 5.1. Potential Medical and Surgical Strategies used for Treatment of Non-alcoholic Steatohepatitis

Lifestyle Changes	Exercise/Dietary Change
Obesity	Weight Loss Program, Orlistat, Sibutramine, Bariatric Surgery
Insulin Sensitizers	Thiazolinediones, Metformin
Anti-oxidants	Vitamin E / ± Vitamin C, Betaine
Cytoprotective agents	Ursodeoxycholic acid (UCDA), Silymarin
Antihyperlipidemic Agents	HMG CoA reductase inhibitors, Fibric Acid Derivative Omega-3 fatty acids
Novel treatments	Pentoxifylline, ACE inhibitor/ARB, Probiotics, Nateglinide

---

of diabetes were independent predictors of advanced fibrosis.[42] None of the patients who were younger than 45 years and who were nondiabetic had advanced fibrosis.[42] Dixon and coworkers found that insulin resistance, raised ALT, and the presence of hypertension were independent predictors of NASH in morbidly obese patients with NAFLD undergoing bariatric surgery.[99] In overweight persons, age $\geq$ 50 years, BMI $\geq$ 28 kg/m^2, ALT $\geq$ 2ULN, and serum triglycerides $\geq$ 1.7 mmol/L were independently associated with advanced fibrosis.[43]

Marchesini and colleagues showed that the presence of metabolic syndrome is associated with a high risk of NASH among NAFLD subjects. Moreover, metabolic syndrome is associated with a high risk of severe fibrosis.[4] The presence of multiple metabolic risk factors is associated with a potentially progressive and more severe form of liver disease. A cohort of NAFLD patients showed that the NAFLD patients with diabetes were more likely to develop cirrhosis, have higher liver-related mortality, and overall mortality compared to nondiabetic patients with NAFLD.[100]

Palekar and colleagues recently proposed a diagnostic model to distinguish patients with simple steatosis and those with NASH. They found that patients with three or more of the following characteristics were more likely to have NASH: female gender, age $\geq$ 50 years, BMI $\geq$ 30 kg/m^2, serum AST $\geq$ 45 IU/L, AST/ALT ratio $\geq$ 0.8, and plasma hyaluronic acid concentration $\geq$ 55μg/l.[101]

Large-scale prospective studies are needed to study long-term outcomes such as the development of clinical cirrhosis, liver-related mortality, and overall mortality in patients with NAFLD. It is also important to study the long-term economic impact of this disease.

More recently, markers of apoptosis, adipokines, protein profiling, and gene expression have been used to develop diagnostic and prognostic biomarkers for NASH.

Treatment

Currently, there is no approved therapy for NAFLD.[102] Moreover, the criteria for who will need therapy has not been well defined. Several medical and surgical treatments are listed in Table 5.1 and discussed below. Weight reduction has shown promising results for obese patients with NAFLD. Weight reduction strategies aim at life style modifications, which include diet with or without exercise or surgical interventions. Most studies suggest that weight loss can be associated with biochemical improvement.

Lifestyle Changes

Lifestyle changes include nutritional counseling with or without exercise. The pathophysiological basis for this approach is that weight reduction results in the loss of adipose tissue, which decreases insulin resistance. Exercise improves muscular insulin sensitivity.[103,104] Several studies have shown that weight reduction with a calorie restricted diet with or without exercise results in significant biochemical improvement, that is, improvement in unexplained elevated serum ALT values presumably related to NAFLD in the overweight and obese adults and children.[105,106] A few trials have also shown a significant reduction in ALT values in patients with biopsy proven NAFLD when they were placed on calorie-restricted diet with or without exercise.[82,107,108,109,110] Lifestyle changes lead to weight loss but it usually is short lived and the long-term data on the histological improvement is lacking. Of some concern is the finding of portal inflammation and fibrosis in obese patients when undergoing rapid weight loss of more than 1.6 kg/week with a very strict diet.[82] If weight reduction is adopted, gradual loss not exceeding 1.6 kg/week should be emphasized through the combination of dietary restrictions and regular aerobic exercise regimen including at least 30 minutes of exercise three to five times per week. However, the validity of this recommendation in the era of bariatric surgery has still not been established.

Medications for Weight Loss

A clinical trial using Orlistat, an enteric lipase inhibitor, showed a mean decrease in body weight by 10.3 kg and significant reductions in serum transaminase levels in obese patients with NASH.[111] One pilot study involving 25 patients compared orlistat with sibutramine (a serotonin and norepinephrine reuptake inhibitor that increases satiety and energy expenditure) for six months and found drug-induced weight loss in both groups, reduced insulin resistance, improved biochemical markers, and improved sonographic findings of steatosis.[112] These findings are promising but long-term patient tolerance to these drugs and the ability to achieve sustained weight reduction need to be addressed.

Bariatric Surgery

Surgical interventions for obesity can be broadly categorized as "restrictive," "malabsorptive," or "mixed restrictive – malabsorptive surgeries."[113] Restrictive surgeries include laparoscopic adjustable gastric banding (LAGS) and vertical banded gastroplasty, which decrease the capacity of the stomach and limit the amount of food consumed. Malabsorptive surgeries, such as roux-en-Y gastric bypass and duodenal switch procedures, work by bypassing a large portion of small intestine to prevent the absorption of fats and nutrients. A recent study from the Swedish Obese Study Group suggests that bariatric surgery can be associated with better long-term outcomes in terms of cardiovascular risk factors such as diabetes, hypertriglyceridemia, and hypertension when compared to a conventional weight loss group.[114]

A recent study by Dixon and coworkers showed that NASH resolved in 82% of patients undergoing laparoscopic adjustable gastric banding (LAGB) after they lost 34 ± 17 kg.[115] Patients who had metabolic syndrome showed a greater improvement in liver histology with weight loss. These and additional studies suggest a positive impact of bariatric surgery on metabolic syndrome and NAFLD.

Drugs Targeting Insulin Resistance

Insulin resistance is an important pathophysiologic factor in NASH. More than 80% of patients with NASH meet the criteria for the metabolic syndrome and nearly all patients have insulin resistance. These findings have led to treatments that target insulin resistance and components of metabolic syndrome. Such treatment strategies aim to improve insulin resistance and protect the liver from oxidative stress. The insulin sensitizing agents, thiazolidinediones and metformin, are the focus of the several ongoing studies.

Thiazolidinediones have been used to improve insulin sensitivity in patients with NASH. This group of drugs improve insulin sensitivity in adipose tissue by activating the nuclear transcription factor peroxisome-proliferator activated-receptor (PPAR-gamma) by binding selective ligands.[116] Tetri and colleagues treated 30 patients with biopsy proven NASH with 4 mg of rosiglitazone twice a day for 48 weeks. These patients showed improvements in insulin resistance as well as biochemical and histological improvements at the end of therapy.[117] Another study by Promrat and coworkers used 30 mg of pioglitazone in 18 patients for 48 weeks and reported improved aminotransferases as well as histologic and radiologic endpoints.[118] Almost two-thirds of patients gained some weight and improvements in biochemical abnormalities were reversed after treatment was discontinued. Further randomized placebo controlled trials are needed to study the effects of these drugs. Pioglitazone and rosiglitazone are currently approved for the treatment of diabetes mellitus (DM). The results of adequately powered, histologically driven studies such as the ongoing trial of pioglitazone under the NASH Clinical Research Network, may be able to better define the efficacy and safety profile of these drugs. In addition, they may provide insights into the future potential use of these drugs in clinical practice.

Metformin is a biguanide that improves insulin resistance and hyperinsulinemia by decreasing hepatic glucose production and increasing peripheral glucose uptake by muscles.[119,120] One of the mechanisms of the action of metformin is to reverse TNF-alpha induced insulin resistance.[121] Small trials using metformin report improved serum ALT values compared to baseline.[122,123,124] A pilot study using up to 2 gm per day of metformin reported initial improvements in ALT levels after three months of therapy, but there was no difference after 12 months of therapy.[125] A large open-label study in nondiabetic subjects randomized subjects to metformin 2 gm daily, weight reducing diet, or vitamin E 800 IU daily.[126] A significantly higher number of subjects taking metformin showed normalized ALT levels compared to the diet or Vitamin E group. Moreover, these subjects showed significant improvements in steatosis, inflammation, and fibrosis compared to baseline, but there was no follow-up histology for the control arm.

Although metformin was well tolerated in all studies with improved ALT levels in the majority of subjects, data regarding its beneficial effects on liver histology remain limited. Additional, well-controlled trials are needed to assess the efficacy and safety of metformin in patients with NAFLD.

LIPID-LOWERING MEDICATIONS

NAFLD treatment strategies aiming to reduce and treat metabolic risk factors have been the focus of therapeutic studies due to the lack of a single effective therapy. Hypertriglyceridemia and low HDL are components of metabolic syndrome; as a result several investigators have attempted to lower lipids and explore the potential role of lipid-lowering agents in the management of NAFLD. A clinical trial using gemfibrozil, a fibric acid with lipid-lowering activity, showed some biochemical improvements in patients with NAFLD when given at the dose of 600 mg per day for four weeks.[127] On the contrary, clofibrate produced no improvements in serum ALT levels or liver histology.[128]

Small pilot trials using HMG-CoA reductase inhibitors (statins) have shown reductions in serum ALT levels.[129,130] A pilot study using pravastatin at 20 mg for six months normalized liver enzymes and improved hepatic inflammation in patients with NASH.[131]

Another pilot study using atorvastatin showed improved serum aminotransferase levels as well as lipid levels in patients with NAFLD and showed that atorvastatin was both effective and safe.[132] Nevertheless, the use of statins is hampered by potential heptotoxicity, especially in patients with active liver disease and those with persistent, unexplained, elevated aminotransferases. However, mounting evidence now suggests that the use of standard doses of these drugs in patients with elevated liver enzymes may not be necessarily associated with an increased risk of serious hepatotoxicity.[133] Large, randomized, controlled trials of these agents with histological follow-up are required to establish the role of these agents in the treatment of NASH, and more importantly, in the subgroup of NASH patients with dyslipidemia.

Antioxidants

Given the role of oxidative stress in the pathogenesis of NASH, considerable effort has focused on the use of antioxidants for the treatment of NAFLD. The effect of Vitamin E as an antioxidant has been evaluated in several studies. The rationale is that it may protect cellular structures against damage from oxygen free radicals and from reactive products of lipid peroxidation. The results so far have been controversial. Two small pilot trials show improved liver enzymes with Vitamin E treatment.[134,135] But two subsequent small, randomized, controlled trials failed to show benefit.[108,136] A randomized study comparing Vitamin E (1000 IU/day) and vitamin C (1000 mg/day) to placebo for six months showed no differences in ALT, hepatic inflammation, or fibrosis at the end of the study.[137] Recently, some reports have raised concerns about the safety of long term high dose Vitamin E use.[138]

Other potential therapies for NASH include betaine, N-acetylcysteine, and pentoxifyllin.[139,140] Betaine is a naturally occurring metabolite of choline that increases S-adenosylmethionine (SAMe) levels. A small, uncontrolled pilot study involving 10 patients with NASH showed that when betaine was given for one year, serum AST and ALT levels decreased significantly and grades of steatosis, necroinflammation, and the stage of fibrosis showed some biochemical improvement in patients with NAFLD.[139]

Pentoxifylline, a TNF-alpha inhibitor, is a potential therapeutic modality because TNF-alpha has been widely implicated in the pathogenesis of NASH. Two pilot studies evaluating the role of pentoxyfylline in NASH reported significant improvements in AST and ALT levels. Moreover, one study showed a reduction in insulin resistance.[91,92]

A recent review on the use of antioxidants supplements for non-alcoholic fatty liver disease and/or steatohepatitis concluded that data is insufficient to support their use, requiring further large prospective randomized clinical trials to assess the efficacy of these agents.[141]

Ursodeoxycholic Acid

Open label studies show that ursodeoxycholic acid (UDCA), a potentially cyto-protective agent, has beneficial effects in patients with NAFLD.[128,142] A small pilot study involving 24 patients using UDCA 13–15 mg/kg/day for 48 weeks showed improvements in serum aminotransferases as well as some improvement in steatosis.[128] On the other hand, Lindor and colleagues conducted a random-ized, double-blind, placebo controlled trial involving 166 patients, 126 of whom completed two years of therapy with UDCA at 13–15 mg/kg/day. The researchers found that UDCA was safe and well tolerated, but was not better than placebo for patients with NASH. UDCA was not associated with improvements in serum liver biochemistries or histology when compared with placebo.[143] Despite these contradictory results, ongoing studies using high dose UDCA with or without other agents are currently underway.

Angiotensin Converting Enzyme Inhibitor/Angiotensin Receptor Blockers

Suppressing the renin-angiotensin system with angiotensin converting enzyme inhibitor (ACEI) or angiotensin receptor blockers (ARB) produce metabolic effects that could prevent type II diabetes mellitus in patients with systemic hypertension or congestive heart failure.[144] The ARBs, telmisartan and irbe-sartan, activate PPAR-gamma and decrease insulin resistance.[145,146] A study of seven patients with hypertension and NASH who were treated with losartan (an ACEI) for 48 weeks, reported histological improvement in necroinflammatory activity in five subjects and a reduction of fibrosis in four patients.[147]

Folic Acid

An open-label pilot study in 10 patients with biopsy proven NASH used 1 mg/day of folic acid for six months and found no significant biochemical improvement after six months of therapy.[148]

OTHER NOVEL AGENTS

Several studies have suggested that intestinal bacterial overgrowth plays a role in the pathogenesis of NASH. Bacterial endotoxins can stimulate hepatic inflam-matory cytokine production and increase oxidative stress leading to subsequent liver injury.[93,149] A recent study involving 22 NAFLD patients using probiotic VSL#3 showed improvement in ALT levels as well as other markers of lipid peroxidation.[150]

A small pilot study in seven patients with NASH using an insulin-type fructan, oligofructose, for eight weeks showed decreased serum levels of ALT and AST compared to placebo group.[151] Interestingly, decreased serum insulin levels were apparent after four weeks of therapy. Nateglinide, an insulin secretagogue, was used in five diabetic patients with NASH for 20 weeks and showed improved biochemical and histological parameters compared to the control group.[152] Muraglitizar, a dual PPAR alpha and gamma agonist, and Rimonabant, a selective cannabinoid-1 receptor blocker, have shown promising results in obese and diabetic patients with metabolic syndrome but these studies lack liver-related outcome data.[153,154]

Summary

NAFLD is one of the most common cause of chronic liver disease worldwide, and its subtype, NASH, can potentially progress to cirrhosis, liver failure, and hepatocellular carcinoma. NAFLD can have a major economic impact on the health care costs due to liver-related morbidity and mortality. Extensive investigations over the last two decades have led to a better understanding of the natural history, epidemiology, and pathophysiology of this disease. Despite the large number of agents that have been tested, no single agent or combination of agents stand out as therapy with proven efficacy. Effective preventive and therapeutic strategies still need to be developed to tackle this evolving global epidemic of nonalcoholic fatty liver disease. A multidisciplinary approach using lifestyle modification and optimizing metabolic risk factors is the best option for the future until the results of ongoing randomized, double blind, placebo controlled trials investigating multiple therapeutic options become available.

REFERENCES

1. Ludwig J, Viggiano TR, McGill DB, et al. Nonalcoholic steatohepatitis: mayo Clinic experience with a hitherto unnamed disease. Mayo Clin Proc 1980;55(7):434–438.
2. Chitturi S, Farrell G, George J. Non-alcoholic steatohepatitis in the Asia-Pacific Region: Future Shock? J Gastroenter Hepatol 2004;19:368–374.
3. Chitturi C, George J. NAFLD/NASH is not just a "Western" problem: Some perspectives on NAFLD/NASH from the east. In: Fatty Liver Disease: NASH and related disorders. Eds. GC Farell, J George, P Hall, AJ McCullough. Blackwell Publishing, Oxford; 2005, pp. 219–228.
4. Marchesini G, Forlani G. NASH: from liver diseases to metabolic disorders and back to clinical hepatology. Hepatology 2002;35:497–9.
5. Marchesini G, Brizi M, Bianchi G, Tomassetti S, Bugianesi E, Lenzi M, McCullough AJ, Natale S, Forlani G, Melchionda N. Nonalcoholic fatty liver liver disease. A feature of the metabolic syndrome. Diabetes 2001;50:1844–50.
6. Caldwell SH, Hespenheide EE. Subacute liver failure in obese women. Am J Gastroenterol 2002;97:2058–67
7. Bugianesi E, Leone A, Vanni E, Marchesini G, Brunello F, Carucci P, Musso A, DePaolis P, Carussoti L, Salizzoni M, Rizzeto M. Expanding the natural history of nonalcoholic

steatohepatitis: From cryptogenic cirrhosis to hepatocellular cancer. Gastroenterology 2002;123:134–40.

8. Caldwell SH, Oelsner DH, Iezzoni JC, Hespenheide EE, Battle EH, Driscoll CJ. Cryptogenic cirrhosis: clinical characterization and risk factors for underlying disease. Hepatology 1999;29(3):664–9.

9. Nair S, Mason A, Eason J, Loss G, Perrillo RP. Is obesity an independent risk factor for hepatocellular carcinoma in cirrhosis? Hepatology 2002;36:150–5.

10. Ong J, Younossi ZM, Reddy V, Price LL, Gramlich T, Mayes J, Boparai N. Cryptogenic cirrhosis and posttransplantation nonalcoholic fatty liver disease. Liver Transpl 2001;7:797–801.

11. Adams LA, Lymp J, St Sauver J, et al. The natural history of nonalcoholic fatty liver disease: a population based cohort study. Gastroenterology 2005;129;113–21.

12. Prevalence of Overweight and Obesity Among Adults: United States, 1999–2002. National Center for Health Statistics Web site: http://www.cdc.gov/nchs/products/pubs/pubd/hestats/obese/obse99.htm. Accessed and Modified August 9, 2007.

13. Prevalence of Diabetes and NAFLD, United States 1980–2005. Data & Trends, National Diabetes Surveillance System. Center for Disease Control and Prevention Web site: http://www.cdc.gov/diabetes/statistics/prev/national/figpersons.htm. Accessed and modified August 9, 2007.

14. Tarantino G, Saldalamacchia G, Conca P, Arena A. Non-alcoholic Fatty Liver Disease: Further Expression of the Metabolic Syndrome. J Gastroenterol Hepatol. 2007;22(3): 293–303.

15. Browning JD, Szczepaniak LS, Dobbins R, Nuremberg P, Horton JD, Cohen JC, Grundy SM, Hobbs HH. Prevalence of hepatic steatosis in an urban population in the United States: impact of ethnicity. Hepatology. 2004;40:1387–95.

16. Clark JM, Brancati FL, Diehl AM. The prevalence and etiology of elevated aminotransferase levels in the united states. Am J gastroenterol 2003;98(5):960–67.

17. Ruhl CE, Everhart JE. Determinants of the association of overweight with elevated serum alanine aminotransferase activity in the united states. Gastoenterology 2003;124(1):71–9.

18. Ioannou GN, Boyko EJ, Lee SP. The prevalence and predictors of elevated serum aminotransferase activity in the united states in 1999–2002. Am J Gastroenterol 2006;101(1):76–82.

19. Mccullough AJ. The epidemiology and risk factors of NASH. In: Fatty Liver Disease: NASH and related Disorders. Eds. GC Farrell, J George, P Hall and AJ Mc Cullough. Blackwell Publishing, Oxford. 2005, pp. 23–37.

20. Weston SR, Leyden W, Murphy R, Bass NM, Bell BP, Manos MM, Terrault NA. Racial and ethnic distribution of nonalcoholic fatty liver in persons with newly diagnosed chronic liver disease. Hepatology 2005;41(2):372–79.

21. Caldwell SH, Harris DM, PatrieJT, Hespenheide EE. Is NASH underdiagnosed among African Americans? Am J Gastroenterol 2002;97(6):1496–1500.

22. Lobstein T, Baur L, Uauy R. Obesity in children and young people: a crisis in public health. Obes Rev. 2004; Suppl 1): 4–104.

23. Ogden CL, Carroll MD, Curtin LR, et al. Prevalence of overweight and obesity in the United States, 1999–2004. JAMA. 2006;295(13):1549–55.

24. Kinugasa A, Tsunamoto K, Furukawa N, et al. Fatty liver and its fibrous changes found in simple obesity of children. J Pediatr Gastroenterol Nutrit 1984;3(3): 408–14.

25. Schwimmer JB, Deutsch R, Rauch JB, et al. Obesity, insulin resistance, and other clinicopathological correlates of pediatric nonalcoholic fatty liver disease. J Pediatr. 2003;143(4):500–5.

26. Talvensaari KK, Lanning M, Tapanainen P, et al. Long-term survivors of childhood cancer have an increased risk of manifesting the metabolic syndrome. J Clin Endocrinol Metab. 1996;81(8):3051–5.

27. Adams LA, Feldstein A, Lindor KD, et al. Nonalcoholic fatty liver disease among patients with hypothalamic and pituitary dysfunction. Hepatology. 2004;39(4):909–14.

28. Srinivasan S, Ogle GD, Garnett SP, et al. Features of the metabolic syndrome after childhood craniopharyngioma. J Clin Endocrinol Metab. 2004;89(1)81–6.

29. Yigit S, Estrada E, Bucci K et al. Diabetic Ketoacidosis secondary to growth hormone treatment in a boy with Prader-Willi syndrome and steatohepatitis. J Pediatr Endocrinol Metab. 2004;17(3):361–4.

30. Setji TL, Holland ND, Sanders LL, et al. Nonalcoholic steatohepatitis and nonalcoholic fatty liver disease in young women with polycystic ovary syndrome. J Clin Endocrinol Metab. 2006.

31. Powell EE, Searle J, Mortimer R. Steatohepatitis associated with limb lipodystrophy. Gastroenterology. 1989;97(4):1022–4.

32. Cauble MS, Gilroy R, Sorrell MF, et al. Lipoatrophic diabetes and end-stage liver disease secondary to nonalcoholic steatohepatitis with recurrence after liver transplantration. Transplantation. 2001;71(7):892–5.

33. Willner IR, Waters B, Patil SR, et al. Ninety patients with nonalcoholic steatohepatitis: insulin resistance, familial tendency, and severity of disease. Am J Gastroentero. 2001;96(10):2957–61.

34. Matteoni CA, Younossi ZM, Gramlich T, Bopari N, Liu YC, McCullough AJ. Nonalcoholic fatty liver disease: A spectrum of clinical and pathological severity. Gastroenterology 1999;116: 1413–19.

35. Teli MR, James OFW, Burt AD, Bennett MK, Day CP. The natural history of nonalcoholic fatty liver. A follow-up study. Hepatology 1995;22:1714–19.

36. Dam-larsen S, Franzmann M, Anderson IB, Christoffersen P, Jensen LB, Surensen TIA, Becker U, Bendsten F. Long term prognosis of fatty liver disease and death. GUT 2004;53:750–5.

37. Powell EE, Cooksley WG, Hanson R, et al. The natural history of nonalcoholic steatohepatitis: a follow-up study of forty-two patients for up to 21 years. Hepatology 1990;11:74–80.

38. Ratziu V, Bonyhay L, Di Martino V, Charlotte F, Cavallaro L, Sayegh-Tainturier MH, Giral P, et al. Survival, liver failure, and hepatocellular carcinoma in obesity-related cryptogenic cirrhosis. Hepatology 2002;35(6):1485–93.

39. Hui JM, Kench JG, Chitturi S, Sud A, Farrell GC, Byth K, Hall P, et al. Long-term outcomes of cirrhosis in nonalcoholic steatohepatitis compared with hepatitis C. Hepatology 2003;38(2):420–7.

40. Cotrim HP, Parana R, Braga E, Lyra L. Nonalcoholic steatohepatitis and hepatocellular carcinoma: Natural history? Am j Gastroenterol 2000;95.10):3018–19.

41. Zen Y, Katayanagi K, Tsuneyama K, Harada K, Araki I, Nakanuma Y. Hepatocellular carcinoma arising in non-alcoholic steatohepatitis. Pathol Int 2001;51(2):127–31.

42. Shimada M, Hashimoto E, Taniai M, Hasegawa K, Okuda H, Hayashi N, Takasaki K, et al. Hepatocellular carcinoma in patients with non-alcoholic steatohepatitis. J Hepatol 2002;37(1):154–60.

43. Ong JP, Younossi ZM. Is Hepatocellular carcinoma part of the natural history of nonalcoholic steatohepatitis? Gastroenterology 2002;123.1):375–78.

44. Angulo P, Keach JC, Batts KP, Lindor KD. Independent predictors of liver fibrosis in patients with nonalcoholic steatohepatitis. Hepatology 1999;30:1356–1366.

45. Ratziu V, Giral P, Charlotte F, Bruckert E, Thibault V, Theodorou I, Khalil L, Turpin G, Opolon P, Poynard T. Liver Fibrosis in overweight patients. Gastroenterology 2000;118:1117–23.

46. Lonardo A, Adinolfi LE, Loria P, et al. Steatosis and Hepatitis c virus: mechanisms and significance for hepatic and extrahepatic disease. Gastroenterology. 2004;126(2):586–97.

47. Czaja AJ, Carpenter HA, Santrach PJ, et al.Host- and disease-specific factors affecting steatosis in chronic hepatitis C. J hepatol. 1998;29(2):198–206.

48. Hourigan LF, Macdonald GA, Purdie D, et al. Fibrosis in chronic hepatitis C correlates significantly with body mass index and steatosis. Hepatology. 1999;29(4):1215–19.

49. Jonsson JR, Edwards-Smith CJ, Purdie D et al. Body composition and hepatic steatosis as precursors of fibrosis in chronic hepatitis C patients. Hepatology. 1999;30:1531–2.

50. Guidi M, Muratori P, Granito A, et al. Hepatic steatosis in chronic hepatitis C: impact on response to anti-viral treatment with peg-interferon and ribavirin. Aliment Pharmacol Ther. 2005;22(10):943–9.

51. Bressler BL, Guindi M, Tomlinson G, et al. High body mass index is an independent risk factor for nonresponse to antiviral treatment in chronic hepatitis C. Hepatology. 2003;38(3):639–44.

52. Powell EE, Jonsson JR, Clouston AD. Steatosis: co-factor in other liver diseases. Hepatology. 2005;42(1):5–13.

53. Powell EE, Ali A, Clouston AD, et al. Steatosis is a cofactor in liver injury in hemochromatosis. Gastroenterology 2005;129(6):1937–43.

54. Falck-Ytter Y, Younossi ZM, Marchesini G, et al. Clinical features and natural history of nonalcoholic steatosis syndromes. Seminars in Liver Disease. 2001;21(1):17–26.

55. Yousseff WI, McCullough AJ. Steatohepatitis in obese individuals. Best Pract Res Clin Gastoenterol 2002;16:733–47.

56. Lee RG, Nonalcoholis Steatohepatitis: a study of 49 patients. Hum pathol 1989;20: 594–8.

57. Hamaguchi M, Kojima T, Takeda N, Nakagawa T, Taniguchi H, Fujii K, Omatsu T, et al. The metabolic syndrome as a predictor of nonalcoholic fatty liver disease. Ann Intern Med 2005;143(10);722–8.

58. Suzuki A, Angulo P, Lymp J, St Sauver J, Muto A, Okada T, Lindor K. Chronological development of elevated aminotransferases in a nonalcoholic population. Hepatology 2005;41(1):64–71.

59. Adams LA, Angulo P. Treatment of non-alcoholic fatty liver disease. Postgrad Med J 2006;82:315–22.

60. Fong DG, Nehra V, Lindor K, Buchman AL. Metabolic and nutritional considerations in nonalcoholic fatty liver. Hepatology 2000;32:3–10.

61. Younossi ZM. Nonalcoholic fatty liver disease. Current Gastroenterology Reports. 1999;1(1):57–62.

62. Sheth SG, Gordan FD, Chopra S. Nonalcoholic steatohepatitis. Ann Intern Med 1997;126: 136–45.

63. Leevy CM. Fatty Liver: a study of 270 patients with biopsy proven fatty liver and a review of the literature. Medicine. 1962;4:249–58.

64. Mathieson NL, Franzen LE, Fryden A, Fuberg U, Bodenar G. The clinical significances of slightly to moderately increased liver transaminase values in asymptomatic patients. Scand J Gastroenterol 1999;34:55–91.

65. Mofrad P, Contos M, Haque M, Sargeant C, Fisher RA, Luketic VA. Clinical and histologic spectrum of nonalcoholic fatty liver disease with normal ALT values. Hepatology 2003;37:1286–92.

66. Sorrentino P, Tarantino G, Conca P, et al. Silent nonalcoholic fatty liver disease-a clinical-histological study. J Hepatol 2004;41:751–57.

67. Prati D, Taioli E, Zanella A, Torre ED, Butelli S, DelVecchio E, et al. Updated definitions of health ranges for serum amino transferase levels. Ann Intern Med 2002;137:1–9.

68. Bacon BR, farahvash MJ, Jannay CG, Neuschwander-Tetri BA. Nonalcoholic steatohepatitis: an expanded clinical entity. Gastroenterology 1994;107:1103–9.

69. Kumar KS, Malet PF. Nonalcoholic steatohepatitis. Mayo Clin Proc 2000;75:733–9.

70. Sadeeh S, Younossi ZM, Remer EM, et al. The utility of radiological imaging in nonalcoholic fatty liver disease. Gastroenterology. 2002;123(3):745–50.

71. Mottin CC, Moretto M, Padoin AV, et al. The role of ultrasound in the diagnosis of hepatic staetosis in morbidly obese patients. Obes surg 2004;14:635–7.

72. Siegelman ES, Rosen MA. Imaging of hepatic steatosis. Seminars Liver Disease. 2001;21:71–80.

73. Fishbein MH, Mogren C, Gleason T, Stevens WR. Relationship of hepatic steatosis to adipose tissue distribution in paediatric nonalcoholic fatty liver disease. J Pediatr Gastroenterol Nutr. 2006;42:83–8.

74. Foucher J, Chanteloup E, Vergniol J, et al. Diagnosis of cirrhosis by transient elastography (Fibroscan): a prospective study. Gut. 2006;55: 403–8.

75. Ziol M, Handra-Luca A, Kettaneh A, Christidis C, et al. Noninvasive assessment of liver fibrosis by measurement of stiffness in patients with chronic hepatitis C. Hepatology. 2005;41: 48–54.

76. Promrat K, Lutchman G, Uwaifo GI, et al. A pilot study of pioglitazone treatment for nonalcoholic steatohepatitis. Hepatology. 2004;39:188–96.

77. Cairns SR, Peters T. Biochemical analysis of hepatic lipid in alcoholic and diadetic and control subjects. Clin Sci.Lond) 1983;65:645–2.

78. Wanless IR, Lentz JS. Fatty liver hepatitis (steatohepatitis) and obesity: an autopsy study with analysis of risk factors. Hepatology 1990;12:1106–10.

79. Adams LA, Sanderson S, Lindor KD, Angulo P. The histological course of nonalcoholic fatty liver disease: A longitudinal study of 103 patients with sequential liver biopsies. J Hepatol 2005;42(1):132–38.

80. Kleiner DE, Brunt EM, Nonalcoholic Steatohepatitis Clinical Research Network et al. Design and validation of a histological scoring system for nonalcoholic fatty liver disease. Hepatology 2005;41: 1313–21

81. Bugianesi E, Gastaldelli A, Vanni E, et al. Insulin resistance in non-diabetic patients with non-alcoholic fatty liver disease: sites and mechanisms. Diabetologia 2005;48(4):634–42.

82. Anderson T, Gluud C, Franzmann MB, Christoffersen P. hepatic effects of dietary weight loss in morbidly obese subjects. J Hepatol 1991;12(2):224–9.

83. Ota T, Takamura T, et al. Insulin Resistance Accelerates a Dietary Rat Model of Nonalcoholic Steatohepatitis. Gastroenterology 2007;132(1): 282–93.

84. Kim JK, Fillmore JJ, Chen Y, Yu C, Moore IK, Pypaert M, Lutz EP, Kako Y, Velez-Carrasco W, Goldberg IJ, Breslow JL, Shulman GI. Tissue specific overexpression of lipoprotein lipase cause tissue specific insulin resistance. PNAS 2001;98:7522–27.

85. Pessayre D, Mansouri A, Hauzi D, et al. Hepatotoxicity due to mitochondrial dysfunction. Cell Biology and Toxicology. 1999;15(6):367–73.

86. Leclercq IA, Farrell GC, Field J, et al. CYP2E1 and CYP4A as microsomal catalysts of lipid peroxides in murine nonalcoholic steatohepatitis. Journal of Clinical Investigation. 200;10598):1067–75.

87. Chitturi S, Farell GC. Etiopathogenesis of nonalcoholic steatohepatitis. Seminars in Liver Disease. 2001;21(1):27–41.5.

88. Tilg H, Diehl AM. Cytokines in alcoholic and nonalcoholic steatohepatitis. N Engl J Med 2000;343(20):1467–76.

89. Edmison J, McCullough AJ. Pathogenesis of Non-alcoholic Steatohepatitis: Human Data;Clinics in Liver Disease. 2007;11(1):75–104.

90. Warne JP. Tumour necrosis factor alpha: A key regulator of adipose tissue mass. J Endocrinol 2003;177: 351–5.

91. Satapathy SK, Garg S, Chauhan R, et al. Beneficial effects of tumor necrosis factor-alpha inhibition by pentoxifylline on clinical, biochemical, and metabolic parameters of patients with nonalcoholic steatohepatitis. Am J Gastrenterol 2004;99:1946–52.

92. Adams LA, Zien CO, Angulo P, et al. A pilot trial of pentoxifylline in nonalcoholic steatohepatitis. Am J Gastroenterol 2004;99:2365–8.

93. Wigg AJ, Roberts-Thomson IC, Dymock RB, McCarthy PJ, Grose Rh, Cummins AG. The role of small intestinal bacterial overgrowth, intestinal permeability, endotoxaemia, and tumour necrosis factor alpha in the pathogenesis of non alcoholic steatohepatitis. Gut 2001;48(2):206–11.

94. Saxena NK, Ikeda K, Rockey DC, Freidman SL, Anania FA. Leptin in hepatic fibrosis: evidence for increased collagen production in stellate cells and lean littermates of ob/ob mice. Hepatology 2002;35:762–71.

95. Honda H, Ikejima K, Hirose M, Yoshikawa M, Lang T, Enomoto N, Kitamura T et al. leptin is required for fibrogenic responses induced by thiocacetamide in the murine liver. Hepatology 2002;36:12–21.

96. Leclercq IA, Farrell GC, Schriemer R, et al. Leptin is essential for the hepatic fibrogenic response to chronic liver injury. J Hepatol 2002;37:206–13.

97. Angulo P, Alba LM, Petrovic LM, et al. Leptin, insulin resistance, and liver fibrosis in human nonalcoholic fatty liver disease. J hepatol 2004;41:943–9.

98. Piccino F, Sangnelli E, Pasquale G, et al. Complications following percutaneous liver biopsy. A multicentre retrospective study on 68,276 biopsies. J Hepatol !986;2:165–73.

99. Dixon JB, Bhathal PS, O'Brien PE. Nonalcoholic fatty liver disease: predictors of nonalcoholic steatohepatitis and liver fibrosis in the severly obese. Gastroenterology 2001;121: 91–100.

100. Younossi ZM, Gramlich T, Matteoni CA, Boparai N, McCullough AJ. Nonalcoholic fatty liver disease in patients with type 2 diabetes. Clin gastroenterol Hepatol 2004;2:262–5.

101. Palekar NA, Naus R, Larson SP, Ward J, Harrison SA. Clinical model for distinguishing nonalcoholic steatohepatitis from simple steatosis in patients with nonalcoholic fatty liver disease. Liver Int 2006;26: 151–6.

102. Kadayifci A, Merriman R, Bass N. Medical treatment of non-alcoholic steatohepatitis;Clinics in Liver Disease. 2007;11(1):119–40.

103. Menshikova EV, Ritov VB, Toledo FG, Ferrell RE, Goodpaster BH, Kelly DE. Effects of weight loss and physical activity on skeletal muscle mitochondrial function in obesity. Am J Physiol Endocrinol Metab 2005;288(4):818–25.

104. Saris WH, Blair SN, Van Baak MA, et al. How much physical activity is enough to prevent unhealthy weight gain? Outcome of the IASO 1st stock conference and consensus statement. Obes Rev 2003;4(2):101–14.

105. Palmer M, Schaffer F. Effect of weight reduction on hepatic abnormalities in overweight patients. Gastroenterology 1990;99(5):1408–13.

106. Vajro P, Fontanella A, Perna C, Orso G, Tedesco M, De VincenZo A. Persistent hyper-aminotransferasemia resolving after weight reduction in obese children. J Pediatr 1994;125(2):239–41.

107. Ueno T, Sugawara H, Sujaka K, Hashimoto O, Tsuji R, Tamaki S et al. Therapeutic effects of restricted diet and exercise in obese patients with fatty liver. J Hepatol 1997;27(1):103–7.

108. Kugelmas M, hill DB, Vivian B, et al. Cytokines and NASH: a pilot study of the effects of lifestyle modification and vitamin E. Hepatology 2003;38:413–19.

109. Hickman IJ, Jonsson JR, Prins JB, Ash S, Purdie DM, Clouston AD, et al. Modest weight loss and physical activity in overweight patients with chronic liver disease results in sustained improvements in alanine aminotransferase, fasting insulin, and quality of life. Gut 2004;53(3):413–9.

110. Huang MA, Greenson JK, Chao C, Anderson L, Peterman D, Jacobson J, et al. One-year intense nutritional counseling results in histological improvements in patients with non-alcoholic steatohepatitis: a pilot study. Am J Gastroenterol 2005;100(5):1072–81.

111. Harrison SA, Ramrakhiani S, Brunt EM, et al. Orlistat in the treatment of NASH: a case series. American journal of Gastroenterology. 2003;98(4):926–30.

112. Sabuncu T, Nazligul Y, Karaoglanoglu M, et al. The effects of sibutramine and orlistat on the ultrasonographic findings, insulin resistance and liver enzyme levels in obese patients with non-alcoholic steatohepatitis. Romanian Journal of Gastroenterology. 2003;98(4):926–30.

113. Brolin RE. Bariatric surgery and long-term control of morbid obesity. Jama 2002;288:2793–6.

114. Sjostrom L, Lindroos AK, Peltonen M, Torgerson J, Bouchard C, Carlsson B, Dahlgren S, Larsson B, Narbro K, Sjostrom CD, Sullivan M, Wedel H, Group SOSSS. Lifestyle, diabetes, and cardiovascular risk factors 10 years after bariatric surgery. N Engl J Med 2004;351:2683–93.

115. Dixon JB, Bhathal PS, Hughes NR, O'Brien PE. Nonalcoholic fatty liver disease: Improvement in liver histological analysis with weight loss. Hepatology 2004;39:1647–54.

116. Yki-Jarvinen H. Thiazolidinediones. N Engl J Med 2004;351(11)1106–18.

117. Neuschwander-Tetri BA, Brunt EM, Wehmeier KR, Oliver D, Bacon BR. Improved nonalcoholic steatohepatitis after 48 weeks of treatment with the PPAR-gamma ligand rosiglitazone. Hepatology 2003;38:1008–17.

118. Promrat K, Lutchman G, Uwaifo GI, Freedman RJ, Soza A, Heller T, Doo E, Ghany M, Premkumar A, Park Y, Liang Tj, Yanovski JA, Kleiner DE, Hoofnagle JH. A pilot study of pioglitazone treatment for nonalcoholic steatohepatitis. Hepatology 2004;39:188–96.

119. Minassian C, Tarpin S, Mithieux G. Role of glucose-6 phosphatase, glucokinase, and glucose-6-phosphatase in liver insulin resistance and its correction by metformin. Biochem Pharmacol 1998;55(8):1213–9.

120. Arslanian SA, Lewy V, Danadian K, Saad R. Metformin therapy in obese adolescents with polycystic ovary syndrome and impaired glucose tolerance: amelioration of exaggerated adrenal response to adrenocorticotropin with reduction of insulinemia/insulin resistance. J Clin Endocrinol Metab 2002;87(4):1555–9.

121. Solomon SS, Mishra SK, Cwik C, Rajanna B, Postlethwaite AE, Pioglitazone and metformin reverse in sulin resistance induced by tumor necrosis factor-alpha in liver cells. Horm Metab Res 1997;29(8):379–82.

122. Marchesini G, Brii M, Bianchi G, et al. Metformin in non-alcoholic steatohepatitis. Lancet 2001;358;893–4.

123. Schwimmer JB, Middleton MS, Deutsch R, et al. A phase 2 clinical trial of metformin as a treatment for non-diabetic paediatric non-alcoholic steatohepatitis. Aliment Pharmacol Ther 2005;21:871–9.

124. Magalotti D, Marchesini G, Ramilli s, et al. splanchnic haemodynamics in non-alcoholic fatty liver disease: effect of a dietary/pharmacological treatment. A pilot study. Dig Liver Dis 2004;36;406–11.

125. Nair S, Diehl Am, Wiseman M, et al. Metformin in the treatment of non-alcoholic steatohepatitis: a pilot open label trial. Aliment Pharmacol Ther 2004;20:23–8.

126. Bugianesi E, Gentilcore E, Manini R, et al. A randomized controlled trial of metformin versus vitamin E or prescriptive diet in nonalcoholic fatty liver disease. Am J Gastroenterol 2005;100:1082–90.

127. Basaranoglu M, Acbay O, Sonsuz A. A controlled trial of gemfibrozil in the treatment of patients with nonalcoholic steatohepatitis. J Hepatol 1999;31(2):384.

128. Laurin J, Lindor KD, Crippin JS, Gossard A, Gores GJ, Ludwig J, et al. Ursodeoxycholic acid or clofibrate in the treatment of non-alcohol-induced steatohepatitis: a pilot study. Hepatology 1996;23(6):1464–7.

129. Kiyici M, Gulten M, Gurel S, Nak SG, Dolar E, Savci G, et al. Ursodeoxycholic acid and atorvastatin in the treatment of nonalcoholic steatohepatitis. Can J Gastroenterol 2003;17(12):713–8.

130. Hatzitolios A, Savopoulos C, Lazaraki G, et al. Efficacy of omega-3 fatty acids, atarvastatin and orlistat in non-alcoholic fatty liver disease with dyslipidemia. Indian J Gastrenterol 2004;23: 131–4.

131. Rallidis LS, Drakoulis CK, Parasi AS. Pravastatin in patients with nonalcoholic steatohepatitis: results of a pilot study. Atherosclerosis 2004;174:193–6.

132. Dominguez E.G., Gisbert J.P., et al. A pilot study of atorvastatin treatment in dyslipemid, non-alcoholic fatty liver patients. Alimentary Pharmacology &Therapeutics. 2006;23(11):1643–7.

133. Chalasani N. Statins and hepatotoxicity: focus on patients with fatty liver. Hepatology 2005;41:690–5.

134. Hasegawa T, Yoneda m, Nakamura K, et al. Plasma transforming growth factor-beta 1 level and efficacy of alpha-tocopherol in patients with non-alcoholic steatohepatitis: a pilot study. Aliment Pharmacol Ther 2001;15:1667–72.

135. Lavine JE. Vitamin E treatment of nonalcoholic steatohepatitis in children: a pilot study. Journal of Peadiatrics. 2000;136(6):734–8.

136. Vajro P, Mandato C, Franzese A, et al. Vitamin treatment in paediatric obesity-related liver disease: a randomized study. J Pediatr Gastroenterol Nutr 2004;38:48–55.

137. Harrison SA, Torgerson S, Hayashi P, et al. Vitamin E and Vitamin C treatment improves fibrosis in patients with nonalcoholic steatohepatitis. American journal of Gastroenterology. 2003;98(11):2485–90.

138. Guallar E, Hanley DF, Miller ER 3rd. n editorial update:Annus horribilis for vitamin E. Ann Intern Med 2005;143: 143–5.

139. Abdelmalek MF, Angulo P, Jorgensen RA, et al. Betaine, a promising new agent for patients with nonalcoholic steatohepatitis: results of a pilot study. American journal of Gastroenterology.2001;96(9):2711–7.

140. Gulbahar O, Karasu ZA, Ersoz G, et al. Treatment of nonalcoholic steatohepatitis with N-acetylcysteine. Abstract Gastroenterology. 2000;118:A1444.

141. Lirussi F, Azzalini L, Orlando S et al. Antioxidant supplements for non-alcoholic fatty liver disease and/or steatohepatitis. Cochrane Database Syst Rev. 2007 Jan 24(1).

142. Kiyici M, Gulten M, Gurel S, et al. Ursodeoxycholic acid and atorvastatin in the treatment of nonalcoholic steatohepatitis. Can J Gastroenterol 2003;17:713–8.

143. Lindor KD, Kowdley KV, Heathcote EJ et al. Ursodeoxycholic acid for treatment of nonalcoholic steatohepatitis: results of a randomized trial. Hepatology 2004;39:770–8.

144. Scheen AJ. Renin-angiotensin system inhibition prevents type 2 diabetes mellitus. Part 1. A metaanalysis of randomized clinical trials. Diabetes Metab 2004;30(6):487–96.

145. Vitale C, Mercuro G, Castiglioni C, Cornoldi A, TulliA, Fini M et al. Metabolic effects oftelmisartan and losartan in hypertensive patients with metabolic syndrome. Cardiovasc Diabetol 2005;4:6–14.

146. Sloniger JA, Saengsirisuwan V, Diehl CJ, Kim JS, Henriksen EJ. Selective angiotensin II receptor antagonism enhances whole-body insulin sensitivity and muscle glucose transport in hypertensive TG(mREN2)27 rats. Metabolism 2005;54(12):1659–68.

147. Yokohama S, Yoneda M, Haneda M, et al. Therapeutic efficacy of an angiotensin II receptor antagonist in patients with non alcoholic steatohepatitis. Hepatology 2004;40: 1222–5.

148. Charatcharoenwitthaya P, Levy C, Angulo P, et al. Open-label pilot study of folic acid in patients with nonalcoholic steatohepatitis. Liver Int. 2007;27(2):220–6.

149. Solga SF, Diehl AM. Non-alcoholic fatty liver disease: lumen-liver interactions and possible role for probiotics. J Hepatol 2003;38(5):681–7.

150. Loguercio C, Federico A, Tuccillo C, Terracciano F, D'Auria MV, De Simone C, et al. Beneficial effects of a probiotic VSL#3 on parameters of liver dysfunction in chronic liver diseases. J Clin Gastroenterol 2005;39(6):540–3.

151. Daubioul CA, Horsmans Y, Lambert P, Danse E, Delzenne NM. Effects of oligofructose on glucose and lipid metabolism in patients with nonalcoholic steatohepatitis: results of a pilot study. Eur J Clin Nutr 2005;59(5):723–6.

152. Morito Y, Ueno T, Sasaki N, Tateishi Y, Nagata E, Kage M, et al. Nateglinide is useful for nonalcoholic steatohepatitis. (NASH) patients with type 2 diabetes. Hepatogastroenterology 2005;52(65):1338–43.

153. Despres JP, Golay A, Sjostrom L;Rimonabant in Obesity-Lipids Study Group. Effects of rimonabant on metabolic risk factors in overweight patients with dyslipidemia. N Engl J Med 2005;353(20):2121–34.

154. Pershadsingh HA. Dual Peroxisome Proliferator-Activated Receptor-alpha/gamma Agonists: In the Treatment of Type 2 Diabetes Mellitus and the metabolic Syndrome. Treat Endocrinol 2006;5(2):89–99.

Alcoholic Liver Disease

Robert O'Shea, MD, Srinivasan Dasarathy, MD,
and Arthur J. McCullough, MD

I. INTRODUCTION

Alcohol is a socially accepted hepatotoxin and its abuse costs approximately
$200 billion annually. In the U.S. population, 7–10% meets the diagnostic cri-
teria for alcohol abuse or alcoholism.[1] Alcohol accounts for 40–50% of all the
deaths due to cirrhosis and remains the most common cause of liver-related
mortality.[2,3] However, alcoholic liver disease (ALD) represents a spectrum of
histologic changes as shown in Table 6.1 with different clinical outcomes.[4]

The mortality rate of alcoholic fatty liver is insignificant,[5] while the age
adjusted death rate for alcoholic cirrhosis is 3.8 per 100,000.[6] The five- and 10-
year survival rates for alcoholic cirrhosis without liver transplantation are 23%
and 7%, respectively, which is significantly less than other forms of cirrhosis (see
Table 6.2).

II. RISK FACTORS

However, it has been estimated that although 75–100% of heavy drinkers show
evidence of fatty liver, only 8–20% of patients will develop cirrhosis.[4] Therefore,
other factors must play a role in placing these individuals at risk for developing
more severe forms of ALD.[4] A number of risk factors have been proposed as
shown in Figure 6.1, but none of them can either singly or in combination
completely explain the reason why only a minority of individuals ingesting large
amounts of alcohol develop ALD.

A. Quantity of Alcohol Ingested

The quantity of alcohol ingested is the most important risk factor (Table 6.3).
Although most investigators[7,8] agree that those who drink heavily (4–5 drinks
per day) are at risk for ALD, others.[9] believe as few as 2–3 drinks may place an
individual at risk.

Table 6.1. Histological Characteristics of ALD

	Fatty Liver	Alcohol Hepatitis	Cirrhosis	Cirrhosis Alcoholic Hepatitis
Ballooning degeneration withPMN's	73%	97%	76%	35%
Mallory Bodies	0	76%	19%	95%
Mega mitochondria	100%	32%	8%	13%
Sclerosing Hyaline Necrosis	4%	68%	3%	44%
Fibrosis	31%	54%	100%	100%
Fat (moderate to severe)	69%	82%	27%	43%
Perivenular Fibrosis	4.9	19%	–	–

These data were obtained and modified from reference 31.

Table 6.2. Survival of Different Types of Cirrhosis

Etiology	(N)	5 year	10 year
Alcohol	(82)	23%*	7%*
Cryptogenic	(13)	33%	20%
HCV	(62)	38%	24%
HBV	(42)	48%	20%
Hemochromatosis	(20)	41%	22%
Autoimmune	(16)	46%	23%
PBC	(36)	56%	39%

* = p < .05 vs other forms of cirrhosis

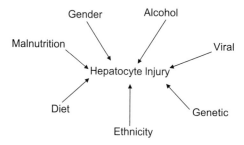

Figure 6.1. Risk factors for hepatic injury in alcoholic liver disease.

   The type of alcohol,[9] binge drinking,[10,11] and mealtime drinking[12] may also all be additional factors impacting of the amount of ALD as a risk factor. A large Danish study observed that beer or spirits were more likely than wine to promote ALD.[9] Investigators from China reported that individuals who consumed spirits outside mealtime developed ALD 2.7 times more often than those who drank only at mealtime.[12] Binge drinking increases the risk for alcoholic hepatitis[10] particularly in women.[11] The basis of liver injury with binge drinking may be related to severe reperfusion injury[13] and damage to mitochondrial DNA.[14]

Table 6.3. Relative Risk of ALD at Different Levels of Alcohol Intake

Weekly Units Alcohol	Alcoholic Cirrhosis		Alcoholic Liver Disease	
	Men	Women	Men	Women
<1	3.7	1.09	1.8	1.0
1–6	1.0	1.0	1.0	1.0
7–13	0.9	4.1*	1.1	2.9*
14–27	1.6	3.1*	1.4	2.9*
28–41	7.0*	16.8*	3.8*	7.3*
42–69	13.0*	NR	5.9*	NR
≥70	18.1*	NR	9.1	NR

These results were estimated from Figure 6.1 in reference 16.
*Represents a statistically significant increased risk of having ALD.
NR = not reported.

B. Gender

Women have been found to be twice as sensitive to alcohol and develop more severe ALD, at lower doses and with shorter duration of alcohol consumption than men.[15,16] As compared to men, in whom 80 gm of daily alcohol was considered to be a hazardous amount, early data suggested the hazardous level to be 60 gm daily in women. Because the majority of those individuals developing ALD ingested more than 35 units per week, a "safe" limit of alcohol intake had been suggests to be 21 units per week in men and 14 units per week in women.[17] However, more recent data from the Copenhagen City study suggest that a lower quantity, more than 7 units per week, may be toxic in women.[16] As shown in Table 6.3, these data confirm the association between increased alcohol intake and ALD, the lower threshold toxic dose and the increased female susceptibility for ALD.

This increased female susceptibility has been related to gender-dependent differences in the hepatic metabolism of alcohol and has been reviewed elsewhere.[18]

C. Virus

Multiple studies have demonstrated that HCV plus alcohol predisposes to more advanced liver injury than alcohol alone.[4] Compared to ALD patients without HCV infection, ALD patients with HCV infection have more severe histological features, have decreased survival, and develop their disease at a younger age.[19–21] The progression of fibrosis is most rapid in male patients who continue to abuse alcohol. Although a daily dose of >50 gm of alcohol has been shown to be a risk factor for fibrosis, even a moderate dose (<50 gm/d) consumption of alcohol has been shown to result in a dose dependent increase in liver disease in patients with HCV.[22,23] Despite these observations, the precise toxic threshold is not known and may be lower and non-uniform amongst patients at risk.[22,24,25,26] The prevalence of HCV also increases proportionally as the liver injury becomes more severe with the relative risk for developing cirrhosis estimated at 8.7 in those ALD patients with anti-HCV.[27] In patients with alcoholic cirrhosis the 10-year absolute cumulative occurrence risk of Hepatocellular Carcinoma (HCC) has been reported to be as high as 81% in anti-HCV positive alcoholic cirrhotics as compared to 19% in anti-HCV negative patients.[28,29,30] Patients with hepatitis C should therefore be strongly urged to abstain from alcohol even in moderate quantities unless further evidence to the contrary becomes available.

D. Malnutrition and Diet

Dietary habits and nutritional status may also be important risk factors.[31] Early studies conducted in hospitalized chronic alcoholic patients with liver disease led to the misconception that malnutrition was a necessary risk factor for ALD. However, alcohol is directly hepatotoxic and does not require pre-existing malnutrition to result in liver injury.

Nutritional disorders including obesity and dietary habits are important risk factors.[32,33,34] Data from France suggest that obesity may be an independent risk factor for developing ALD.[34] In alcoholic patients from China, excess body weight was associated with a five-fold increase in risk of ALD.[35] Increased tumor necrosis factor activity and hepatic insulin resistance that are associated with obesity seem to contribute to the aggravation of alcoholic liver disease. Obesity also makes the liver susceptible to alcohol mediated injury by metabolic activation of CYP2E1, oxidant stress, and immune hyper reactivity in the liver. It is currently unclear whether the hepatotoxic consequences of obesity and ethanol ingestion are additive or synergistic. High-fat diets are necessary to promote alcohol-induced liver disease in animals. In addition, the incidence of cirrhosis appears lower than expected in countries with high intakes of saturated fat; an epidemiological finding which is independent from other risk factors and supported by animal data.[36]

III. TREATMENT

A. Alcoholic Hepatitis

i. PROGNOSIS

The mortality rate of hospitalized patients with alcoholic hepatitis varies widely. Based on clinical experience and many clinical trials, it is clear that patients with mild disease need not be treated with extraordinary measures. It is also likely that patients with severe disease *in extremis* may be too ill to respond to any form of therapy. Currently, alcoholic hepatitis is not a routine indication for orthotopic liver transplantation; with particular cases considered on a case by case basis.[37] Therefore, it is important to identify those patients who might benefit from aggressive intervention, as well as for those for whom the therapeutic benefit risk ratio is favorable.

ii. PROGNOSTIC SCORING SYSTEMS

Although several clinical scoring systems have been derived in patients with cirrhosis, relatively few have been specifically tested in alcoholic hepatitis. These severity of illness scores for ALD include the Child-Truscott-Pugh (CTP) score, which is used commonly to estimate the severity of cirrhosis,[38] the combined

Table 6.4. Discriminant Function Associated with Prognosis in Alcoholic Liver Disease

	Discriminant Function	Score Indicating Poor Prognosis
Initial	[4.6 × prothrombin time (seconds)] + Serum bilirubin (mg/dL)	>93
Modified	4.6 (patient's prothrombin time-control time) + Serum bilirubin (mg/dL)	≥32

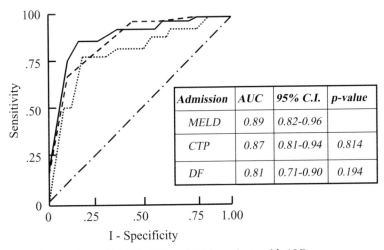

Admission	AUC	95% C.I.	p-value
MELD	0.89	0.82-0.96	
CTP	0.87	0.81-0.94	0.814
DF	0.81	0.71-0.90	0.194

Figure 6.2. Comparison of MELD, CTP, and DF in patients with ALD.

clinical laboratory index of the University of Toronto,[39] and the Maddrey Discriminate Function[40] (MDF) as shown in Table 6.4, the Beclere model,[41] the MELD score,[42] and most recently the ASH test.[43]

The MDF score was derived from clinical trials of patients with AH, and has since been widely applied clinically to managing patients with this disease. It has been used to stratify patients' severity of illness for most of the research involving the use of steroids in patients with AH. A "discriminate function score" of ≥32 is highly correlated with a >50% short-term mortality rate in patients with AH. One review compared the CTP score and the Orrego score with the MDF in a Veterans Administrative Cooperative AH Study, evaluating their ability to predict 30-day mortality.[44] All correlated with survival, but the less complex Maddrey criteria had the best correlation and the highest positive predictive value. Furthermore, the prognostic value of the MDF criteria has been confirmed prospectively. More recently, investigators have applied the MELD score to predict the outcome in patients with AH. In a comparison of the use of the MDF in patients with AH, the MELD score was shown to predict the outcome as well as the discriminate factor[42,45] as shown in Figure 6.2. Using the usual cut-off (<32 or ≤32, versus a MELD score of >18), the two indices have similar sensitivities, although the MELD score may have had a higher specificity.

Dynamic models, which incorporate the changes in laboratory studies over time, have also been used to estimate the outcome in this patient population. Recently a French group identified the changes in bilirubin in the first week of

Table 6.5. Clinical Trials of Corticosteroids for Alcoholic Liver Disease

Author	Date	Number of Patients	Deaths: Placebo (with 95% CI)	Deaths: Steroid (with 95% CI)	RR
Porter	1972	20	7/9 (0.77) (0.44–0.93)	6/11 (0.55) (0.28–0.79)	1
Helman	1971	37	6/17 (0.35) (0.14–0.62)	1/20 (0.05) (0.0013–0.25)	0.143
Campra	1973	45	9/25 (0.36) (0.2–0.56)	7/29 (0.35) (0.18–0.57)	1
Blitzer	1977	33	5/16 (0.31) (0.14–0.56)	6/12 (0.5) (0.25–0.75)	1
Lesesne	1978	14	7/7 (1.0) (0.63–1.0)	2/7 (0.29) (0.09–0.65)	0.29
Shumaker	1978	27	7/15 (0.47) (0.25–0.75)	6/12 (0.5) (0.25–0.75)	1
Maddrey	1978	27	6/31 (0.194) (0.09–0.36)	1/24 (0.042) (0.009–0.20)	0.22
Depew	1980	28	7/13 (0.54) (0.29–0.77)	8/15 (0.53) (0.3–0.75)	1
Theodossi	1982	55	16/28 (0.57) (0.39–0.74)	17/27 (0.63) (0.44–0.79)	1
Mendenhall	1984	178	50/88 (0.57) (0.46–0.67)	55/90 (0.61) (0.51–0.71)	1
Bories	1987	45	2/21 (0.095) (0.029–0.29)	1/24 (0.42) (0.0098–0.20)	1
Carithers	1989	66	11/31 (0.36) (0.21–0.53)	2/35 (0.057) (0.108–0.19)	0.16
Ramond	1992	61	16/29 (0.55) (0.37–0.72)	4/32 (0.125) (0.05–0.28)	0.23

hospitalization to be significantly associated with outcome of patients with AH treated with prednisolone.[46]

iii. PATHOPHYSIOLOGY BASED TREATMENT

Although a number of different treatments have been tested in alcoholic hepatitis, only those that focus on immunosuppressives and cytokines have had any success. Therefore, the focus of this discussion is treatment as it relates to immunosuppression, oxidative stress, and anti-cytokines.

B. Corticosteroids

Corticosteroids have been used in the treatment of this disorder for seven decades, and are thus the most extensively studied treatment modality.[47–59] The efficacy however, remains controversial. As shown in Table 6.5, five randomized clinical trials suggested that corticosteroids reduce mortality compared with placebo, where eight others found no difference in outcomes.

Although the results are not consistent, multiple differences in trial design may explain the different outcomes. These include differences in dose and duration of therapy, selection of patients (e.g., varying time intervals before randomization or inconsistent use of disease severity scoring), possible misclassification bias (e.g., differing percentages of patients who underwent liver biopsy to confirm the diagnosis), severity of illness, concomitant medical problems or medications, as well as undiagnosed chronic viral hepatitis infections. Despite these differences, three separate meta-analyses have found a benefit to the use of steroids.[60,61,62] The results of the combined data from one of these meta-analyses[62] indicate that corticosteroids should be targeted to specific subsets of patients with severe disease. In response to the meta-analyses, a reanalysis of pooled data from three placebo-controlled randomized trials using the MDF as a measure of disease severity[63] concluded that corticosteroid treated patients had a significantly higher survival rate than patients given placebo: 84.6% versus

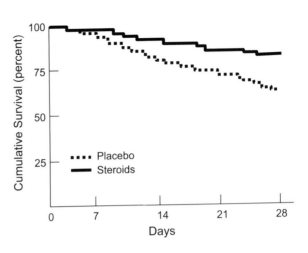

Figure 6.3. Survival of Patients with an MDF[3] from Three Randomized controlled trials of corticosteroids.[46,48,49]

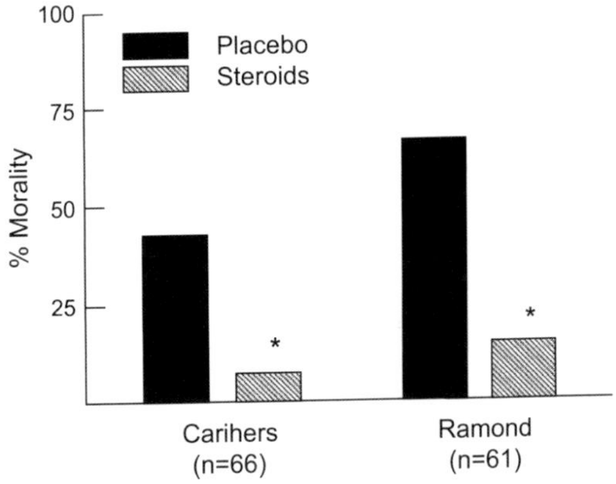

Figure 6.4. The Effect of Steroids vs. Placebo on Mortality in Patients with Alcoholic Hepatitis.

65% (Figure 6.3). Extrapolating from this result, a number needed to treat of five (i.e., five patients treated to prevent one death) was calculated.

The efficacy of corticosteroids is substantiated by the fact that the two prospective studies[58,59] which stratified patients according to disease severity quantified by the DF, both showed significant benefit in terms of 30-day hospital survival for patients with severe AH (Figure 6.4). In addition, a follow-up study of Mathurin[64] showed that steroids improved the survival at one year but not two years in these patients.

These combined data provide a number of tangible suggestions for the management of these patients. First, only patients with severe disease (as defined by the presence of hepatic encephalopathy, the MDF, or possibly the MELD score) should be treated with corticosteroids. Secondly, approximately 5–7 patients need to be treated to avoid one death. This latter point emphasizes the importance of careful selection to avoid the side effects of corticosteroids in the other 4–6 patients who will derive no clinical benefits from corticosteroids. In general, this means excluding patients with active infection and being certain of the diagnosis (liver biopsy may be necessary) because histologically confirmed alcoholic hepatitis may correlate poorly with the clinical impression of alcoholic hepatitis[64,65] and up to as many as 28% of patients with a clinical picture of alcoholic hepatitis do not have histological features of alcoholic hepatitis on

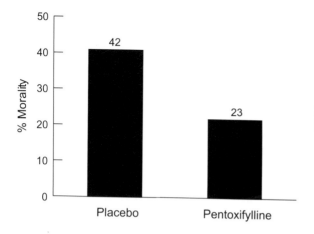

Figure 6.5. Pentoxifylline Decreased Morality in AH.

liver biopsy. Third, while such treatment reduces mortality risk by 25%, there is still up to 44% mortality in patients receiving corticosteroids. Therefore, other therapies or combination of therapies need to be considered. Consistent with this latter point the use of corticosteroids for AH is infrequent[66] despite the fact that the 1998 recommendation of the American Society of Gastroenterology that corticosteroids should be used in the treatment of severe AH.[67]

C. Anti-Cytokine Therapy

i. PENTOXIFYLLINE

Several recent studies have focused on the use of pentoxifylline, a phosphodiesterase inhibitor initially used in the treatment of peripheral vascular disease, based on its ability to increase erythrocyte flexibility, reduce blood viscosity, and inhibit platelet aggregation. Phosphodieterase inhibition, however, has also been shown to have multiple effects on immune markers. In particular, pentoxifylline has been shown to reduce the production of TNF-α, IL-5, IL-10, and IL-12. It also has been shown to decrease the transcription of IL-2 and TNF-α promoters in transiently transfected normal T-cells, to inhibit the activation of nuclear factor KB (NF-κB) and nuclear factor of activated T-cells, and stimulate activation of protein-1 and cAMP response element-binding proteins.[68] In an animal model it has been shown to reduce portal pressure in an experimental model of cirrhosis.[69]

Based on these data, a clinical trial using pentoxifylline in 101 patients with severe AH was undertaken.[70] Patients were randomized to receive either pentoxifylline 400 mg three times a day or placebo. In hospital mortality was significantly lower in pentoxifylline recipients, as compared with controls 24.5% versus 46.1% of patients (Figure 6.5) yielding a relative risk of 0.59. Of the patients who died, hepatic failure with hepatorenal syndrome developed in significantly fewer pentoxifyllone recipients, compared with controls (50% versus 91%). Lastly, new onset renal impairment developed in significantly fewer pentoxifylline recipients, compared with controls; further progression in hepatorenal syndrome occurred in 4 of 18 patients in their respective treatment groups, yielding a relative risk of 0.3. The difference in mortality between the two groups suggests a number needed to treat of 4.7, which is almost identical to the number arrived by Mathurin et al. comparing the use of steroids to placebo. The mechanism whereby pentoxifylline decreased the development of hepatorenal syndrome is unclear, but could be related to either direct effects on the liver (although any of the above possible mechanisms) or alternatively, by direct renal effect.

ii. ANTI-TNF TREATMENT

These data along with more recent studies that inhibit particular cytokines have recently generated interest in this type of treatment. Two small uncontrolled pilot studies using infliximab (IgG-1 monoclonal antibody to TNF) suggested a benefit in AH.[71,72] On the basis of these studies, a clinical trial using infliximab (10 mg/kg) in combination with prednisolone (40 mg/d) versus prednisolone alone was begun in France.[73] A concern regarding the likelihood of infection using this form of treatment[74] was indeed verified. A total of 36 patients were randomized before the trial was stopped prematurely by the data safety monitoring board, based on a substantially higher death rate in the infliximab group (39% vs. 11%).

Most of these were related to a very significant increase in the risk of infection in patients on active treatment compared to controls who had been treated with prednisolone alone. However, this study was criticized both based on the specifics of the study design[75] as well as the premise for the use of such therapy.[76]

iii. ETANERCEPT

Etanercept, a P75 soluble TNF receptor: FC fusion protein, neutralizes soluble TNF and excludes an effect on membrane bound TNF. It has been used in a variety of rheumatologic disorders including rheumatoid and psoriatic arthritis, as well as ankylosing spondylitis. The only published report in patients with liver disease treated 13 patients with moderate or severe alcoholic hepatitis for a two-week duration.[77] The 30-day survival rate for patients receiving etanercept was 92%. Adverse events (including an infection, hepatorenal decompensation, and gastrointestinal bleeding) required premature discontinuation of etanercept in 23% of patients. Based on this study, a larger multicenter clinical trial is now underway.

Although these results are intriguing, the lack of a control arm, the inclusion of patients with more moderate disease (making interpretation of survival statistics uncertain), and the high drop-out rate temper the enthusiasm for the use of etanercept. In addition, questions have been raised regarding the extent to which TNF inhibition is useful in this disease, as TNF has been shown to be important in hepatic regeneration.[78]

D. Antioxidants

i. VITAMIN E

Vitamin E when used along was not shown to be significantly beneficial in either AH[79] or alcoholic cirrhosis.[80] However, neither of these studies were optimally designed and there are data suggesting that vitamin E when combined with other antioxidants may improve outcome in AH.[81]

ii. S-ADENOSYL-L-METHIONINE

A trial of 62 patients with alcoholic cirrhosis treated with SAMe and followed for up to two years was not able to detect a difference in overall mortality in treated patients versus controls. The subgroup with Childs A or B cirrhosis

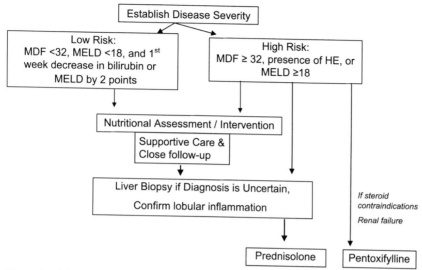

Figure 6.6. Therapeutic Algorithm for the Management of Alcoholic Hepatitis.

receiving supplementations, however, showed a significant improvement in the rate of liver transplant or mortality.[82] Although a systematic review failed to show any significant differences in outcomes in patients treated with alcoholic liver disease with SAMe[83], the number of patients studied was low and there is a pressing need for further trials in this area.[84]

E. Potential New Therapies

Thalidomide,[85] misoprostol,[76] adiponectin,[86] and probiotics[87] have all been shown in preliminary reports to have anti-cytokine properties. Emerging data suggest that a role for TNF-α mediated apoptosis in alcoholic hepatitis[88] and therefore targeting this therapy inhibiting apoptosis may be effective.[89] Finally, aggressive new therapy to remove cytokines via leukocytapheresis[90] or other extracorporeal recirculating systems[91] deserve additional trials.

Figure 6.6 provides a proposed management algorithm based on a number of hypotheses from a therapeutic optimist. Although this algorithm is speculative, its intent is to stimulate discussion and to emphasize several of the following points for both clinicians and clinical investigators.

1. Only patients with severe AH should be treated with more than general supportive therapy. Severity is defined by a MDF $\geq$ 32 or a MELD score > 18. The latter needs to be tested prospectively.
2. Nutritional supplements should be provided to patients with severe AH.
3. Although steroids have been proven to be effective therapy in severe AH, the optimal duration of treatment needs to be reconsidered and predictors of steroid treated response needs to be reconsidered. The efficacy of pentoxifylline needs to be confirmed and compared to steroids in severe AH.
4. Combination therapy with steroids and pentoxifylline may be more beneficial than either agent individually due to their different mechanisms of efficacy.

5. Although infliximab and etanercept may eventually be shown to be effective therapeutic agents in severe AH, less expensive agents with a better safety profile should be also tested in anti-cytokines.

IV. LONG TERM

It is important that the clinician consider the long term of ALD in addition to treatment of acute symptomatic episodes of alcoholic hepatitis.

A. Nutritional Therapy

Protein calorie malnutrition that is widely prevalent in ALD[92] is associated with major complications observed in cirrhosis (infection, encephalopathy, and ascites) and indicates a poor prognosis. It now seems clear that long-term aggressive nutritional therapy is necessary and reasonable for these patients. General goals and practical points for nutritional therapy in chronic liver disease (Table 6.6) have been suggested but three additional points need to be emphasized.[93,94]

First, nutritional assessment should be an ongoing process. Second, multiple feedings emphasizing breakfast and a nighttime snack with a regular oral diet at higher than usual dietary intakes (1.2–1.5 g/kg for protein and 35–40 Kcal/kg for energy) seem indicated. Third, during intermittent acute illness or exacerbations of the underlying chronic liver disease above normal protein (1.5–2.0 gm/kg body weight and energy 40–45 Kcal/kg) improve protein calorie malnutrition.[95]

B. Other Therapies

A number of other therapies have been investigated but to date have not produced convincing evidence that they should be used for the long-term treatment of ALD. These agents include: PTU, SAMe, colchicine, vitamin E, corticosteroids, and anabolic steroids.[96–99] Corticosteroids are used in the therapy of alcoholic cirrhosis only when severe alcoholic hepatitis is also present and it would be essential in this situation to have histological documentation of inflammation superimposed on cirrhosis.

C. Antiviral Therapy

Alcohol use even in moderate quantities has been suggested to worsen the course of hepatitis C. Additionally, it has been shown that response rates to interferon-based treatment protocols are less effective in the presence of active alcohol use.[100] It is therefore recommended that therapy for hepatitis C is started only in patients who have been abstinent for at least six months. If hepatitis C can be eradicated, the long-term prognosis of ALD should improve.

D. Liver Transplantation for ALD

ALD is the second most common indication for orthotopic liver transplantation (OLT) for chronic liver disease in the Western world. A six-month period of abstinence has been recommended as a minimal listing criterion allowing chemical

Table 6.6. Guidelines for the Nutritional Management of Patients with Liver Disease

Assume protein calorie malnutrition is present in all patients with cirrhosis.

Assume an inadequate dietary intake, particularly in hospitalized patients.

Nutritional assessment is useful in all types of cirrhotic patients.

A composite score (emphasizing anthropometry, hand grip strength, and creatinine-height index) combined with overall clinical judgment should be employed.

Determine energy expenditure requirements with indirect calorimetry (if possible) in hospitalized patients or patients listed for liver transplantation. If energy expenditure requirements are estimated from prediction equations, calculate energy need based on ideal weight rather than actual weight if extracellular water (ascites/edema) is present.

The clinician should remember that all the methods for nutritional assessment in cirrhosis are influenced or potentially influenced by the presence of liver disease alone as well as abnormalities associated with liver disease such as renal failure, alcohol ingestion and expansion of the extracellular water compartment.

Treatment of liver disease:

Cirrhotics should never be treated prophylactically with protein restriction to prevent hepatic encephalopathy.

Protein restriction below the required amounts should not be continued for more than 3-4 days.

Neomycin or lactulose may exacerbate malabsorption and this should be considered in the nutritional management plan.

Treat ascites aggressively to decrease energy expenditure.

Diuretic therapy is preferred over large volume paracentesis for the management of ascites in order to minimize protein loss.

Balance the need for sodium restriction with nutritional considerations and diet palatability.

Qualitative stool fat should be done intermittently, especially in patients with alcoholic or cholestatic cirrhosis. If malabsorption is present, determine the cause and treat.

Monitor for hypoglycemia and treat aggressively with concentrated glucose solutions recognizing that these may also decrease serum ammonia levels.

Nutritional management:

Nutritional requirements may vary according to the specific type of patient and/or clinical situation.

Multiple (5–6) small feedings with a carbohydrate-rich evening snack, which consists of approximately 10–15% of caloric needs, should be given. The need for breakfast feeding must also be stressed.

Complex, rather than simple carbohydrates should be used for calories. Lipids should supply 20–40% of caloric needs.

Long term nutritional supplements may be necessary to provide recommended protein and caloric supplements.

Severely malnourished or decompensated cirrhotics should be given oral or enteral supplements.

Patients with severe alcoholic hepatitis should be given supplemental standard protein 1.0 g/kg via an enteral or peripheral parenteral route.

Perioperative nutritional therapy should be given to those cirrhotic patients with significant malnutrition and post-liver transplant patients.

Standard protein or amino acid mixtures should be supplied to meet the measured estimated nitrogen needs. Branched-chain amino acids should be given only if the required amount of protein results in worsening hepatic encephalopathy.

Enteral feedings is the preferred route of feeding patients with insufficient oral intake. Enteral feeding tubes may be used even if non-bleeding varices are present.

Do no use any nutritional product devoid of cysteine or tyrosine as the only nitrogen source for any prolonged period of time.

dependency issues to be resolved during this period. Adherence to the six-month abstinence could result in a resolution of the anti-inflammatory effects of recent alcohol consumption and thus may make OLTx unnecessary in a subset of these patients. The requirement for a fixed abstinence period, the so-called six-month rule, as a predictor of future abstinence is arbitrary but used most often. An evaluation of the peritransplant period in ALD showed that patients were more ill at the time of OLT and likely to have a prolonged intensive care unit stay and increased blood product requirements. Decreased acute and chronic rejection after OLT are also observed. There have been multiple published reports[101–122] on the outcome of liver transplantation in alcoholic patients in over 1,200 patients followed over 11 years.

One-third to one-half of alcoholic liver recipients will report some use of alcohol in the first five years after transplantation. It has been suggested that the consequences for alcohol is minimal for many recipients because the amount consumed is small and occurs infrequently but there is little reliable data to support this contention. Rates of recidivism at 3–5 years after OLT have been reported between 11–49%. It should be emphasized that the rate of recidivism depends on the method used to assess alcohol use and abuse. Higher rates have been reported with objective criteria like urine and blood alcohol levels, carbohydrate-deficient transferin, or a detailed structured interview rather than unstructured questioning of the patients. However, recipients who relapse into alcohol use after OLT have similar or potentially lower graft failure rates compared to non-ALD. Poor follow-up attendance and non-compliance with therapy is observed in only a minority of patients, graft rejection rates are similar for patients with ALD (acute rejection 41% and chronic rejection 5.6%) compared to the non-ALD patients (43.7% acute rejection and 6.2% chronic rejection). Therefore, OLT should be offered to appropriately selected patients with ALD.

In light of a still incomplete understanding of the involved pathophysiologic mechanisms and conflicting data regarding the efficacy of specific interventional therapies of ALD, a conservative approach seems justified. These include general supportive, aggressive nutritional interventions and the judicious use of corticosteroids and pentoxifylline in selected patients with severe alcoholic hepatitis. In addition, abstinence from alcohol, treating the co-morbidities of obesity and hepatitis C, and continuous nutritional monitoring are prudent on a long-term basis with liver transplantation offered for select patients with progressive disease. An algorithm has been proposed for long-term management of ALD (Figure 6.7). Although algorithms are by necessity incomplete, they are provided to stimulate different approaches to this disease and to emphasize several of the following important issues.

The management of the complications of chronic liver disease (ascites, portal hypertension associated bleeding, encephalopathy, and hepatocellular) is similar in alcoholic and non-ALD. However, abstinence remains the cornerstone of therapy for ALD. There is also consensus for the use of corticosteroids and pentoxifylline in severe alcoholic hepatitis, for maintaining good nutritional status, for treating co-morbidities in all forms of ALD, and for liver transplantation in carefully selected patients with end stage ALD. No other therapies can be recommended at the present time, although nascent data suggest that a number of newer therapies may be effective.

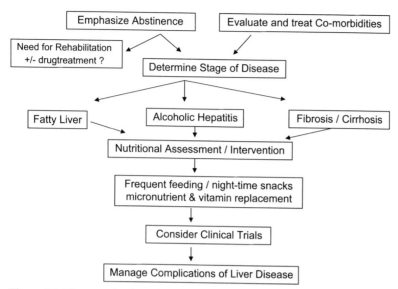

Figure 6.7. Therapeutic Algorithm for the Long-term Management of ALD.

Building on our increased knowledge of the molecular basis of ALD, a greater understanding of the pathophysiology of ALD and the interactive role of other co-factors in causing hepatotoxicity needs to remain a major focus of alcohol research.

REFERENCES

1. Dawson DA, Grant BF, Chou SP, Pickering RP. Subgroup variation in the U.S. drinking patterns: Results of the 1992 National Longitudinal Alcohol Epidemiologic Study. J Subst Abuse 1995;7:331–4.
2. Mandavam S. Jamal MM, Morgan TR. Epidemiology of alcoholic liver disease. Semin Liver Dis 2004;24:217–32.
3. Jamal MM, Morgan TR. Liver disease in alcohol and hepatitis C. Best Pract Res Clin Gastroenterol 2003;17:649–62.
4. O'Shea RS, McCullough AJ. Treatment of alcoholic hepatitis. Clin Liver Dis 2005;9:103–34.
5. Dam-Larsen S, Franzmann M, Andersen IB, Christoffersen P, et al. Long-term prognosis of fatty liver: Risk of chronic liver disease and death. Gut 2004;53:750–5.
6. Singh GK, Hoyert DL. Social epidemiology of chronic liver disease and cirrhosis mortality in the United States 1935–1977: Trends and differentials by ethnicity, socioeconomic status and alcohol consumption. Hum Biol 2000;72:801–20.
7. Bellentani S, Saccoccio G, Costa G, Tiribelli C, et al. Drinking habits as cofactors of risk for alcohol induced liver damage. Gut 1997;41:845–50.
8. Kamper-Jorgensen M, Gronbaek M, Tolstrup J, Becker U. Alcohol and cirrhosis: dose-response or threshold effect? J Hepatol 2004;41:25–30.
9. Becker U, Gronbaek M, Johansen D, Sorensen TI. Lower risk for alcohol-induced cirrhosis in wine drinkers. Hepatology 2002;35:868–75.
10. Barrio E, Tome S, Rodriguez I, Gude F, et al. Liver disease in heavy drinkers with and without alcohol withdrawal syndrome. Alcohol Clin Exp Res 2004;28:131–36.
11. Tolstrup JS, Jensen MK, Tjonneland A, Overvad K, Gronback, M. Drinking pattern and mortality in middle-aged men and women. Addiction 2004;99:323–30.

12. Lu XL, Luo JY, Tao M, Gen Y, Zhao P, et al. Risk factors for alcoholic liver disease in China. World J Gastroenterol 2004;10:2423–6.

13. French SW. The role of hypoxia in the pathogenesis of alcoholic liver disease. Hepatol Res 2004;29:69–74.

14. Mansouri A, Gaou I, DeKerguenec C, Amsellem S, et al. An alcoholic binge causes massive degradation of hepatic mitochondrial DNA in mice. Gastroenterology 1999;117:181–90.

15. Loft S, Olesen KL, Dossing M. Increased susceptibility to liver disease in relation to alcohol consumption in women. Scand J Gastroenterol 1987;22:1251–6.

16. Becker U, Deis A, Sorensen TI, Gronbaek M, et al. Prediction of risk of liver disease by alcohol intake, sex, and age: A prospective population study. Hepatology 1996;23:1025–9.

17. Lelbach WK. Epidemiology of alcoholic liver disease. Prog Liv Dis 1976;5:494–515.

18. Crabb DW. Pathogenesis of alcoholic liver disease: Newer mechanisms of injury. Keio J Med 1999;48:184–8.

19. Poynard T, Bedossa P, Opolon P. Natural history of liver fibrosis progression in patients with chronic hepatitis C. The OBSVIRC, METAVIR, CLINIVIR, and DOSVIRC groups. Lancer 1997;349:825–32.

20. Bellentani S, Pozzato G, Saccoccio G, Crovatto M, Croce LS, et al. Clinical course and risk factors of hepatitis C virus related liver disease in the general population: Report from the Dionysos study. Gut 1999;44:874–80.

21. Corrao G, Arico S. Independent and combined action of hepatitis C virus infection and alcohol consumption on the risk of symptomatic liver cirrhosis. Hepatology 1998;27:914–19.

22. Hezode C, Lonjon I, Roudot-Thoraval F, Pawlotsky JM, Safrani ES, Shumeaux D. Impact of moderate alcohol consumption on histological activity and fibrosis in patients with chronic hepatitis C, and specific influence of steatosis: a prospective study. Aliment Pharmacol Ther 2003;17:1031–7.

23. Monto A, Patel K, Bostrom A, Pianko S, et al. Risks of a range of alcohol intake on hepatitis C-related fibrosis. Hepatology 2004;39:826–34.

24. Freeman AJ, Dore GJ, Law MG, Thorpe M, et al. Estimating progression to cirrhosis in chronic hepatitis C virus infection. Hepatology 2001 Oct;34(4 Pt1):809–16.

25. Hutchinson SJ, Bird SM, Goldberg DJ. Influence of alcohol on the progression of hepatitis C virus infection: A meta-analysis. Clin Gastroenterol Hepatol 2005;3(11):1150–9.

26. Tsui JI, Pletcher MJ, Vittinghoff E, Seal K, Gonzales R. Hepatitis C and hospital outcomes in patients admitted with alcohol-related problems. J Hepatol 2006;44:262–6.

27. Yokoyama H. Ishii H, Moriya S, Magata S, Watanabe T, Kamegaya K, et al. Relationship between hepatitis C virus subtypes and clinical features of liver disease seen in alcoholics. J Hepatol 1995;22:130–4.

28. Fasani P, Sangiovanni A, DeFazio C, Borzio M, Bruno S, Ronchi G, et al. High prevalence of multinodular hepatocellular carcinoma in patients with cirrhosis attributable to multiple risk factors. Hepatology 1999;29:1704–7.

29. Marsano LS, Pena LR. The interaction of alcoholic liver disease and hepatitis C. Hepatogastroenterology 1998;45:331–9.

30. Monto A, Wright TL. The epidemiology and prevention of hepatocellular carcinoma. Semin Oncol 2001;28:441–9.

31. Sarin SK, Dhingra N, Bansal A, Malhotra S, Guptan RC. Dietary and nutritional abnormalities in alcoholic liver disease: A comparison with chronic alcoholics without liver disease. Am J Gastroenterol 1997;92:777–83.

32. Leevy CM, Moroianu SA. Nutritional aspects of alcoholic liver disease. Clin Liver Dis 2005;9:67–81.

33. Iturriaga H, Bunont D, Hirsch S, Ugarte G. Overweight as a risk factor or a predictive sign of histological liver damage in alcoholics. Am J Clin Nutri 1988;47:235–8.

34. Naveau S, Giraud V, Borotto E, Aubent A, Capron F, Chaput JC. Excess weight as a risk factor for alcoholic liver disease. Hepatology 1997;25:108–11.

35. Lu XL, Luo JY, Tao M, Gen Y, Zhao P, Zhao HL. Risk factors for alcoholic liver disease in China. World J Gastroenterol 2004;10:2433–66.

36. Mezey E. Dietary fat and alcoholic liver disease. Hepatology 1998;28:901–9.

37. Mathurin P, Is alcoholic hepatitis an indicator for transplantation? Current management and outcomes. Liver Transplantation 2005;11(suppl 1): 21–4.

38. Kurner T, Kropf J, Kosche R, Kristal H, Jaspersen D, Gressner AM. Improvement of prognostic power of the Child-Pugh classification of liver cirrhosis by hyaluronan. J Hepatol 2003;39:947–53.

39. Orrego H, Israel Y, Blake JE, Medline A. Assessment of prognostic factors in alcoholic liver disease toward a global quantitative expression of severity. Hepatology 1983;3:896–905.

40. Maddrey WC. Alcoholic hepatitis: Clinicopathologic features and therapy. Semin Liv Dis 1988;8:91–102.

41. Mathurin P, Duchatelle V, Ramond MJ, Degott C, Bedossa P, et al. Survival and prognostic factors in patients with severe alcoholic hepatitis treated with prednisolone. Gastroenterology 1996;110:1847–53.

42. Sheth M, Riggs M, Patel T. Utility of the Mayo end-stage liver disease.MELD) score in assessing prognosis of patients with alcoholic hepatitis. BMC Gastroenterol 2002;2:1–5.

43. Thabut D, Navean S, Charlotte F, Massard J, et al. The diagnostic value of biomarkers.Ash test) for the prediction of alcoholic steato-hepatitis in patients with chronic alcoholic liver disease. J Hepatol 2006;44:1175–85.

44. Mendenhall CK. Alcoholic hepatitis. In: Schiff L, Schiff ER, editors. Diseases of the liver. 6th edition. Philadelphia: JB Lippincott Co, 1987, pp. 669–685.

45. Srikureja W, Kyola NL, Runyon R, Hu KQ. Meld score is a better prognostic model than Child-Turcotte-Pugh score on discriminant function score in patients with alcoholic hepatitis. J Hepatol 2005;42:700–6.

46. Mathurin P, Abdelnour M, Ramond MJ, Carbonell N, Fartoux L, et al. Early change in bilirubin levels is an important prognostic factor in severe alcoholic hepatitis treated with prednisolone. Hepatology 2003;38:1363–9.

47. Helman RA, Temko MH, Nye SW, Fallon HU. Natural history and evaluation of prednisolone therapy. Ann Intern Med 1971;74:311–21.

48. Porter HP, Simon FR, Pope CE, Volwiler W, Fenster LF. Corticosteroid therapy in severe alcoholic hepatitis. N Engl J Med 1971;284:1350–5.

49. Campra JL, Hamlin EM Jr, Kirshbaum RJ, Olivier M, Redeker AG, Reynolds TB. Prednisone therapy of acute alcoholic hepatitis. Ann Intern Med 1973;79:625–31.

50. Blitzer BL, Mutchnick MG, Joshi PH, Phillips MM, Fessel JM, Conn HO. Adrenocorticosteroid therapy in alcoholic hepatitis: A prospective, double-blind randomized study. Am J Dig Dis 1977;22:477–84.

51. Lesesne HR, Bozymski EM, Fallon JH. Treatment of alcoholic hepatitis with encephalopathy. Comparison of prednisolone with caloric supplements. Gastroenterology 1978;74:169–73.

52. Maddrey WC, Boitnott JK, Bedine MS, Weber FL Jr, Mezey E, White RI Jr. Corticosteroid therapy of alcoholic hepatitis. Gastroenterology 1978;75:193–9.

53. Shumaker JB, Resnick RH, Galambos JT, Makopour H, Iber FL. A controlled trial of 6-methylprednisolone in acute alcoholic hepatitis. Am J Gastroenterol 1978;69:443–9.

54. Depew W, Boyer T, Omata M, Redeker A, Reynolds T. Double-blind controlled trial of prednisolone therapy in patients with severe acute alcoholic hepatitis and spontaneous encephalopathy. Gastroenterology 1980;78:524–9.

55. Theodossi A, Eddleston ALWF, Williams R. Controlled trial of methylprednisolone therapy in severe acute alcoholic hepatitis. Gut 1982;23:75–9.

56. Mendenhall CL, Anderson S, Garcia-Pont P, Goldberg S, et all. Short-term and long-term survival in patients with alcoholic hepatitis treated with oxandrolone and prednisolone. N Engl J Med 1984;311:1464–70.

57. Bories P, Guedj JY, Mirouze D, Yousfi A, Michel H. Traitement de L'hépatite alcoolique aiguë par la prednisolone. Presse Med 1987;16:769–72.

58. Carithers RL Jr, Herlong HF, Diehl AM, Shaw EW, Combes B, Fallon HJ, Maddrey WC. Methylprednisolone therapy in patients with severe alcoholic hepatitis: A randomized multicenter trial Ann Intern Med 1989;11:685–90.

59. Ramond MJ, Poynard T, Rueff B, Mathurin P, et al. A randomized trial of prednisolone in patients with severe alcoholic hepatitis. N Engl J Med 1992;326:507–12.

60. Daures JP, Peray P, Bories P, Blanc P, Yousfi A, Michel H, Gremy F. Place de la corticotherapyie dans le traitement des hépatite alcoolique aiguë. Resultats dune métaanalyse. Gastroenterol Clin Biol 1991;15:223–28.

61. Reynolds TB, Benhamou JP, Blake J. Treatment of alcoholic hepatitis. Gastroenterol Int 1989;2:208–16.

62. Imperiale TF, McCullough AJ. Do corticosteroids reduce mortality from alcoholic hepatitis. Ann Intern Med 1990;113:299–307.

63. Mathurin P, Mendenhall CL, Carithers RL Jr, Ramond MJ, et al. Corticosteroids improve short term survival in patients with severe alcoholic hepatitis.AH): Individual data analysis of the last three randomized placebo controlled double-blind trials of corticosteroids in severe AH. J Hepat 2002;36:547–8.

64. Mathurin P, Duchatelle V, Ramond MJ, Degott C, et al. Survival and prognostic factors in patients with severe alcoholic hepatitis treated with prednisolone. Gastroenterology 1996;110:1847–55.

65. Schicting D, Juhl E, Poulsen H, Winkel P, and the Copenhagen Study Group for Liver Diseases. Alcoholic hepatitis superimposed on cirrhosis, clinical significance of long term prednisolone treatment. Scan J Gastroenterol 1976;22:305–12.

66. O'Keefe C, McCormick PA. Severe acute alcoholic hepatitis: an audit of medical treatment. Med J 2002;95:108–111.

67. McCullough AJ, O'Connor JFB. Alcoholic liver disease: Proposed recommendations for the American College of Gastroenterology. Am J Gastroenterol 1998;93:2022–36.

68. Jimenez JL, Punzon C, Navarro J, Munoz-Fernandez MA, Fresno M. Phosphodiesterase 4 inhibitors prevent cytokine secretion by T lymphocytes by inhibiting nuclear factor KB and nuclear factor of activated T cells activation. J Pharmacol Exp Ther 2001;299:753–59.

69. Sanchez S, Albornoz L, Bandi JC, Gerona S, Mastai R. Pentoxifylline, a drug with rheological effects, decreases portal pressure in an experimental model of cirrhosis. Eur J Gastroenterol Hepatol 1997;9:27–31.

70. Akriviadis E, Botla R, Briggs W, Han S, Reynolds T, Shakil O. Pentoxifylline improves short-term survival in severe acute alcoholic hepatitis: a double-blind, placebo-controlled trial. Gastroenterology 2000;119:1787–91.

71. Spahr L, Rubbia-Brandt L, Frossard JL, Giostra E, et al. Combination of steroids with infliximab or placebo in severe alcoholic hepatitis: a randomized controlled pilot study. J Hepatol 2002;37:448–55.

72. Tilg H, Jalan R, Kaser A, Davies NA, Offner FA, Hodges SJ, Ludwiczek O, et al. Anti-tumor necrosis factor-alpha monoclonal antibody therapy in severe alcoholic hepatitis. J Hepatol 2003;38:518–20.

73. Naveau S, Chollet-Martin S, Dharancy S, Mathurin P, Jouet P, Piquet MA, et al. Foie-Alcool group of the Association Française pour l'Etude du Foie. A double-blind randomized controlled trial of infliximab associated with prednisolone in acute alcoholic hepatitis. Hepatology 2004;39:1488–90.

74. Poynard T, Thabut D, Chryssostalis A, Taieb J, Ratziu V. Anti-tumor necrosis factor-alpha therapy in severe alcoholic hepatitis: are large randomized trials still possible? J Hepatol 2004;38:419–25.

75. Mookerjee RP, Tilg H, Williams R, Jalan R. Infliximab and alcoholic hepatitis. Hepatology 2004;40:499–500.

76. McClain CJ, Hill DB, Barve SS. Infliximab and prednisolone: Too much of a good thing? Hepatology 2004;39:1488–90.

77. Menon KV, Stadheim L, Kamath PS, Wiesner RH, et al. A pilot study of the safety and tolerability of etanercept in patients with alcoholic hepatitis. Am J Gastroenterol 2004;99:255–60.

78. Akerman PA, Cote PM, Yang SG, McClain C, et al. Long-term ethanol consumption alters the hepatic response to the regenerative effects of tumor necrosis factor alpha. Hepatology 1993;17:1066–73.

79. Mezey E, Potter JJ. A randomized placebo controlled trial of vitamin E for alcoholic hepatitis. J Hepatol 2004:40:40–6.

80. de la Maza MP, Peterman M, Bunout D, Hirsh S. Effects of long-term vitamin supplementation in alcoholic cirrhotics. J Am Coll Nutri 1995;14:192–6.

81. Wenzel G, Kuklinski B, Ruhlmann C, Ehrhardt D. Alcohol-induced toxic hepatitis—a "free radical" associates disease. Lowering facility by adjuvant antioxidant therapy. Z Gesamte In Med 1993;48:490–6.

82. Mato JM, Camara J, Fernandez de Pas J, Caballeria L, Coll S, Caballero A, et al. S-adenosylmethionine in alcoholic liver cirrhosis: A randomized, placebo-controlled, double-blind, multicenter clinical trial. Hepatol 1999;30:1081–9.

83. Rambaldi A, Gluud C. S-Adenosyl-L-methionine for alcoholic liver diseases. Cochrane Database Syst Rev 2004:3

84. Purohit V, Russo D. S-adenosyl-L-methionine in the treatment of alcoholic liver disease: introduction and summary of the symposium. Alcohol 2002;27:151–4.

85. Austin AS, Mahida YR, Clark D, Ryder SD, Freeman JG. A pilot study to investigate the use of oxypentifylline (pentoxifylline) and thalidomide in portal hypertension secondary to alcoholic cirrhosis. Aliment Pharmacol Ther 2004;19:78–82.

86. Yokota T, Oritani K, Takahashi I, Ishikawa J, Maatsuyama A, Ouchi N, et al. Adiponectin, a new member of the family of soluble defense collagens, negatively regulates the growth of myelomonocytic progenitors and the functions of macrophages. Blood 2000;96:1723–32.

87. Li Z, Yang S, Lin H, Huang J, Watkins PA, et al. Probiotics and antibiotics to TNF inhibit inflammatory activity and improve non-alcoholic fatty liver disease. Hepatology 2003;37:347–50.

88. Natori S, Rust C, Stadheim LM, Srinivasan A, Burgart LJ, Gores CJ. Hepatocyte apoptosis is a pathologic feature of human alcoholic hepatitis. J Hepatol 2001;34:330–3.

89. Day CP. Apoptosis in alcoholic hepatitis: A novel therapeutic target? J Hepatol 2001;34:248–53.

90. Mutimer DJ, Burra P, Neuberger JM, Hubscher S, Byuckels JA, et al. Managing severe alcoholic hepatitis complicated by renal failure Q J Med 1993;86:649–56.

91. Jalan R, Sen S, Steiner C, Kapoor D, Alisa A, Williams R. Extracorporeal liver support with molecular adsorbents recirculating system in patients with severe acute alcoholic hepatitis. J Hepatol 2003;38:104–6.

92. Mendenhall CL, Anderson S, Weesner RE, Goldberg SJ, Crolic KA. Protein-calorie malnutrition associated with alcoholic hepatitis. Veterans Administration Cooperative Study Group on Alcoholic Hepatitis. Am J Med 1984;76:211–22.

93. Nompleggi DJ, Bonkovsky HL. Nutritional supplementation in chronic liver disease: an analytical review. Hepatology 1994;19:518–33.

94. Lochs H, Plauth M. Liver cirrhosis: rationale and modalities for nutritional support—the European Society of Parenteral and Enteral Nutrition consensus and beyond. Curr Opin Clin Nutri Metab Care 1999;2:345–9.

95. McCullough AJ, Bugianesi E. Protein-calorie malnutrition and the etiology of cirrhosis. Am J Gastroenterol 1997;92:734–8.

96. Rambaldi A, Gluud C, Rambaldi A. Propylthiouracil for alcoholic liver disease. Cochrane Database Syst Rev 2005;(4):CD002800.

97. Rambaldi A, Gluud. S-adenosyl-L-methionine for alcoholic liver diseases.Cochrane Review Cochrane Database Syst Rev 2001;4:CD002235.

98. Rambaldi A, Gluud C. Colchicine for alcoholic and non-alcoholic liver fibrosis and cirrhosis. Cochrane Database Syst Rev 2005;(2):CD002148.

99. Rambaldi A, Iaguinto G, Gluud C. Anabolic-androgenic steroids for alcoholic liver disease. Cochrane Database Syst Rev 2003;(1):CD003045.

100. Safdar K, Schiff ER. Alcohol and hepatitis C. Semin Liver Dis 2004;24:305–15.

101. Mackie J, Groves K, Hoyle A, et al. Orthotopic liver transplantation for alcoholic liver disease: a retrospective analysis of survival, recidivism, risk factors predisposing to recidivism. Liver Transplant 2001;7:418–27.

102. Burro P, Lucy MR. Liver transplantation in alcoholic patients. Transpl Int 2005;18:491–8.

103. Bellamy CO, DiMartini AM, Ruppert K, et al. Liver transplantation for alcoholic cirrhosis: long term follow-up and impact of disease recurrence. Transplantation 2001;72:619–26.

104. Gish RG, Lee A, Brooks L, et al. Long-term follow-up of patients diagnosed with alcohol dependence or alcohol abuse who were evaluated for liver transplantation. Liver Transpl 2001;7:581–7.

105. Stefanini GF, Biselli M, Grazi GL, et al. Orthotopic liver transplantation for alcoholic liver disease: rates of survival, complications and relapse. Hepatogastroenterology 1997;44:1356–9.

106. Zibari GGB, Edwin D, Wall L, et al. Liver transplantation for alcoholic liver disease. Clin Transplant 1996;10(6 Pt 2):676–9.

107. Howard L, Fahy T. Liver transplantation for alcoholic liver disease. Br J Psychiatry 1997;171:497–500.

108. Lucey MR, Brown KA Everson GT, et al. Minimal criteria for placement of adults on the liver transplant waiting list: a report of a national conference organized by the American Society of Transplant Physicians and the American Association for the Study of Liver Diseases. Liver Transpl Surg 1997;3:628–37.

109. Osorio RW, Ascher NL, Avery M, et al. Predicting recidivism after orthotopic liver transplantation for alcoholic liver disease. Hepatology 1994;20(1 Pt 1):105–10.

110. Pageaux GP, Michel J, Coste V, et al. Alcoholic cirrhosis is a good indication for liver transplantation, even for cases of recidivism. Gut 1999;45:421–6.

111. Goldar-Najafi A, Gordon FD, Lewis WD, et al. Liver transplantation for alcoholic liver disease with or without hepatitis C. Int J Surg Pathol 2002;10:115–22.

112. Jain A, DiMartini A, Kashyap R, et al. Long-term follow-up after liver transplantation for alcoholic liver disease under tacroimus. Transplantation 2000;70:1335–42.

113. Pereira SP, Williams R. Alcohol relapse and functional outcome after liver transplantation for alcoholic liver disease. Liver Transpl 2001;7:204–5.

114. Dhar S. Omran L, Bacon BR, et al. Liver transplantation in patients with chronic hepatitis C and alcoholism. Dig Dis Sci 1999;44:2003–7.

115. Tang H, Boulton R, Gunson B, et al. Patterns of alcohol consumption after liver transplantation. Gut 1998;43:140–5.

116. Fabrega E, Crespo J, Casafont F, et al. Alcoholic recidivism after liver transplantation for alcoholic cirrhosis. J Clin Gastroenterol 1998;26:204–6.

117. Kumar S, Stauber RE, Gavaler JS, et al. Orthotopic liver transplantation for alcoholic liver disease. Hepatology 1990;11:159–64.

118. Bird GL, O'Grady JG, Harvey FA, et al. Liver transplantation in patients with alcoholic cirrhosis: selection criteria and rates of survival and relapse. BMJ 1990;301:15–17.

119. Knechtle SJ, Fleming MF, Barry KL, et al. Liver transplantation for alcoholic liver disease. Surgery 1992;112:694–701.

120. Platz KP, Mueller AR, Spree E, et al. Liver transplantation for alcoholic cirrhosis. Transpl Int 2000:13(Suppl 1):S127–30.

121. Gerhardt TC, Goldstein RM, Urschel HC, et al. Alcohol use following liver transplantation for alcoholic cirrhosis. Transplantation 1996;62:1060–3.

122. Berlakovich GA, Steininger R, Herbst F, et al. Efficacy of liver transplantation for alcoholic cirrhosis with respect to recidivism and compliance. Transplantation 1994;58:560–5.

Genetic Hemochromatosis and Iron Overload

Bruce R. Bacon, MD

BACKGROUND

Hereditary hemochromatosis (HH) is a common inherited disorder of iron metabolism that can lead to excess iron deposition in the liver, heart, pancreas, joints, and skin leading to functional insufficiency and organ damage. Much has been learned about the phenotypic expression of hemochromatosis over the last several years and our knowledge of cellular iron metabolism has advanced considerably since the discovery of *HFE*, the gene mutated in the majority of patients with HH. Also, it has become increasingly apparent that patients with other common liver diseases (chronic viral hepatitis, alcoholic liver disease, nonalcoholic fatty liver disease) frequently are complicated by mild to moderate degrees of secondary iron overload. A high prevalence of patients with the genetic defect for hemochromatosis (either C282Y or H63D mutation) has been found in patients with porphyria cutanea tarda (PCT) consistent with the knowledge for many years that iron reduction has played a role in the treatment of PCT.

In this chapter, I will describe the epidemiology and pathogenesis of hemochromatosis and outline the steps necessary for diagnosis, treatment, and screening for hemochromatosis.

IRON OVERLOAD SYNDROMES

Current classification of iron overload syndromes divides these patients into three groups: (1) those who have inherited causes of iron overload, (2) those who have various causes of secondary iron overload, and (3) a small miscellaneous group. Approximately 85–90% of patients who have inherited forms of iron overload are homozygous for the C282Y mutation in *HFE* or are compound heterozygotes, meaning that one allele has the C282Y mutation and one allele has the H63D mutation.[1] The remaining 10–15% of patients who have inherited forms of iron overload most likely have mutations in other genes involved in iron homeostasis such as hemojuvelin, transferrin receptor 2, hepcidin, and ferroportin. Further, there may be some patients with African iron overload for which the majority

Table 7.1. Classification of Iron Overload Syndromes

- Hereditary hemochromatosis
  - *HFE*-related
    - C282Y/C282Y
    - C282Y/H63D
    - Other *HFE* mutations
  - Non-*HFE*-related
    - Hemojuvelin (HJV)
    - Transferrin receptor-2 (TfR-2)
    - Ferroportin (SLC40A1)
    - Hepcidin (HAMP)
    - African iron overload
- Secondary iron overload
  - Iron-loading anemias
    - Thalassemia major
    - Sideroblastic
    - Chronic hemolytic anemia
    - Aplastic anemia
    - Pyruvate kinase deficiency
    - Pyridoxine-responsive anemia
  - Parenteral iron overload
    - Red blood cell transfusions
    - Iron-dextran injections
    - Long-term hemodialysis
  - Chronic liver disease
    - Porphyria cutanea tarda
    - Hepatitis C
    - Hepatitis B
    - Alcoholic liver disease
    - Nonalcoholic steatohepatitis
    - Following portocaval shunt
  - Dysmetabolic iron overload syndrome
- Miscellaneous
  - Neonatal iron overload
  - Aceruloplasminemia
  - Congenital atransferrinemia

seem to have mutations in ferroportin. Other causes of secondary iron overload are divided between those causes related to iron loading anemias, those related to chronic liver disease, transfusional iron overload, and miscellaneous causes. These are outlined in Table 7.1.

HFE-related HH is the most common cause of inherited iron overload and affects approximately 1 in 200 to 250 individuals of northern European descent.[2] With the advent of genetic testing in the late 1990s, *HFE*-linked HH is frequently identified in asymptomatic probands and in presymptomatic relatives of patients who are known to have the disease.[3] Accordingly, a genetic diagnosis can be legitimately applied to individuals who have not yet developed any phenotypic expression. These individuals have a "genetic susceptibility" to developing iron overload but may never do so, for reasons that are still to be determined. Recent population studies have shown that approximately 40% of individuals who are homozygous for the C282Y mutation do not have increased levels of ferritin, meaning that they do not have evidence of increased iron stores.[2,4–7] This observation and recognition has changed the way we think about hemochromatosis. Twenty years ago, it was felt that all individuals who were genetically susceptible would have evidence of phenotypic expression. Now we know that phenotypic expression only occurs in about half of C282Y homozygotes, and fewer than 10% of C282Y homozygotes will develop severe iron overload accompanied by organ damage and all of the clinical manifestations of hemochromatosis. These observations have led to a definition of different stages of the recognition of hemochromatosis that were identified at a consensus conference of the European Association for the Study of Liver Diseases several years ago.[8] These are defined as follows:

- Stage 1 refers to those patients with the genetic disorder with no increase in iron stores who have "genetic susceptibility."
- Stage 2 refers to those patients with the genetic disorder who have phenotypic evidence of iron overload but who are without tissue or organ damage.
- Stage 3 refers to those individuals who have the genetic disorder and have iron overload and have iron deposition to the degree that tissue and organ damage occurs.

This recognition is important to allow clinicians to categorize patients who have positive genetic test results.

GENETICS OF *HFE*-LINKED HEMOCHROMATOSIS

HFE encodes for a major histocompatibility complex (MHC) class I-like molecule that requires interaction with β_2-microglobulin (β_2m) for normal presentation to the extracellular surface of cells.[3] The protein has a signal peptide binding domain, an immunoglobulin-like domain, a single transmembrane region, and a short cytoplasmic tail. Several missense mutations have been identified in *HFE*. Clearly, the most important mutation results in a change of cysteine to tyrosine at amino acid position 282 (cys 282 → tyr, C282Y). This single mutation is responsible for the majority of patients with iron overload. The second results in a change of histidine to aspartate at amino acid position 63 (his 63 → asp, H63D), and the third results in a change of serine to cysteine at amino acid position 65 (ser 65 → cys, S65C). In 1996, in the original study by Feder et al., 83% (148 of 178) of patients who had typical phenotypic hemochromatosis were found to be C282Y homozygotes.[3] An additional 4% of patients were found to be compound heterozygotes, wherein they had one allele with the C282Y mutation and one with the H63D mutation. Numerous additional studies have confirmed these results and on average about 85–90% of patients with typical phenotypic hemochromatosis are found to be C282Y homozygotes. These studies are summarized in Table 7.2. For those 10–15% of patients who have typical hemochromatosis but who are C282Y negative, it is expected that they may have mutations in ferroportin, transferrin receptor 2, hepcidin, or hemojuvelin, but at the present time, we do not have commercially available genetic testing for any of these mutations.

In prospective population studies, C282Y homozygosity is found in about 1 in 250 individuals or 0.4% of the population (see Table 7.3). The compound

Table 7.2. HFE Genotype in Patients with Typical Phenotypic HH

Study	Feder et al.[3]	Beutler et al.[4]	Jouanolle et al.[28]	Jazwinksa et al.[29]	Carella et al.[30]	Adams and Chakrabarti[31]	Bacon et al.[32]
Country	USA	USA	France	Australia	Italy	Canada	USA
No. of Patients	178	147	65	112*	75	128	66
Genotype *n*(%)							
C282Y C282Y	148 (83)	121 (82)	59 (91)	112 (100)	48 (64)	122 (95)	60 (91)
C282Y** H63D	8 (4)	8 (5)	3 (5)	0	2 (2.27)	2 (1.6)	1 (1.5)
C282Y Wild type	1 (0.5)	2 (1)	0	0	2 (2.27)	2 (1.6)	1 (1.5)
H63D H63D	1 (0.5)	2 (1)	1 (1.5)	0	1 (1.3)	0	0
H63D Wild type	7 (4)	4 (3)	2 (3)	0	3 (4)	0	2 (3)
Wild type Wild type	13 (7)	10 (7)	0	0	16 (21)	4 (3.1)	1 (1.5)

*All patients had a family history of iron overload.
**Compound heterozygote.

Table 7.3. Screening for HH in the General Population

Population Sample	Country	*n*	Prevalence of Homozygotes	C282Y Homozygotes with Normal Ferritin (%)
Electoral roll	New Zealand	1,064	1 in 213	40
Primary care	USA	1,653	1 in 276	50
Epidemiological survey	Australia	3,011	1 in 188	25
Blood donors	Canada	4,211	1 in 327	81
General public	USA	41,038	1 in 270	33
Primary care	North America	44,082	1 in 227	25
Total		**95,059**	**1 in 250**	**42**

heterozygote genotype is found in about 1% to 2% of the population, and of these patients, only a small percentage (<5%) develop any significant degree of iron overload.

PATHOPHYSIOLOGIC MECHANISMS IN *HFE*-RELATED HH

The first link between HFE protein and cellular iron metabolism resulted from the observation that HFE protein along with β_2m forms a complex with transferrin receptor (TfR-1).[9] This physical association was observed in cultured cells and in duodenal crypt enterocytes which is considered the site of regulation of dietary iron absorption. The observation that HFE protein and TfR-1 were physically associated led to a number of investigations on the effect of HFE protein on TfR-1-mediated iron uptake and cellular iron stores. This so-called "crypt hypothesis" is now thought to be less important since hepcidin has been discovered.[10,11] Hepcidin is a 25 amino acid peptide that influences systemic iron status. Hepcidin is considered to be the principal iron regulatory hormone. Alterations in the regulation of hepcidin expression are thought to play a role in the pathogenesis of hemochromatosis. Accordingly, patients with *HFE*-linked HH have reduced hepatic expression of hepcidin, as do *HFE* knockout mice, despite excess hepatic iron stores. Conversely, over-expression of hepcidin in *HFE* knockout mice prevents the hemochromatosis phenotype. The molecular mechanisms by which hepcidin expression is regulated by body iron status have not been fully determined. However, it has been hypothesized that TfR-2 in hepatocytes may act as an iron sensor. Also, hemojuvelin appears to be involved within the liver and is necessary for hepcidin expression. Mutations in TFR-2 and in hemojuvelin cause rare forms of hemochromatosis in humans and TfR-2 mutant mice have a hemochromatosis phenotype.[12] It is expected that over the next several years an understanding of how hepcidin is regulated in the hepatocyte will become apparent, elucidating this pathophysiological mechanism in the regulation of iron uptake, both in the normal situation and in hemochromatosis. It is still not clear how mutated HFE impacts hepatocellular hepcidin production.

CLINICAL PRESENTATION

Hemochromatosis is increasingly being recognized by astute clinicians, yet it is still underdiagnosed, mainly because it is thought to be a rare disorder that can only be manifested by the clinical findings seen in fully established disease, wherein there is increased skin pigmentation, diabetes, and cirrhosis. Genetic susceptibility (C282Y homozygosity) for hemochromatosis is seen in about 1 in 250 individuals, however, fully expressed disease with end organ manifestations is seen in fewer than 10% of these individuals. This explains the discrepancy between how common the disease is felt to be (1 in 250) versus how commonly we see end-stage disease (1 in 2,500). The heterozygote (C282Y/wt) frequency is found in approximately 1 in 10 individuals, demonstrating how common this inherited abnormality is in Caucasian populations.

Clinical manifestations from patients reported in series from the 1950s up to the 1980s demonstrates that most patients had classic symptoms and findings of advanced hemochromatosis[13] (see Table 7.4). By the 1990s, HH was increasingly being identified by evaluating patients who had abnormal iron studies on routine chemistry panels or by patients having been identified by family screening.[14,15] When HH patients were identified in this way, approximately 75% of them were without symptoms and did not exhibit any of the end-stage manifestations of the disease.[15] Currently, in large population screening studies, only about 60% of C282Y homozygotes are found to have an elevated ferritin level and, as mentioned previously, only a small percentage of these people have clinical consequences of iron storage disease.[2,4] Nonetheless, it is still important for clinicians to be aware of the symptoms that patients may exhibit and the physical findings with which they can present.

Table 7.4. Clinical Features of HH by Series by Year

Features	Milder et al. 1980[13]	Edwards et al. 1980[33]	Niederau et al. 1985[34]	Adams et al. 1991 [35]
Number of subjects	34[†]	35*	163*	37[‡]
Symptoms (#)				
Weakness, lethargy	73	20	83	19
Abdominal pain	50	23	58	3
Arthralgias	47	57	43	40
Loss of libido, impotence	56	29	38	32
Cardiac failure symptoms	35	0	15	3
Physical and Diagnostic Finding (%)				
Cirrhosis (biopsy)	94	57	69	3
Hepatomegaly	76	54	83	3
Splenomegaly	38	40	13	–
Loss of body hair	32	6	20	–
Gynecomastia	12	–	8	–
Testicular atrophy	50	14	–	–
Skin pigmentation	82	43	75	9
Clinical diabetes	53	6	55	11

* Patient selection occurred by both clinical features and family screening.
† Only symptomatic index cases were studied.
‡ Discovered by family studies.

Table 7.5. Symptoms in Patients with Hereditary Hemochromatosis

Asymptomatic
- Abnormal serum iron studies on routine screening chemistry panel
- Evaluation of abnormal liver tests
- Identified by family screening

Non-specific, systemic symptoms
- Weakness
- Fatigue
- Lethargy
- Apathy
- Weight loss

Specific, organ-related symptoms
- Abdominal pain (hepatomegaly)
- Arthralgias (arthritis)
- Diabetes (pancreas)
- Amenorrhea (cirrhosis)
- Loss of libido, impotence (pituitary, cirrhosis)
- Congestive heart failure (heart)
- Arrhythmias (heart)

When patients present with symptoms, consideration of hemochromatosis should be given when there are complaints of fatigue, right-upper quadrant abdominal pain, arthralgias-or, typically of the second and third MCP joints, impotence, decreased libido and symptoms of heart failure or diabetes (Table 7.5). Similarly, physical findings of an enlarged liver, particularly in the

> **Table 7.6. Physical Findings in Patients with Hereditary Hemochromatosis**
>
> **Asymptomatic**
> - No physical findings
> - Hepatomegaly
>
> **Symptomatic**
> - Liver
>   - Hepatomegaly
>   - Cutaneous stigmata of chronic liver disease
>   - Splenomegaly
>   - Liver failure: ascites, encephalopathy, etc.
> - Joints
>   - Arthritis
>   - Joint swelling
> - Heart
>   - Dilated cardiomyopathy
>   - Congestive heart failure
> - Skin
>   - Increased pigmentation
> - Endocrine
>   - Testicular atrophy
>   - Hypogonadism
>   - Hypothyroidism

presence of cirrhosis, extrahepatic manifestations of chronic liver disease, testicular atrophy, signs of congestive heart failure, skin pigmentation or arthritis, should raise the suspicion of hemochromatosis (Table 7.6). Many of these signs and symptoms are certainly indicative of disease processes other than hemochromatosis, but the thoughtful clinician will make sure that hemochromatosis is investigated when seeing patients who exhibit these symptoms. Currently, most new patients with HH come to medical attention because of screening, either by family studies or by astute and conscientious primary care physicians. Finally, in older series of patients with HH, when patients were identified by symptoms or physical findings of the disease, women typically presented about 10 years later than men and there were about 10 times the number of men presenting as women. This is presumably because of the effects of menstrual blood loss and iron loss during pregnancy, having a "protective" effect for women. More recently, with a greater proportion of patients identified by population screening studies or by family screening studies, the age of diagnosis for women is about the same as that for men, and the number of men identified was roughly equivalent to the number of women found. Clinicians should not wait for symptoms when they see abnormal iron studies and should be definitive in evaluating patients for hemochromatosis.

DIAGNOSIS

Once the diagnosis is considered, either in the context of family studies or abnormal screening iron studies or if the patient is found to have an abnormal genetic test or has any of the above-mentioned symptoms or findings, then definitive diagnosis is relatively easy. Once HH is considered, fasting transferrin saturation (serum iron divided by total iron binding capacity (TIBC) or transferrin × 100%) and ferritin levels should be obtained. Both of these will be elevated in symptomatic patients. It has been stated for years that transferrin saturation should be measured in the morning as a fasting sample, but recent studies from the HEIRS trial have shown less importance of this recommendation.[16] The sensitivity and specificity of both transferrin saturation and ferritin become problematic when young individuals are being evaluated or when patients have abnormal iron studies in the context of other liver diseases, specifically chronic viral hepatitis, NASH, or alcoholic liver disease. Additionally, it is known that ferritin is an acute phase reactant and other inflammatory disorders, such as arthritis or some cancers, can cause elevated serum ferritin levels in the absence of iron overload. Thus, there are many false-positive and false-negative results when serum iron studies are obtained, and these determinations must be put in context. The development of a widely available genetic test (*HFE* mutation analysis) has contributed to a much better characterization of those patients with underlying liver disease and abnormal serum iron studies. Regardless, in the absence of any other medical illness, the combination of an elevated transferrin saturation level and an elevated ferritin level is highly sensitive and specific for a diagnosis of hemochromatosis.

Currently, if either a fasting transferrin saturation or ferritin level is elevated, *HFE* mutation analysis should be performed. If the patient is a C282Y homozygote or a compound heterozygote with normal liver enzymes and abnormal iron studies, then *HFE*-linked HH is the diagnosis, and phlebotomy therapy can be initiated. If the liver enzymes (ALT or AST) are elevated or if the ferritin is >1000 ng/ml, then patients should be considered for liver biopsy.[17] This is recommended to identify patients with advanced fibrosis so as to screen them appropriately if they have cirrhosis. When liver biopsy is performed, the Perls' Prussian blue stain should be utilized, and it is reasonable to determine the hepatic iron concentration (HIC). Liver biopsy will provide an assessment of the degree of fibrosis and whether or not cirrhosis is present and if there are any other histologic abnormalities, such as steatosis.[18] From a prognostic standpoint, it is important to determine if there is advanced fibrosis or cirrhosis because the risk of hepatocellular cancer is significantly increased in those patients who have cirrhosis.

When iron stains are done on liver biopsies, iron deposition is found in higher levels in periportal (zone 1) hepatocytes, and there is a periportal to pericentral (zone 3) gradient.[18] At higher power, iron is seen predominantly in parenchymal cells with very little in Kupffer cells (reticuloendothelial cells). When patients progress to advanced liver disease, the cirrhosis is characteristically micronodular. In symptomatic patients, the hepatic iron concentration is typically above 10,000 mcg/g dry weight (normal <1500 mcg/g, dry weight), and values as high as 40,000 mcg/g can be seen, although this is uncommon. In patients with secondary iron overload related to alcoholic liver disease, chronic viral hepatitis or fatty liver disease, the hepatic iron concentration is rarely as high as 10,000 mcg/g and is more commonly in the 2,000–3,000 mcg/g range. Genetic testing is now very helpful in determining whether these patients have HH along with a second liver disease or a liver disease with secondary iron overload (Table 7.7).

Table 7.7. Laboratory Findings in Patients with Hereditary Hemochromatosis

Measurements	Normal Subjects	Patients with Hereditary Hemochromatosis	
		Asymptomatic	Symptomatic
Blood (fasting)			
Serum iron level (μg/dL)	60–80	150–280	180–300
Serum transferrin level (mg/dL)	220–410	200–280	200–300
Transferrin saturation (%)	20–50	45–100	80–6000
Serum ferritin level (ng/mL)			
Men	20–200	150–1000	500–6000
Women	15–150	120–1000	500–6000
Genetic (*HFE* mutation analysis)			
C282Y/C282Y	wt/wt	C282Y/C282Y	C282Y/C282Y
C282Y/H63D*	wt/wt	C282Y/H63D	C282Y/H63D
Liver			
Hepatic iron concentration			
μg/g, dry weight	300–1500	2000–10,000	8000–30,000
μmol/g, dry weight	5–27	36–179	140–550
Hepatic iron index**	<1.0	>1.9	>1.9
Liver histology			
Perls' Prussian blue stain	0–1+	2+ to 4+	3+, 4+

* Compound heterozygote
** Hepatic iron index (HII) is calculated by dividing the hepatic iron concentration (in μmol/g, dry weight) by the age of the patient (in years). With increased knowledge of genetic testing results in patients with iron overload, the utility of HII has diminished.

MANAGEMENT

Once the diagnosis of HH is established, physicians are responsible for adequate treatment of the proband, and for recommending family screening. Treatment is simple, effective, inexpensive and safe. Patients should initially have weekly therapeutic phlebotomy of 500 ml of whole blood, which is equivalent to approximately 200–250 mg of iron, depending on the hemoglobin concentration of the blood. Some patients can tolerate twice weekly phlebotomy and some can only tolerate one-half unit removed every other week. Therapeutic phlebotomy should be performed until patients develop iron-limited erythropoiesis, which is identified by the failure of the hematocrit/hemoglobin to recover before the next phlebotomy. It is reasonable to routinely monitor transferrin saturation and ferritin levels every three months to provide some prediction of the return to normal iron stores and to provide a method of encouraging patients who are undergoing phlebotomy. Therapeutic phlebotomy is continued until the transferrin saturation is <50% and the serum ferritin is <50 ng/ml. It is not necessary for patients to become iron deficient and/or anemic. Rather, the desired endpoint is for these patients to be depleted of their excess iron stores. Therapeutic phlebotomy is tolerated well by most patients, and some individuals actually have a sense of improved well-being after the initial phlebotomies have been

---

Table 7.8. Response to Phlebotomy Treatment in Patients with HH

- Reduction to normal tissue iron stores.
- Improved survival if diagnosis and treatment before development of cirrhosis and diabetes.
- Improved sense of well-being, energy level.
- Improved cardiac function.
- Improved control of diabetes.
- Reduction in abdominal pain.
- Reduction in skin pigmentation.
- Normalization of elevated liver enzymes.
- Reversal of hepatic fibrosis (approximately 30% of cases).
- No reversal of established cirrhosis.
- Reduction in portal hypertension in cirrhotics.
- No (or minimal) improvement in arthropathy.
- No reversal of testicular atrophy.

---

completed. Abnormal liver enzymes will become normal once iron stores have been depleted, however, established cirrhosis will not reverse. Recent studies have shown that increased fibrosis (other than advanced cirrhosis) will reverse with phlebotomy therapy.[19] Further, parameters of portal hypertension improve with phlebotomy. Other benefits of phlebotomy include reduction in skin pigmentation, improvement in cardiac function, reduction in insulin requirements for those patients who are diabetic, loss of abdominal pain, and an improved energy level. Conditions that characteristically do not improve with phlebotomy include testicular atrophy, established cirrhosis and the arthropathy of hemochromatosis (Table 7.8). It must be recognized that the risk of hepatocellular carcinoma does not decrease with phlebotomy if the patient already has cirrhosis.

Once the initial therapeutic phlebotomy has been successfully completed and patients no longer have increased iron stores, then patients should be considered for maintenance phlebotomy. Not all patients require maintenance phlebotomy. In those who show evidence of reaccumulation of iron (increasing ferritin levels over time), then maintenance phlebotomy is usually done every 2–3 months. Because most patients with HH absorb approximately 2–3 mg of iron per day in excess of their daily requirements, they will accumulate an excess of approximately 250 mg or iron over a three-month (90 day) period. This is then balanced by the 250 mg of iron that is removed from a single phlebotomy with these individuals remaining in normal iron balance. Some patients absorb more than 2–3 mg per day and thus require maintenance phlebotomy more often.

SCREENING FOR HH

Family Screening, Population Screening

All first-degree relatives of an identified proband should be screened for hemochromatosis, including siblings, parents, and children. These recommendations could be extended to include aunts, uncles, and cousins, as well. Genetic testing with *HFE* mutation analysis along with transferrin saturation and ferritin is usually recommended. If there is an elevated ferritin level in a C282Y homozygote or a compound heterozygote, then it is reasonable to proceed with therapeutic phlebotomy as long as liver enzymes are normal and ferritin levels are not >1000 ng/ml. If patients have submitted to a prospective population screening survey outside the context of a family history and are identified as being C282Y homozygotes, then iron studies should be performed and patients should be treated accordingly. Currently, population screening on a wide-scale basis is not being recommended because so few people have fully established disease or evidence of significant degrees of iron overload. Unfortunately, genetic discrimination can occur in individuals with a genetic diagnosis, even though they may have no phenotypic expression.[20]

IRON AND OTHER LIVER DISEASES

Many patients with liver disease have abnormalities in serum markers of iron metabolism. These abnormalities are more commonly seen in patients with hepatocellular liver diseases than in those with cholestatic liver diseases. Several clinical studies have shown that approximately 50% of patients with alcoholic liver disease,[21] chronic viral hepatitis C,[22] and fatty liver disease[23] have abnormalities in serum iron studies. Generally, this is an elevation in serum ferritin, but occasionally, an elevated transferrin saturation can be seen as well. When liver biopsy is performed, increased iron deposits can be seen usually in a pan-lobular distribution (rather than a periportal distribution) with iron in both hepatocytes and sinusoidal lining cells (Kupffer cells), rather than in hepatocytes predominantly.[18] Hepatic iron concentrations may be slightly increased or normal.

When *HFE* mutations have been evaluated in patients with alcoholic liver disease (ALD), there has been no increased incidence of either C282Y or H63D over that of control populations.[24] Furthermore, there is no increase in *HFE* mutations in patients with alcoholic liver disease who had an increased amount of fibrosis. Thus, the abnormal iron studies frequently seen in patients with ALD are most likely due to mechanisms other than mutations in *HFE*.

In chronic hepatitis C, the relationship of abnormal iron studies and elevated hepatic iron concentrations with treatment response to interferon monotherapy has been known for several years.[25] Several studies have shown that patients who failed to respond to interferon monotherapy had a higher hepatic iron concentration than in those who responded. The follow-up to this observation involved therapeutic phlebotomy to deplete iron stores in an effort to enhance their response to therapy. Reduced iron stores by therapeutic phlebotomy did result in improved liver enzymes and had some marginal benefit on histology, but there was no effect on HCV RNA levels. When similar studies were done in hepatitis C patients treated with interferon and ribavirin or PEG-interferon and ribavirin, there was no relationship between hepatic iron concentration and response to therapy.

When *HFE* mutation analysis has been investigated in patients with chronic hepatitis C, the frequency of C282Y and H63D mutations has been equivalent to that of control populations (as seen in alcoholic liver disease). However, most studies have shown that, when *HFE* mutations are present, they do in fact correlate with increased iron stores seen histologically, and some studies have shown a synergistic effect with the development of increased hepatic fibrosis when increased iron levels were present.[25] Currently, it is recommended that *HFE* mutation analysis be done when abnormal iron studies are seen in patients with chronic hepatitis C. Iron stains are performed on liver biopsy samples when biopsies are done for grading and staging, and if iron stores are increased, it is reasonable to perform therapeutic phlebotomy to deplete excess iron prior to initiating antiviral treatment.

In patients with NAFLD, several studies have provided conflicting results with some showing an increase in *HFE* mutations in patients with NASH, whereas others show no difference from control populations.[26] When there has been an increased prevalence of *HFE* mutations in NASH, there has been good correlation between abnormal iron studies and hepatic iron concentrations. Furthermore, some studies have shown an increase in fibrosis in NASH patients with *HFE* mutations and increased iron stores. These observations have not been confirmed by others, and more investigation in this area is necessary. Finally, in one study, iron depletion in fatty liver disease did lead to improved liver enzymes and reduced insulin resistance.

In porphyria cutanea tarda (PCT), the relationship between abnormalities in iron metabolism and the role of therapeutic phlebotomy in the treatment of this disorder has been known for many years.[27] Also, it has been shown that as many as 70% of patients with PCT are infected with hepatitis C and many patients with PCT drink excessive amounts of alcohol. Also, an increased prevalence of *HFE* mutations has been shown in both European and American studies of PCT patients, and the use of phlebotomy to deplete excess iron stores is still recommended. Therefore, when seeing someone with PCT, hepatitis C testing should be performed and *HFE* mutation analysis, as well as iron studies, should be done.

SUMMARY

In summary, the discovery of *HFE* has led to an enhanced ability for clinicians to accurately diagnose patients with HH. Liver biopsy is much less important currently in the evaluation of patients with hemochromatosis, and great reliance is placed on *HFE* mutation analysis. In patients with elevated liver enzymes (ALT or AST) or a very high ferritin level (>1000 ng/ml), liver biopsy should be performed. At some point, it is expected that genetic testing will be commercially available for mutations in ferroportin, transferrin receptor-2, hepcidin, hemojuvelin, and still other genes not yet identified in iron metabolism. Treatment of HH remains straightforward, inexpensive, effective, and simple. Interactions between iron and hepatitis C and NAFLD are still being clarified, and the pathophysiological mechanisms that occur in HH are increasingly being understood. At some time in the future, it will be possible to apply this information to liver diseases complicated by secondary iron overload.

REFERENCES

1.   Harrison SA, Bacon BR. Hereditary hemochromatosis: Update for 2003. Journal of Hepatology 2003;38:S14–S23.

2. Adams PC, Reboussin DM, Barton JC, McLaren CE, Eckfeldt JH, McLaren GD, Dawkins FW, Acton RT, Harris EL, Gordeuk VR, Leiendecker-Foster C, Speechley M, Snively BM, Holup JL, Thomson E, Sholinsky P. Hemochromatosis and Iron Overload Screening (HEIRS) Study Research Investigators. Hemochromatosis and iron-overload screening in a racially diverse population. New England Journal of Medicine 2005;352:1769–78.

3. Feder JN, Gnirke A, Thomas W, Tsuchihashi Z, Ruddy DA, Basava A, Dormishian F, Domingo Jr R, Ellis MC, Fullan A, Hinton LM, Jones NL, Kimmel BE, Kronmal GS, Lauer P, Lee VK, Loeb DB, Mapa FA, McClelland E, Meyer MC, Mintier GA, Moeller N, Moore T, Morikang E, Prass CE, Quintana L, Starnes SM, Schatzman RC, Brunke KJ, Drayna DT, Risch NJ, Bacon BR, Wolff RK. A novel MHC class I-like gene is mutated in patients with hereditary haemochromatosis. Nature Genetics 1996;13:399–408.

4. Beutler E, Felitti VJ, Koziol JA, Ho NJ, Gelbart T. Penetrance of 845G-A (C282Y) HFE hereditary haemochromatosis mutation in the USA, Lancet 2002;359:211–18.

5. Merryweather-Clarke AT, Pointon JJ, Sherman JD, Robson KJ. Global prevalence of putative haemochromatosis mutations. Journal of Medical Genetics 1997;34:275–8.

6. Olynyk JK, Cullen DJ, Aquilia S, Rossi E, Summerville L, Powell LW. A population-based study of the clinical expression of the hemochromatosis gene. New England Journal of Medicine 1999;341:718–24.

7. Ombiga J, Adams LA, Tang K, Trinder D, Olynyk JK. Screening for HFE and iron overload. Seminars in Liver Disease 2005;25:402–10.

8. Adams P, Brissot P, Powell LW. EASL International Consensus Conference on Haemochromatosis. Journal of Hepatology 2000;33:485–504.

9. Waheed A, Parkkila S, Saarnio J, Fleming RE, Zhou XY, Tomatsu S, Britton RS, Bacon BR, Sly WS. Association of HFE protein with transferrin receptor in cryptal enterocytes of human duodenum. Proceedings of the National Academy of Sciences, USA 1999;96:1579–84.

10. Fleming RE, Britton RS, Waheed A, Sly WS, Bacon BR. Pathogenesis of hereditary hemochromatosis. Clinics in Liver Disease 2004;8:755–73.

11. Fleming RE, Bacon BR. Orchestration of iron homeostasis. New England Journal of Medicine 2005;352:1741–1744.

12. Fleming RE, Migas MC, Holden CC, Waheed A, Britton RS, Tomatsu S, Bacon BR, Sly WS. Transferrin receptor 2: Continued expression in mouse liver in the face of iron overload and in hereditary hemochromatosis. Proceedings of the National Academy of Sciences, USA 2000;97:2214–9.

13. Milder MS, Cook JD, Stray S, Finch CA. Idiopathic hemochromatosis, an interim report. Medicine (Baltimore) 1980;59:34–49.

14. Adams PC, Deugnier Y, Moirand R, Brissot P. The relationship between iron overload, clinical symptoms, and age in 410 patients with genetic hemochromatosis. Hepatology 1997;25:162–6.

15. Bacon BR, Sadiq SA. Hereditary hemochromatosis: Presentation and diagnosis in the 1990s. American Journal of Gastroenterology 1997;92:784–9.

16. Adams PC, Reboussin DM, Press RD, Barton JC, Acton RT, Moses GC, Leiendecker-Foster C, McLaren GD, Dawkins FW, Gordeuk VR, Lovato L, Eckfeldt JH. Biological variability of transferrin saturation and unsaturated iron-binding capacity. American Journal of Medicine 2007;20:999.e1–7.

17. Bacon BR, Olynyk JK, Brunt EM, Britton RS, Wolff RK. HFE genotype in patients with hemochromatosis and other liver diseases. Annals of Internal Medicine 1999;130:953–62.

18. Brunt EM. Pathology of hepatic iron overload. Seminars in Liver Disease 2005;25:392–401.

19. Powell LW, Dixon JL, Ramm GA, Purdie DM, Lincoln DJ, Anderson GJ, Subramaniam VN, Hewett DG, Searle JW, Fletcher LM, Crawford DH, Rodgers H, Allen KJ, Cavanaugh JA, Bassett ML. Screening for hemochromatosis in asymptomatic subjects with or without a family history. Archives of Internal Medicine 2006;166:294–301.

20. Shaheen NJ, Lawrence LB, Bacon BR, Barton JC, Barton NH, Galanko J, Martin CF, Burnett CK, Sandler RS. Insurance, employment, and psychosocial consequences of a diagnosis of hereditary hemochromatosis in subjects without end organ damage. American Journal of Gastroenterology 2003;98:1175–80.

21. Fletcher LM, Dixon JL, Purdie DM, Powell LW, Crawford DH. Excess alcohol greatly increases the prevalence of cirrhosis in hereditary hemochromatosis. Gastroenterology 2002;122:281–9.

22. Di Bisceglie AM, Axiotis CA, Hoofnagle JH, Bacon BR. Measurement of iron status in patients with chronic hepatitis. Gastroenterology 1992;102:2108–13.

23. Bacon BR, Farahvash MJ, Janney CG, Neuschwander-Tetri BA. Nonalcoholic steato-hepatitis: An expanded clinical entity. Gastroenterology 1994;107:1103–9.

24. Chapman RW, Morgan MY, Laulicht M, Hoffbrand AV, Sherlock S. Hepatic iron stores and markers of iron overload in alcoholics and patients with idiopathic hemochro-matosis. Digestive Disease and Sciences 1982;27:909–16.

25. Olynyk JK, Bacon BR. Hepatitis C and iron. In: Liang TJ, Hoofnagle JH, eds. Hepatitis C. New York: Academic Press; 2000:415–26.

26. Neuschwander-Tetri BA, Bacon BR. Nonalcoholic steatohepatitis. Medical Clinics of North America, 1996;80:1147–66.

27. Alla V, Bonkovsky HL. Iron in nonhemochromatotic liver disorders. Seminars in Liver Disease 2005;25:461–72.

28. Jouanolle AM, Gandon G, Jézéquel P, Blayau M, Campion ML, Yaouanq J, Mosser J, Fergelot P, Chauvel B, Bouric P, Carn G, Andrieux N, Gicquel I, Le Gall JY, David V. Haemochromatosis and HLA-H. Nat Genet 1996;14:251–2.

29. Jazwinska EC, Cullen LM, Busfield F, Pyper WR, Webb SI, Powell LW, Morris CP, Walsh TP. Haemochromatosis and HLA-H. Nat Genet 1996;14:249–51.

30. Carella M, D'Ambrosio L, Totaro A, Grifa A, Valentino MA, Piperno A, Girelli D, Roetto A, Franco B, Gasparini P, Camaschella C. Mutation analysis of the HLA-H gene in Italian hemochromatosis patients. Am J Hum Genet 1997;60:828–32.

31. Adams PC, Chakrabarti S. Genotypic/phenotypic correlations in genetic hemochro-matosis: evolution of diagnostic criteria. Gastroenterology 1998;114:319–23.

32. Bacon BR, Britton RS. Hemochromatosis and other iron storage disorders. In: Schiff ER, Sorrell MF, Maddrey WC, eds. Diseases of the Liver. 10th edition. Baltimore: Lippincott, Williams, & Wilkins, 2007;1041–61.

33. Edwards CQ, Cartwright GE, Skolnick MH, Amos DB. Homozygosity for hemochro-matosis: clinical manifestations. Ann Intern Med 1980;93:519–25.

34. Niederau C, Fischer R, Sonnenberg A, Stremmel W, Trampisch HJ, Strohmeyer G. Survival and causes of death in cirrhotic and noncirrhotic patients with primary hemochromatosis. N Engl J Med 1985;313:1256–62.

35. Adams PC, Kertesz AE, Valberg LS. Clinical presentation of hemochromatosis: a chang-ing scene. Am J Med 1991;90:445–9.

8

Wilson's Disease

Jamile Wakim-Fleming, MD, FACG, and
Kevin D. Mullen, MD, FRCPI

BACKGROUND

Wilson's disease or hepatolenticular degeneration, is an autosomal-recessive disorder in which the primary biochemical abnormality resides in the liver, leading to the accumulation of copper in various tissues notably the hepatocytes and the basal ganglia. Its clinical presentation ranges from asymptomatic abnormal elevations of liver enzymes to fulminant liver failure, psychological and neurological disturbances. Although the disorder is uncommon occurring in 1/30,000 individuals, early diagnosis is important because effective therapy with chelating agents is available to prevent permanent liver and brain damage. Liver transplantation corrects the primary biochemical abnormality, thus curing the liver disease and is lifesaving in fulminant hepatic failure. Although it could improve the neurological manifestations, liver transplantation has not shown to reverse advanced brain damage.

PATHOPHYSIOLOGY

Copper is an essential trace element involved in key enzyme activities. However, the excess of copper is toxic and postulated to cause free oxygen radical formation, mitochondrial damage, lipid peroxidation, and triglyceride accumulation in the cells.

In the normal state, copper is absorbed in the duodenum and jejunum and transported in the portal circulation to the liver. In the Golgi apparatus of the liver, copper binds to various proteins or metallothioneins such as apoceruloplasmin to form ceruloplasmin the major copper binding protein synthesized in the liver. The synthesis of ceruloplasmin and the excretion of copper in bile, its main route of elimination, are essential in maintaining copper homeostasis. Any disruption along this pathway would result in copper accumulation and disease.[1,2]

Wilson's disease stems form mutations in the Wilson's disease gene ATP7B located on chromosome 13. This gene encodes for an ATPase, a protein situated in the Golgi apparatus of the hepatocyte and is involved in the incorporation of copper into apoceruloplasmin during the synthesis of ceruloplasmin. Mutations in the ATP7B gene results in decreased biliary excretion of copper, reduced circulating serum level of ceruloplasmin and increased hepatic copper. As toxic copper accumulates in the liver, the level of circulating non-ceruloplasmin bound copper increases and copper deposits in other organs of the body such as the brain, kidneys, and eyes, and its excretion in the urine increases.[1,3]

More that 200 distinct mutations have been described in the Wilson's gene. Such mutations manifest in various phenotypic expressions that can be severe resulting in disease early in childhood or less severe resulting in disease in adulthood. Homozygote patients inherit disease-specific mutation of both alleles of the ATP7B gene and present with severe disease. In such cases measurements of hepatic copper is not necessary. Most patients are compound heterozygotes for the ATP7B gene mutation meaning that they have two different ATP7B mutations. One mutation in one single allele does not lead to disease.[2]

Even though low ceruloplasmin levels are a distinct feature of this disease this protein is not directly involved in biliary copper excretion. Patients with hereditary absence of ceruloplasmin have normal hepatic copper excretion.[4] The hepatic Wilson's ATPase seems to be the most important ATPase even though this protein is expressed in many tissues as evidenced by the recovery from copper overload after successful liver transplantation.

On liver biopsy, the early stages of copper accumulation are associated with micro and macrosteatosis. With progression of copper accumulation, inflammatory and mononuclear cells infiltrate portal and periportal areas leading to lobular necrosis and bridging fibrosis. As the disease continues to progress in the absence of appropriate therapy, micro- and macronodules of cirrhosis start to develop.[5,6]

In the brain, neurological changes include an increase in the number of astrocytes in the lenticular nuclei, swelling of the ganglia giving the appearance of spongiform degeneration and neuronal loss.[6]

CLINICAL PRESENTATION

Liver disease is the most common presentation in childhood. The average age at the time of presentation is the 10–13 year age group. However, the diagnosis must be considered in any individual between the ages of 3 and 40 years who present with unexplained hepatic, neurologic, or psychiatric manifestations. Reflecting the belief that neurological disease is virtually always preceded by extensive liver disease, the typical age of presentation for neurological manifestations of Wilson's disease is in the twenties. Some cases, however, only came to light in the fifth or sixth decade. Approximately half of the patients with Wilson's disease present with a liver problem whereas neurological presentations are seen in 30–35% of patients. Other less common presentations are psychiatric illness (10%) and hemolytic anemia or jaundice. Unusual presentations due to copper deposition in other organs have been described.[7,8]

Sunflower cataracts and the Kaiser Fleischer ring result from the deposition of copper in the anterior capsule of the lens and in Descemet membrane of the cornea respectively. Both gradually disappear with effective therapy and reaccumulate with noncompliance with therapy but they do not affect the vision. Kaiser Fleischer ring is a golden-brown or greenish discoloration that is best seen by slit-lamp examination of the eye and is almost always present in individuals with neurological manifestations.[1]

Abnormal laboratory values include low total serum copper and ceruloplasmin levels.

HEPATIC PRESENTATIONS

Wilson's disease may present as (1) an asymptomatic elevation of liver transaminases; (2) a chronic active hepatitis type picture mimicking autoimmune hepatitis with arthropathy, rash, elevation of IgG and positivity for antinuclear antibodies, and smooth muscle antibodies; (3) fulminant liver failure with hemolysis and acute renal failure as well as (4) cirrhosis.[1,4] Except in the asymptomatic cases of the young which are found during family screening and where the serum level of liver transaminases is usually normal, in cases of fulminant hepatic failure and in cirrhosis, the level of serum transaminases may rise only mildly thus not reflecting the severity of the disease. Sometimes the only biochemical indication of underlying cirrhosis is thrombocytopenia. Herewithin is one of the real problems in early detection of Wilson's disease. At times cirrhosis is recognized with the onset of variceal bleeding, ascites, or hepatic encephalopathy. Fulminant liver failure because of Wilson's disease poses all sorts of difficulties in trying to pinpoint the etiology.[9] It is commonly associated with a hemolytic anemia assumed to be due to the rapid release of copper from the liver. Emergency liver transplantation is needed to ensure survival in patients who present with this form of Wilson's disease.

NEUROLOGICAL PRESENTATIONS

Although the goal is to identify Wilson's disease before neurological manifestations appear, more than half of Wilson's disease patients present with neurological signs and symptoms usually in the second or third decade of life. Early symptoms of neurological disease can be subtle and feature behavioral changes or loss of scholarly prowess. Dysarthria, drooling, dystonia, chorea, tremor, and loss of facial expressions are frequently seen as basal ganglia degeneration become prominent.[10,11] Clearly a family history of early onset Parkinson type symptoms should raise the possibility of Wilson's disease. As the basal ganglia degeneration worsens, patients can exhibit severe spasticity, severe movement disorders, and seizures. At this point, Magnetic Resonance Imaging of the basal ganglia is grossly abnormal in most patients showing general atrophy and pontine myelinolysis.[12,13] Resolution of some of these changes has been observed with successful chelation therapy.[12] However, when chelation therapy is only instigated after the onset of neurological symptoms and signs there can be major worsening of the neurological status of some patients (See Treatment).

Table 8.1. Less Common Manifestations of Wilson's Disease

- Sunflower Cataracts
- Osteomalacia
- Pancreatitis
- Amenorrhea
- Rhabdomyolysis
- Hypothyroidism
- Cardiac Rhythm Disorder
- Osteoarthritis
- Chondrocalcinosis

Table 8.2. Where Wilson's Disease Must Be Ruled Out

- Idiopathic cirrhosis – by clinical biochemical radiological or histologic criteria
- Coombs negative hemolytic anemia
- Transaminase elevations with low serum ceruloplasmin
- Neuropsychiatric disease associated with liver disease
- Fulminant liver failure

PSYCHIATRIC PRESENTATIONS

Dramatic psychiatric illness can be the initial presentation for patients with Wilson's disease in about one-third of the cases. Although psychiatrists are to some extent aware of the association of psychiatric disease with Wilson's disease, the underlying liver disorder can often be missed. It has been recommended that all patients with progressive psychiatric disease should be specifically screened for the presence of Wilson's disease. Behavioral changes, schizophrenia, and variable degrees of cognitive impairment can be seen without the more recognized basal ganglia symptoms. Reduction of reliance on old psychiatric drugs with extrapyramidal side effects is resulting in better recognition of some cases of neurological Wilson's disease. As in all the manifestations of Wilson's disease, there is always a major potential reversal of the neuropsychiatric symptoms with chelation therapy.[14]

OTHER PRESENTATIONS

Renal deposition of copper can result in renal tubular acidosis, urinary calculi, and a Fanconi type syndrome with aminoaciduria and glucosuria.[15] An intravascular hemolysis syndrome can be seen in 10% of patients. This has been particularly observed in the acute liver failure presentation of Wilson's disease.[16] Table 8.1 lists some of the less common diseases associated with Wilson's disease but most are seen in conjunction with either hepatic or neurological disease.

DIAGNOSIS

Listed in Table 8.2 are the situations where a diagnosis of Wilson's disease should be seriously entertained. Once the diagnosis is considered, the initial

---

Table 8.3. Other Causes of Low Ceruloplasmin Levels

- Hereditary aceruloplasminemia (homozygotes and heterozygotes)
- Menke disease (X-linked disorder of copper metabolism)
- Malabsorption
- Causes of false "normal" ceruloplasmin levels, (1) patients with Wilson's disease in the presence of acute inflammation of the liver, (2) pregnancy, (3) estrogen supplementation, (4) use of oral contraceptives
- Marked hepatic or splenic inflammation and end stage liver disease
- Assay problems
- Marked renal or enteric protein loss

Table 8.4. Caveats in Diagnosis of Wilson's Disease

Kayser-Fleischer rings may be absent in 50% of patients with liver disease
Low serum ceruloplasmin levels alone does not diagnose disease
Laboratory errors can occur.
24-hour urinary copper output may be normal in asymptomatic patient.
Liver biopsy findings no-specific
Increased hepatic copper >250 µg/g dry weight alone does not diagnose disease

---

biochemical tests to perform are serum ceruloplasmin and total serum copper concentrations. A finding of a serum ceruloplasmin concentration below 20 mg/dl in patients with neurological or hepatic disease and the presence of Kayser-Fleischer rings on slit-lamp exam initially pins down the diagnosis of Wilson's disease in the majority of cases. However, occasionally serum ceruloplasmin levels will rise temporarily because this protein is an acute phase reactant.[4,17,18] Other processes can cause low serum ceruloplasmin levels (Table 8.3). When diagnostic uncertainty exists, a 24-hour urinary copper excretion test (i.e., >100 µg copper excreted in 24 hours) and serum level of non-ceruloplasmin bound copper may help in supporting the diagnosis. Non-ceruloplasmin copper level or free copper level can be calculated from the difference between serum copper concentration and three times the serum concentration of ceruloplasmin. In Wilson's disease, values are typically >25 mg/dl. Quantitative measurement of hepatic copper content will yield the diagnosis in most cases. Untreated Wilson's disease patients will usually have hepatic copper levels greater that 250 µg/g dry weight or considerably higher (normal <50 µg/g). However, one has to use a copper-free biopsy needle and get an adequate sized biopsy to obtain accurate liver copper levels.[19]

The finding of an increased hepatic content in liver biopsy without the other features of Wilson's disease is expected in long-standing cholestatic liver disorders and in idiopathic copper toxicosis syndromes. This occasionally leads to the misdiagnosis of Wilson's disease in a patient without this disorder Table 8.4. In patients for whom the diagnosis remains uncertain molecular genetic studies and mutation analysis become valuable. DNA testing may be done in serum or in liver tissue specimens.

> **Table 8.5. Screening for Wilson's Disease**
>
> - Only recommended for 1st degree relatives and siblings
> - Complete history and physical examination
> - Slit-lamp opthalmoscopy
> - Transaminase level and other standard liver tests
> - Serum ceruloplasmin
> - 24-hour urine copper excretion
> - Liver biopsy done selectively
> - If Proband mutation known direct molecular analysis can be done

SCREENING FOR WILSON'S DISEASE

Table 8.5 lists the tests recommended for screening of first-degree relatives and siblings of patients with documented Wilson's disease. The presence of hereditary deficiency of ceruloplasmin can complicate screening investigation and more sophisticated molecular tests for the Wilson's genes may be needed for clarification.[20]

MANAGEMENT

The mainstay of therapy for Wilson's disease is lifelong pharmacologic treatment that aims at reducing toxic copper levels and at maintaining a reduced level to prevent further intoxications and recurrences. Failure to comply with lifelong therapy could lead to recurrence of symptoms and worsening of disease. Early diagnosis followed by early therapy is critical to avoid permanent liver and brain damage. Thus, preemptive treatment is recommended in asymptomatic patients who are diagnosed during family screening. The prognosis is excellent with early treatment and considerable recovery may occur even after symptoms have developed. Clinical, laboratory and radiological improvements have been described with effective therapy.[21] Three commercially available drugs, Penicillamine, trientene, and Zinc, have been used effectively. Penicillamine and trientene are copper chelators.

Penicillamine promotes urinary excretion of copper, induces metallothioneins that will bind copper, and interferes with collagen cross-linking. It is excreted in kidneys and has a half-life of 1.7–7 h. Its absorption decreases when ingested with meals. Improvement of clinical and biochemical abnormalities occur in the first six months and up to a year of initiation of therapy. However, worsening of neurological symptoms has been reported in up to 50% of cases during the initial phase of therapy.[22] Its use is associated with numerous side effects such as sensitivity reactions (fever, cutaneous reactions, eruptions, lymphadenopathy, neutropenia, thrombocytopenia, and proteinuria). These usually occur in the first few weeks of therapy and require immediate discontinuation. Overall rate of discontinuation of treatment averages 20–30%. Other side effects include lupus like reactions, Goodpasture syndrome and hepatic siderosis, which is a late side effect.[23] The tolerability of penicillamine is enhanced by starting with low doses of 150–500 mg/day and increments of 250 mg a week for a maximum daily dose of 1.5 g in 2–4 divided regimens and regular supplementation with pyridoxine at a dose of 25–50 mg a day.

Trientene hydrochloride another copper chelator forms a stable complex with copper, is better tolerated than penicillamine and has a better safety profile. Similar to penicillamine, when trientene was used as initial therapy for neurological symptoms, neurological worsening was reported in up to 26% of cases.[2] Trientene forms toxic complex with iron leading to reversible sideroblastic anemia and iron overload in the liver. Other side effects include hemorrhagic gastritis, loss of taste, and skin rash. Typical effective dosages are 750–1500 mg a day in 2–3 divided regimens.

Zinc interferes with intestinal absorption of copper. It competes with a carrier of copper into enterocytes and induces metallothioneins forming zinc-copper complexes that will be shed during normal turn over of enterocytes. Zinc has the most favorable safety profile. Its half-life is about 11 days. Its absorption and effectiveness diminish when taken with food. Gastric irritation is its main side effects and worsening of liver and pancreatic biochemical abnormalities have been described.

Treatment of Wilson's disease should be individualized depending on (1) whether the patient is symptomatic or asymptomatic, (2) the severity of symptoms, (3) and whether there is liver disease or neurological disease. The following scenarios describe specific clinical issues related to Wilson's disease:

1. Patients who are diagnosed before symptoms appear, such as during family screenings, should be treated preemptively to maintain a low level of copper, prevent the onset of symptoms and the worsening of disease. Zinc is the preferred first line of therapy due to its effectiveness and good safety profile. The usual dose depends on the type of Zinc preparation (zinc sulfate, zinc acetate, zinc gluconate). The latter two are better tolerated. Zinc is usually given in three divided doses outside meal times. Trientene has also been used preemptively and is preferred over penicillamine.

2. Patients presenting with liver disease, should be treated with either chelator or with combination chelators and zinc in severe cases. Once disease symptoms have regressed and biochemical abnormalities have stabilized, patients should be placed on maintenance doses. These are in order of 30–50% of initial doses. In fulminant liver disease or decompensated liver cirrhosis, liver transplantation becomes the only effective treatment. Liver transplantation corrects the underlying metabolic disorder and restores a normal phenotype and effectively cures the liver disease.

3. Patients presenting with neurological disease or behavioral/psychological symptomatology require chelator therapy.[2] Trientene has been favored over penicillamine given its most favorable safety profile. Whether combination therapy with zinc is effective remains controversial. Improvement of symptoms occurs in the initial 6–24 months of therapy. Although the literature is meager on the response to therapy, not all symptoms are reported to improve and residual neurological and psychological abnormalities were observed. Penicillamine has been reported to cause worsening of neurological disease in up to 50% of cases [24] and newer experimental evidence supports the use of tetrathiomolybdate as the possible treatment of choice because it has not shown to exacerbate neurologic disease. However it is still not approved

for use in the United States.[24] Despite reports of its effectiveness in ameliorating neurological symptoms, liver transplantation is not recommended as primary treatment of neurologic disease because outcome is not always favorable and advanced brain damage has not shown to be reversible.[25,26]

4. Pregnant women receiving therapy for Wilson's disease should continue the treatment throughout pregnancy, but dose reduction in the order of 25–50% of pre-pregnancy state for both chelators penicillamine and trientene is required so that copper is not depleted from the body. Copper depletion is associated with congenital malformations. The dosage of zinc salts should be maintained throughout pregnancy. If initial diagnosis of Wilson's disease is made during pregnancy, then prompt therapy is recommended.[27] Penicillamine is Food and Drug Administration (FDA) Category D. Trientene and zinc are FDA Category C.

Along pharmacologic therapy for Wilson's disease, a lifelong reduction in dietary copper is required. Foods high in copper concentration include shellfish, nuts, chocolate, mushrooms, and organ meets. Supplemental vitamin E as an antioxidant has been suggested and therapy for symptomatic portal hypertension (banding esophageal varices, diuretics, and beta blockers) and neurologic and psychologic support are required.

Due to potential treatment failure and noncompliance with medication, adequacy of therapy should be monitored twice-yearly by using objective testing such as: (1) serum non-ceruloplasmin bound copper level (should be < 10 mg/dl), this being the single best parameter for gauging adequacy of compliance with treatment, (2) urinary copper excretion which is usually higher in patients treated with chelating agents than in patients taking zinc (> 250 μg/24 h versus >150 μg/24 h respectively), (3) regular assessment of hepatic function, (4) periodic slit lamp examinations, and (5) evaluation of somato-sensory and auditory evoked potentials.

SUMMARY

In summary, early diagnosis and treatment of Wilson's disease are essential in order to avoid toxicity and permanent damage to liver and brain. Chelators and zinc are effective in the initial phase and as maintenance. Maintenance therapy is required indefinitely and verification that therapy is adequate and effective should be done twice yearly. Liver transplantation effectively cures the liver disease but may not reverse advanced brain damage. Genetic testing is valuable in screening first-degree relatives of a proband and in situations where the diagnosis remains uncertain. Gene replacement therapy and hepatocytes transplantation are potential future therapies.

REFERENCES

1. Roberts, EA, Cox DW. Zakim and Boyer's Hepatology. Wilson's Disease. Thomas D Boyer, Teresa L. Wright, Michael P Manns, eds. 5th ed., 1221. Saunders, 2006.
2. Ala A, Schilsky ML. (2004) Wilson's disease: pathophysiology, diagnosis, treatment, and screening. Clin Liv Dis 2004;8(4):787–805.

3. Ferenci P. Wilson's Disease. Clin Gastroenterol Hepatol 2005;3:726–33.

4. Meyer LA, Durley AP, Prohaska JR, et al. Copper transport and metabolism are normal in aceruloplasminemic mice. J Biol Chem, 2001;276;36857–61.

5. Schilsky, ML, Tavill, AS. Schiff's Diseases of the Liver. Eugene R Schiff, Michael F. Sorrell, Willis C Maddrey, eds. 10[2], 1023. Lippincott, Williams & Wilkins, 2007.

6. Kitzberger R, Madl C, Ferenci P. Wilson disease. Metab Brain Dis, 2005;20(4):295–302.

7. Brewer GJ, Yuzbasiyan-Gurkan V. Wilson's disease. Medicine, 1992;71:139–64.

8. Lau JYN, Lai CL, Wu PC, et al. Wilson's disease: 35 years experience. QJM 1990; 75(278):597–605.

9. McCullough AJ, Fleming RM, Thistle JL et al. Diagnosis of Wilson's disease presenting as fulminant hepatic failure. Gastroenterology, 1983;84:161–7.

10. Oder W, Grimm G, Kollegger H et al. Neurologic and neuropsychiatric spectrum of Wilson's disease: a prospective study of 45 cases. J Neurolmag, 1991;238:281–7.

11. Aisen AM, Martel W, Gabrielsen TO, et al. Wilson's disease of the brain: MR Imaging. Radiology, 1990;157:137–9.

12. Takahashi W, Yoshii E, Shinohara Y. Reversible magnetic resonance imaging lesions in Wilson's disease: clinical-anatomical correlation. J Neuroimag, 1996;6:246–8.

13. Alanen A, Komu M, Penttinen M, et al. Magnetic resonance imaging and proton MR spectroscopy in Wilson's disease. Br J Radiol, 1999;72:749–52.

14. Dening TR, Berrios GE. Wilson's disease: Psychiatric symptoms in 195 cases. Arch Gen Psychiatry, 1989;46:1126–34.

15. Elias LJ, Hayslett JP, Spargo BH, et al. Wilson's disease with reversible renal tubular dysfunction. Ann Intern Med, 1971;75:427–33.

16. McIntyre N, Clink HM, Levi AJ, et al. Hemolytic anemia in Wilson's disease. N Engl J Med, 1967;276:439–44.

17. Schilsky MI, Sternlieb I. (1997) Overcoming obstacles to the diagnosis of Wilson's disease. Gastroenterology, 1997;113:350–3.

18. Ferenci P. Pathophysiology and clinical features of Wilson's disease. Metabolic Brain Disease, 2004;19:229–39.

19. Kim TJ, Kim IO, Kim WS, Cheon JE, Moon SG, Kwon JW et al. MR imaging of the brain in Wilson's disease of childhood: findings before and after treatment with clinical correlation. ANJR Am J Neuroradiol, 2005;27(6):1373–8.

20. Brewer GJ, Terry CA, Aisen AM, Hill GM. Worsening of neurologic syndrome in patients with Wilson's disease with initial penicillamine therapy. Arch Neurol, May 1987;44(5):490–3.

21. Kim TJ, Kim IO, Kim WS, Cheon JE, Moon SG, Kwon JW et al. MR imaging of the brain in Wilson's disease of childhood: findings before and after treatment with clinical correlation. ANJR Am J Neuroradiol, 2006;27(6):1373–8.

22. Brewer GJ, Terry CA, Aisen AM, Hill GM. Worsening of neurologic syndrome in patients with Wilson's disease with initial penicillamine therapy. Arch Neurol, May 1987;44(5):490–3.

23. Merle U, Schaefer M, Ferenci P, Stremmel W. Clinical presentation, diagnosis and long-term outcome of Wilson's disease: a cohort study. Gut, 2007;56(1):115–20.

24. Brewer GJ, Askari F, Lorincz MT, Carlson M, Schilsky M, Kluin KJ et al. Treatment of Wilson's disease with ammonium tetrathiomolybdate: IV. Comparison of tetrathiomolybdate and trientene in a double-blind study of treatment of the neurologic presentation of Wilson's disease. Arch Neuro, 2006;63(4):521–7.

25. Eghtesad B, Nezakatgoo N, Geraci LC et al. Liver transplantation for Wilson's disease: a single-center experience. Liver Transpl Surg, 1999;5(6):467–74.

26. Wang XH, Cheng F, Zhang F et al. Living-related liver transplantation for Wilson's disease. Transpl Int, 2005;18(6):651–6.

27. Roberts EA, Schilsky ML. A practice guideline on Wilson's disease. Hepatology, 2003;37(6);1475–92

Alpha-1 Antitrypsin Deficiency and the Liver

Steven D. Nathan, MD,[1] and James K. Stoller, MD, MS[2]

BACKGROUND

Alpha-1 antitrypsin (AAT) deficiency is a common genetic disorder characterized by low levels of serum AAT, a plasma protein with antiproteolytic activity. Although the primary clinical manifestation of AAT deficiency is lung disease, the liver is the second most common organ to be involved. Lung disease manifests primarily as emphysema, while liver disease can manifest as cirrhosis and/or liver cancer. This chapter will review the history of AAT deficiency; the genetics and pathophysiology of AAT deficiency; clinical features; and the management of AAT deficiency with a specific focus on the liver.

Alpha-1 antitrypsin deficiency was first described in 1963 when Drs. Laurell and Eriksson in Malmo, Sweden recognized that five individuals lacking a protein in the alpha band on serum protein electrophoresis also demonstrated early-onset COPD and a family history of emphysema.[1] Six years later, Sharp and colleagues described the association of AAT deficiency with neonatal cirrhosis.[2] Since the initial description of AAT deficiency as a genetic disease, over 100 different alleles coding for the AAT protein have been described. Through the 1980s, the pathogenesis of liver disease in individuals with the most common severe deficient AAT variant, PI*ZZ, became better understood; specifically, polymerization of the protein within the hepatocyte (so-called "loop-sheet polymerization") interferes with secretion of AAT into the bloodstream, thereby causing serum levels of AAT to be low and causing the accumulation of the unsecreted protein within the hepatocyte. In 1987, the first pooled human plasma preparation for intravenous infusion, which is called augmentation therapy, became available in the United States as Prolastin (Talecris Biotherapeutics, Research Triangle, NC). Two preparations of pooled human plasma-derived purified AAT – Zemaira (CSL Behring, State College, PA) and Aralast (Baxter Healthcare, Deerfield, Ill) were subsequently approved by the United States Food and Drug Administration in 2003. Also in 2003, the American Thoracic Society and European Respiratory Society approved and published a systematic evidence-based standards document for diagnosing and managing individuals with AAT deficiency which should help to optimize care provided to these individuals.[3]

Table 9.1. *Selected PI Variants with Characteristics Including Type of Mutation, Cellular Defect, and Disease Association*

PI Allele	Type of Mutation	Cellular Defect	Disease Association
Normal Alleles			
M (various)	Substitution (1 bp)	None	Normal
$X_{christchurch}$	Glu363→Lys	None	Normal
Deficiency Alleles			
S	Glu254→Val	IC Degradation	Lung
Z*	Glu342→Lys	IC Accumulation	Lung, liver
M_{malton}	Phe52→delete	IC Accumulation	Lung, liver
S_{iiyama}	Phe53→Ser	IC Accumulation	Lung
$M_{heerlen}$	Pro369→Leu	IC Degradation	Lung
$M_{procida}$	Leu41→Pro	IC Degradation	Lung
$M^{*}_{mineral\ springs}$	Gly67→Glu	IC Degradation	Lung
Null Alleles			
$QO_{granite\ falls}$	1 bp deletion Tyr160→Frame shift	Stop codon at 160; No mRNA	Lung
$QO_{ludwigshafen}$	Ile92→Asn	No protein	Lung, liver
$QO_{hongkong-1}$	2 bp deletion Leu318→Frame shift	Truncated from stop codon at 334; IC Accumulation	Lung
$QO_{isola\ di\ procida}$	17 kb deletion in exons 2–5	Deletion of coding regions; No mRNA	Lung
Dysfunctional Alleles			
F	Arg223→Cys	Defective NE inhibition	Lung
Pittsburgh	Met358→Arg	Antithrombin 3 activity	Bleeding diathesis
$M^{*}_{mineralsprings}$	Gly67→Glu	Defective NE inhibition	Lung
Z*	Glu342→Lys	Defective NE inhibition	Lung, liver

Adapted from Online Mendelian Inheritance in Man, OMIM (TM). Johns Hopkins University, Baltimore, MD. MIM Number: 107400: 3/17/2004: World Wide Web URL: http://www.ncbi.nlm.nih.gov/omim/. DeMeo DL and Silverman EK. Thorax 2004;59: 259;64. Reproduced with permission from the BMJ Publishing Group.
IC = intracellular, bp = base pair(s), NE = Neutrophil elastase
* Note that $M_{mineral\ springs}$ and Z have dysfunctional characteristics described based on altered rates of association and inhibition of neutrophil elastase, as well as deficiency characteristics.

THE ALPHA-1 ANTITRYPSIN PROTEIN AND GENETICS OF AAT DEFICIENCY

Alpha-1 antitrypsin is a genetic disease that is inherited as an autosomal co-dominant condition. The gene that encodes alpha-1 antitrypsin is located on the long arm of chromosome 14 (14q32.1) and, under normal conditions, produces a 52 kilodalton 394 amino acid glycoprotein, which is called M-type AAT. Alpha-1 antitrypsin is a protease inhibitor that confers more than 90% of the protection against breakdown of lung elastin in the interstitium by the neutrophil primary granule enzyme called neutrophil elastase. Alpha-1 antitrypsin is referred to as a member of the serpin family (along with other protease inhibitors like

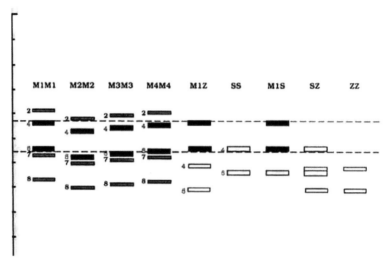

Figure 9.1. Schematic of alpha-1 antitrypsin PI types separated according to their migration on a thin-layer polyacrylamide gel prepared for isoelectric focusing from pH 4 to 5. The band pattern identifies the phenotypes.
From: Brantly M. Alpha-1 antitrypsin genotypes and phenotypes. In: Alpha-1 Antitrypsin Deficiency: Biology, Pathogenesis, Clinical Manifestations, Therapy. Crystal RG (ed). Marcel Dekker, Inc. New York/Basel/Hong Kong, 1996. With permission.

antithrombin III and an alpha-1 antichymotrypsin), where serpin is an acronym for **ser**ine **p**rotease **in**hibitor.

To date, more than 100 variants of the AAT gene have been described (Table 9.1) and have been classified into four groups: normal (e.g., M type and normal variants), deficient, null, and dysfunctional alleles.[3,4] The normal AAT phenotype (so-called PI*MM, where PI stands for "protease inhibitor") characterizes approximately 95% of Caucasian Americans and almost all non-Caucasians. Individuals with this phenotype have normal levels of fully functional alpha-1 antitrypsin.

Alpha-1 antitrypsin variants are commonly identified by the technique of isoelectric focusing. The alleles are named alphabetically based on their mobility in an electrophoretic field of pH 4–5 (Figure 9.1). The predominant normal phenotype is PI*MM (where the M protein migrates in the middle). The moving variants are named in alphabetical order based on the rapidity of their migration on the polyacrylamide gel. The A protein is the most rapidly moving and the Z protein, which is the most common severe deficiency variant causing disease, migrates most slowly because a single amino acid substitution of lysine for glutamic acid at position 342 renders the protein less negatively charged.

Individuals who are homozygous for the deficient allele, Z (called PI*ZZ or Z homozygotes) comprise 95% of those with clinical disease due to AAT deficiency and 2–3% of all individuals with chronic obstructive pulmonary disease. Serum levels of PI*ZZ individuals are 10–15% of normal (i.e., 20–30 mg/dl versus normal levels of 150–350 mg/dl [Table 9.2]) Because the Z protein may polymerize within the hepatocyte (in a process called "loop-sheet polymerization"), individuals with the Z allele (both heterozygotes and PI*ZZ homozygotes) are at risk for liver disease.

Table 9.2. Relationship Between Serum Phenotype, Serum Level of Alpha-1 Antitrypsin, and Risk of Developing Obstructive Lung Disease

Phenotype	AAT Serum Level Using Immunoelectrophoresis (mg/dL)	AAT Serum Level Using Highly Purified Standard (μmol/L)	Risk of Pulmonary Disease
Null-null	0	0	Extremely high risk
ZZ	20–45	2.5–7	High risk
SZ	75–120	8–19	Mild increased risk
SS	100–140	15–33	No increase
MZ	90–210	12–35	No increase
MM	150–350	20–48	No increase

After: Stoller JK, Aboussouan LS. Alpha-1 antitrypsin deficiency. Lancet 2005; 365:2225–36; with permission.

The S allele is another deficient allele that occurs more commonly than Z. This allele has a valine replacing a glutamic acid residue at position 264 (summarized as Glu264Val). Patients who are homozygous for the S mutation (PI*SS) demonstrate a 40% decrease in the serum concentration of alpha-1 antitrypsin. However, this minor decrease by itself does not pose a significant threat to health because the serum levels of PI*SS individuals exceed the protective threshold serum value of approximately 50 mg/dL or 11 micromolar (using a highly purified laboratory standard, Table 9.2). A value below this threshold is associated with a greater risk of emphysema. Therefore, individuals with the PI*SS phenotype are neither at risk for emphysema nor liver disease.[4,5]

Individuals who are mixed heterozygotes with the S and Z alleles (PI*SZ) are at risk for liver disease because the Z-type protein can polymerize and accumulate within the hepatocyte. Approximately 10% of PI*SZ individuals have serum levels below the protective threshold value and are at risk for emphysema, especially if they smoke.[6]

Null and dysfunctional alleles are rare. Null variants cause a defect in transcription or translation and thus produce no alpha-1 antitrypsin. The resultant complete absence of AAT in serum predisposes to severe emphysema but not to liver disease because null-type AAT protein is not produced and therefore does not accumulate within hepatocytes.

Finally, dysfunctional AAT alleles produce alpha-1 antitrypsin with aberrant function. For example, patients with the Pittsburgh variant of alpha-1 antitrypsin present with a bleeding diathesis because the dysfunctional alpha-1 antitrypsin acts as a thrombin inhibitor.[5]

PATHOGENESIS

As a member of the serine protease inhibitor (serpin) family of proteins, AAT is vulnerable to misfolding. A conformational change in AAT impairs both its ability to bind to and neutralize neutrophil elastase function and its ability to be secreted from the hepatocyte. As such, alpha-1 antitrypsin deficiency is an example of a "conformational disease," which is due primarily to the polymerization of some abnormal variant forms of the protein, most notably the Z-type protein.[5]

Although liver and lung disease result from the same genetic abnormality, the pathogenesis of the two organ dysfunctions differs markedly. Emphysema is felt to result from unopposed elastolytic breakdown of lung matrix proteins when serum and lung levels of AAT are insufficient to protect against the neutrophil elastase burden. The burden of neutrophil elastase increases with lung inflammation, as in cigarette smoking, dusty occupational exposure, and pneumonia.

In contrast, liver disease does not result from unopposed proteolytic damage but rather from the accumulation within the hepatocyte of unsecreted AAT protein. Alleles associated with intra-hepatocyte "loop-sheet polymerization" include: Z, M_{malton}, M_{duarte}, and S_{iiyama}. Heterozygotes for these alleles also appear to be at risk for liver disease.[7] Though the precise mechanism of liver damage is incompletely understood, it appears that liver disease results from the net effect of intrahepatocyte polymerization and failure of cellular mechanisms to clear intrahepatocyte protein. Inflammatory cytokines such as interleukin-6, tumor necrosis factor-α, and endotoxin can lead to increased production of AAT, as can increased temperature.

The pathologic hallmark of intra-hepatocyte polymerization is the presence of globules within the hepatocyte (see color plate of Figure 9.2) that stain positively (as eosinophilic granules) with periodic Schiff (PAS) reagent and are resistant to diastase (which excludes glycogen as the cause of the staining).[8]

CLINICAL PRESENTATION

Clinical conditions associated with alpha-1 antitrypsin deficiency include lung disease (especially emphysema and bronchiectasis), liver disease (especially cirrhosis and hepatoma), panniculitis, and antiproteinase 3 antibody-positive (i.e., C-ANCA) vasculitis.[3] Though variably reported, other associations with alpha-1 antitrypsin deficiency (e.g., aneurysms, glomerulonephritis, and inflammatory bowel disease) remain uncertain.

Liver Disease

The liver disease associated with AAT deficiency characteristically affects two distinct age groups: newborns through the first few years of life and adults over the age of 50 years. Indeed, AAT deficiency is the most common genetic cause of neonatal liver disease and the second most common indication for liver transplantation in the United States after primary biliary atresia.[9]

Children who present with AAT deficiency classically present with acute hepatitis and jaundice. These findings occur later than and should be distinguished from the physiologic jaundice of the newborn and other pathologic forms of neonatal liver disease, including infections, metabolic diseases, and inherited hepatobiliary anomalies such as biliary atresia. Alpha-1 antitrypsin deficiency should be suspected if a newborn develops an elevated conjugated bilirubin during the first four months of life. Almost all of these newborns will have hepatomegaly and approximately half of them will have associated splenomegaly.

Sveger et al. conducted the largest available study of the natural history of alpha-1 antitrypsin deficiency by screening 200,000 Swedish newborns for AAT deficiency. One in 1,575 of these infants was PI*ZZ. Of these PI*ZZ newborns who were followed, 11% developed hepatocellular damage which usually began as neonatal hepatitis and cholestasis between four days and four months after birth and persisted for up to one year. Other children manifested hepatomegaly with elevated transaminases but without evidence of hepatic decompensation. Of 14 children with neonatal hepatitis, 21% progressed to cirrhosis by age 7. The rest remained healthy at age 8 with only intermittent elevations of their transaminases.[10]

In the subset of newborns (10–15%) with neonatal hepatitis, 5% remained jaundiced, with cirrhosis and death resulting at one year. The remaining infants displayed one of four clinical patterns (about 25% each):

1) Resolution of hepatitis by age 3–10 years without hepatosplenomegaly,
2) Development of cirrhosis with end-stage liver disease or death between 6 months and 17 years of age,
3) Evidence of cirrhosis by histology but without symptoms for more than 10 years, and
4) Persistence of elevated transaminases without cirrhosis.[10]

As opposed to lung disease (Table 9.2), the development of neonatal liver disease is unrelated to serum levels of AAT in individuals with at-risk alleles. Indeed, patients who are Z heterozygotes may also develop liver disease. Therefore, serum levels of AAT cannot be used to exclude the diagnosis of AAT deficiency-associated liver disease and phenotyping (Table 9.1) is needed to assess undiagnosed neonatal liver disease.[11]

Estimates suggest that 12 to ~34% of AAT deficient individuals develop liver disease through the course of their lifetimes.[13] In a post-mortem analysis of 38 decedents with AAT deficiency, Eriksson et al. reported that cirrhosis was found in approximately one-third of the decedents, of whom a further one-third had concomitant hepatocellular carcinoma.[12] Notably, these investigators suggested that the prevalence of liver disease may be underestimated because AAT deficient smokers may die before their liver disease becomes evident. In other estimates of the frequency of liver disease among AAT deficient individuals, 7.6% of 2,175 individuals in the Alpha-1 Foundation Registry reported a history of jaundice or liver disease. A survey of a subgroup of 104 patients with known liver disease showed that 29% of respondents were diagnosed with liver disease before age 18, of whom 50% had advanced disease. Of the remaining 71% diagnosed after age 18, one-third had advanced disease. Factors that appear to increase the risk of advanced liver disease include male gender and obesity; somewhat surprisingly, neither viral hepatitis nor alcohol consumption appears to be a risk factor.[4]

Individuals with at-risk alleles may develop adult-onset cirrhosis or hepatoma, often without antecedent liver disease in childhood. Interestingly, hepatoma may occur in the absence of cirrhosis; thus, patients identified as deficient in AAT should be monitored accordingly. The risk of hepatoma is greater in males than in females. In an early study of 246 PI*ZZ homozygotes, cirrhosis occurred in 11.8% and hepatoma in 3.3%.[13] Data from the National Heart, Lung and Blood Institute (NHLBI) Registry of Individuals with AAT Deficiency suggest that liver disease was responsible for about 10% of deaths, while 72% of deaths were attributable to emphysema.[14]

Pulmonary Disease

Though individuals with severe alpha-1 antitrypsin deficiency comprise 2–3% of all patients with COPD, many lines of evidence suggest that AAT deficiency is under-recognized.[15] For example, of the estimated 100,000 Americans with severe deficiency of AAT, less than 10,000 are currently clinically recognized. Furthermore, several studies demonstrate long delays (i.e., mean of 5.6 to 8.3 years) between the patient's first symptom of AAT deficiency and the first diagnosis.[13,14] In one study, the mean number of physicians seen before AAT deficiency was first diagnosed was 2.7+/−2.4. One-fifth of these patients saw at least 4 physicians before the diagnosis was established, with approximately 10% seeing at least six physicians.[13] These observations underscore the need for heightened awareness of AAT deficiency by clinicians.

Pulmonary features that should especially prompt the clinician to suspect AAT deficiency include early-onset COPD (e.g., before age 50), development of COPD in a non- or trivial smoker, a panacinar pathologic pattern of emphysema, and a preferentially basilar distribution of emphysema on the chest radiograph or CT scan. As an example of the early age of onset of emphysema, in one large series, the mean age of AAT deficient individuals was 46 years (+/−11 years) versus 60–70 years in AAT-replete COPD patients.[16]

Although having AAT serum levels below the protective value poses a risk for emphysema, not all AAT deficient individuals will develop emphysema. For example, in the NHLBI Registry of Individuals with Severe Deficiency of AAT, approximately 15% of 1,129 participants had values of FEV1 above 80% predicted. Besides cigarette smoking, other risk factors for emphysema include dusty occupational exposure and emphysema in parents.[17] Variability in the development of emphysema between PI*ZZ siblings suggests the presence of other genetic risk modifiers for emphysema which are currently being studied.

Other Clinical Manifestations of Alpha-1 Antitrypsin Deficiency

Alpha-1 antitrypsin deficiency can also be associated with diseases affecting organs other than the lung or liver. Specifically, skin involvement may present as panniculitis, due to unopposed proteolysis in the fatty layer of the skin. The pathogenetic mechanism is felt to resemble that which causes proteolytic damage in the lung. Affected patients may present with inflammatory skin lesions in areas of trauma, e.g., commonly the thighs and buttocks. The skin lesions are characteristically erythematous and painful and may become indurated and necrotic with an oily discharge. Panniculitis is uncommon, with fewer than 100 cases reported to date. Though many phenotypes are implicated, two thirds of reported patients are PI*ZZ.

Vasculitis characterized by antibodies to proteinase 3 (C-ANCA positive) is also associated with AAT deficiency. For example, approximately 2% of all patients with Wegener's granulomatosis are PI*ZZ homozygotes and the frequency of abnormal AAT alleles among Wegener's granulomatosis patients is higher than in the general population. Current views suggest that AAT can bind proteinase 3, the antigen implicated in C-ANCA-positive vasculitis, and that AAT deficiency allows greater antigen expression.

Other conditions for which associations with AAT deficiency have been proposed include vascular disease, such as fibromuscular dysplasia or aneurysms; inflammatory bowel disease; glomerulonephritis; IgA deficiency; and rheumatoid arthritis. However, in none has the association with AAT deficiency been firmly established. Membranoproliferative glomerulonephritis has rarely been associated with the PI*ZZ phenotype; all affected patients have also had cirrhosis, raising the possibility that the development of membranoproliferative glomerulonephritis is due to liver disease.[18]

DIAGNOSIS

Indications for testing for AAT deficiency have been developed by the American Thoracic Society (ATS) and European Respiratory Society (ERS).[3] Settings in which testing is recommended include:

1. Symptomatic adults with emphysema, chronic obstructive pulmonary disease, or asthma with airflow obstruction that is incompletely reversible after aggressive treatment with bronchodilators;
2. Unexplained liver disease (including in neonates, children, and adults);
3. Asymptomatic individuals with persistent obstruction on pulmonary function tests with identifiable risk factors (e.g., cigarette smoking, occupational exposure);
4. Adults with necrotizing panniculitis; and
5. Siblings of an individual with PI*ZZ alpha-1 antitrypsin deficiency.

Importantly, in testing patients with unexplained liver disease for AAT deficiency, it is important to recognize that lung disease may not coexist in the same patient, so that its absence should not discourage testing.

The initial diagnostic test to perform in a patient suspected of having AAT deficiency is a quantitative serum level of alpha-1 antitrypsin, usually performed by nephelometry (Table 9.2). Because some available commercial standards may overestimate alpha-1 antitrypsin levels by 35–40%, highly purified standards in testing are essential.[3] Normal serum levels are ~150–350 mg/dl (using immunoelectrophoresis) or 100–220 mg/dl (or 20–53 micromolar) by nephelometry. Notably, because AAT is an acute phase reactant, serum levels can rise during acute illness, at least in heterozygotes. Thus, testing serum levels during acute illness can mask the diagnosis in heterozygotes (Table 9.2).

Individuals with borderline or low alpha-1 antitrypsin concentrations should also undergo phenotyping to determine their protease inhibitor (PI) type. Protease inhibitor typing is often performed by isoelectric focusing within a narrow pH gradient (pH 4 to 5) in a gel. As noted, bands migrate according to their isoelectric points (Figure 9.1) and the band pattern determines the phenotype. Polymerase chain reaction assays for the common deficient alleles (e.g., Z and S) can also be performed.

Once the diagnosis of AAT deficiency is established, further evaluation should include pulmonary function testing (i.e., with spirometry and post-bronchodilator testing, and measurement of diffusing capacity for carbon monoxide) and liver function tests. Though not routinely indicated in management, liver biopsy can help to stage liver disease, rule out alternate etiologies for liver disease, and identify the alpha-1 antitrypsin polymers within hepatocytes as PAS-positive, diastase-resistant globules.

When performed, liver biopsy of neonates will often show one of three histologic patterns:

1) Hepatocellular damage with normal bile ducts and minimal inflammation,
2) Varying degrees of portal fibrosis with ductal proliferation (often confused with biliary atresia),
3) Hypoplasia of intrahepatic ducts.[8]

A suggestive finding on light microscopy is the presence of PAS-positive, diastase resistant globules in periportal hepatocytes, adjacent to bands of fibrosis (see color plate of Figure 9.2). The globules appear as magenta-colored inclusions that represent aggregated polymers of variant alpha-1 antitrypsin protein. These globules may not be evident during the first 12 weeks of life. Though the size of the globules increases with age, neither the size nor amount of accumulated polymers correlates with the extent of liver disease.

Fibrosis may also be a feature of the liver pathology of alpha-1 antitrypsin deficiency for phenotypes associated with intra-hepatocyte accumulation (e.g., Z, M_{malton}, etc.). The process begins with low-grade inflammation, starting in the portal tracts. Fibrosis characteristically increases as the disease progresses.[8]

MANAGEMENT

Because AAT deficiency is a multi-system, genetic disease, ideal management includes multidisciplinary input that assesses pulmonary, hepatic, dermatologic, and genetic issues. Primary management goals include preventing the progression of emphysema, monitoring for liver damage, and thereby optimizing the quality and duration of patients' lives. Genetic counseling and assessing risk in family members is also important.

For patients with emphysema due to AAT deficiency, therapies that are useful in "usual" COPD apply. These include bronchodilators, supplemental oxygen when indicated, pulmonary rehabilitation, prophylactic vaccination against influenza and pneumococcal infection, and for patients with advanced lung disease, lung transplantation.[19]

Specific therapy for COPD due to alpha-1 antitrypsin deficiency involves the infusion of pooled human plasma alpha 1-antiprotease, called augmentation therapy. The goal of intravenous augmentation therapy is to raise serum levels above the protective threshold of 11 micromolar, so as to prevent the

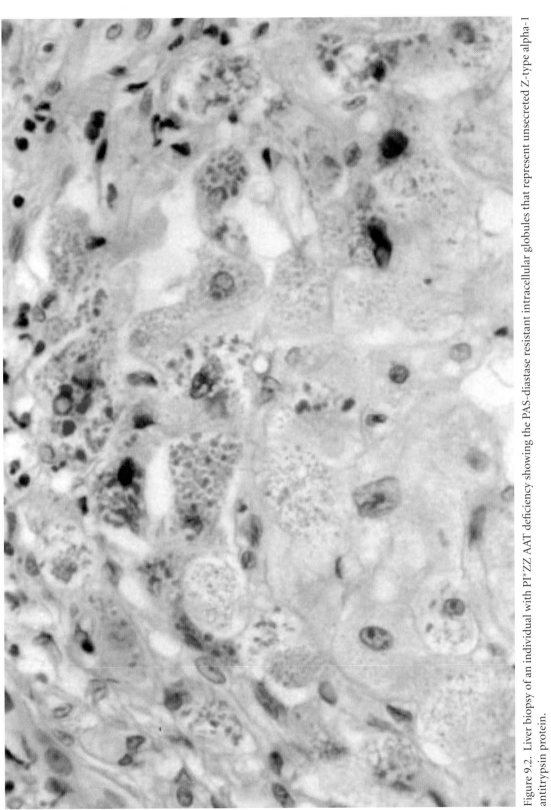

Figure 9.2. Liver biopsy of an individual with PI*ZZ AAT deficiency showing the PAS-diastase resistant intracellular globules that represent unsecreted Z-type alpha-1 antitrypsin protein.

progression of emphysema. Available evidence supports the biochemical efficacy of intravenous augmentation therapy, in that serum levels can be raised and maintained above 11 micromolar for almost the entire dosing interval, which is recommended at once weekly.[20]

The clinical evidence showing that augmentation therapy has efficacy in slowing the rate of lung function decline is provided by several observational cohort studies and a single randomized controlled trial.[21] In this single randomized controlled trial, Dirksen et al. allocated 58 PI*ZZ subjects with moderate emphysema (FEV1 30–80% of predicted) to receive intravenous pooled human plasma AAT or placebo once monthly for at least three years. Though the rates of decline in the FEV1 were similar between the groups, assessment of lung densitometry by chest CT scan showed a trend toward a slower annual loss of lung tissue in augmentation therapy recipients ($p = 0.07$).

Several observational cohort studies have also shown that intravenous augmentation therapy is associated with a slowed rate of decline of lung function in individuals with established emphysema, especially in those with a moderate degree of airflow obstruction.[22–24] The NHLBI Registry of Individuals with Severe Deficiency of AAT also showed a survival advantage among intravenous augmentation therapy recipients.[22]

Based on the best available evidence, current treatment guidelines for AAT deficiency endorse the use of intravenous augmentation therapy in individuals with established emphysema of moderate degree (FEV1 35–60% of predicted).[3] The evidence is less strong for individuals with mild (FEV1 > 60% predicted) or severe airflow obstruction (FEV1 < 35% predicted). Augmentation therapy is not recommended as a preventive strategy in individuals with normal lung function, as not all at-risk individuals develop lung dysfunction. Also, active smoking is considered by some clinicians to be a contraindication to intravenous augmentation therapy because cigarette smoke can inactivate AAT by direct oxidation

Three available products are currently available in the United Stated for intravenous AAT augmentation: Prolastin (Talecris Biotherapeutics, Research Triangle Park, North Carolina), Aralast (Baxter Healthcare, Deerfield, Illinois), and Zemaira (CSL Behring, King of Prussia, Pennsylvania). Each of these products is derived from purified pooled human plasma. The recommended dose is 60 mg/kg once weekly intravenously, though other dosing frequencies and dosages are sometimes prescribed (e.g., 120 mg/kg biweekly or 250 mg/kg once monthly). All available forms of augmentation therapy have small amounts of IgA that can pose a risk for anaphylaxis in IgA-deficient recipients. Therefore, testing patients to rule out IgA deficiency is recommended before intravenous augmentation therapy is initiated. Also, although official recommendations do not require hepatitis vaccinations before augmentation therapy, many clinicians recommend vaccinating hepatitis B-naïve patients before initiating the infusions.

Intravenous augmentation therapy is generally well tolerated, with low rates of adverse events, few of which are severe. In the NHLBI Registry, infusion-related adverse events occurred at a low rate of 0.02 events per patient-month.[4] The most common adverse events include fever, chills, urticaria, nausea, and vomiting.

All currently available preparations of pooled human plasma antiprotease are costly (e.g., estimates ranging from $28,075 to 65,973 per year[4]); therefore, the decision to implement augmentation therapy must also be weighed against the cost. The most recent cost-effectiveness analysis of augmentation therapy concludes that augmentation therapy does not satisfy traditional cost-effectiveness criteria (i.e., of <$50,000 per quality-adjusted life-years).[25] However, Gildea et al. underscore that this finding must be understood in the context that intravenous augmentation therapy is currently the only specific treatment for AAT deficiency-related lung disease.

In the context that intravenous augmentation therapy is inconvenient and expensive, active research is exploring alternative treatment strategies.[26] Current research is examining the effectiveness of administering pooled human plasma antiprotease by inhalation as well as preparing recombinant AAT for inhalation. Other strategies regard the development of small oligomers to bind to deficient-type AAT proteins to prevent polymerization and encourage secretion from the hepatocyte.[27] Gene therapy is also being explored using an adeno-associated vector to transfect the normal human AAT gene by intramuscular injection.[28] With this approach, prolonged expression of serum levels exceeding the protective threshold value have been achieved in mice and human trials are currently under way.[29]

Regarding therapy for the liver disease of AAT deficiency, no specific treatment is currently available. Investigational approaches have been undertaken that include the administration of drugs to prevent the intrahepatic polymerization of the variant AAT protein and/or to encourage its secretion.[7,30] These compounds include chemical chaperones (such as glycerol, trimethylamine oxide, deuterated water and, 4-phenylbutyrate [4-PBA]) and iminosugar compounds (such as castanospermine[7]). However, a recent open label study of 4-PBA administered to 10 AAT deficient patients over two weeks failed to demonstrate a significant increase in AAT serum levels.[31]

Liver transplantation is reserved for individuals with end-stage liver disease and is "curative" of the deficiency in that successful liver transplant recipients will have the normal type and amounts of circulating AAT. Outcomes of liver transplantation for AAT deficient patients are excellent, with reported rates of survival exceeding 92% at five years.[7]

Comprehensive management of the patient with AAT deficiency should also include genetic counseling. The 2003 ATS/ERS standards document, recommends phenotyping all siblings of PI*ZZ homozygote patients, as there is a 25% chance that they will also have severe deficiency.[3] Testing should also be discussed with children, parents, and distant relatives of patients.

As an instructive scenario, each child of a marriage of 2 PI*MZ parents has a 50% chance of inheriting one Z allele. On average, 25% of the offspring of this parentage will be PI*ZZ and PI*MM, with 50% as PI*MZ.

As another common scenario, a PI*ZZ parent may wish to assess his/her child's risk for being a homozygote. In the context that genetic discrimination can affect those with established carriage of the Z allele, parents may wish to spare their children's being tested. If the spouse of a PI*ZZ individual is found to be PI*MM, each child of that pair can be predicted to be PI*MZ without test confirmation. On the other hand, if the spouse is found to be PI*MZ (as are 3% of Americans), then each child has a 50% chance of being either PI*ZZ or PI*MZ and must be phenotyped to determine disease risk.

Table 9.3. Effect of Smoking on the Rate of FEV1 Decline Among Individuals with Alpha-1 Antitrypsin Deficiency

Author (Year)(Ref)	N	FEV1 Slope (ml/yr [SD])*		
		Never Smokers	Ex-smokers	Current Smokers
Janus (1985)[34]	21	−80 (±38)[†]	−61 (±43)[†]	−316 (±43)[†]
Hutchison (1987)[35]	82	−66 (±55)	−44 (±56)	−67 (±46)
Wu (1988)[36]	80	−61 (±100)	−81 (±70)	−61 (±170)
Seersholm (1995)[37]	161	−86 (±107)	−52 (±80)	−132 (±105)
Seersholm (1997)[38‡]	198		−53 (CI 48−58)[§]	
Seersholm (1997)[38¶]	97		−75 (CI 63−87)[§]	
NHLBI Registry (1998)[22]	1129	−67 (CI 56−78)[§]	−54 (CI 46−63)[§]	−109 (CI 81−137)[§]
Piitulainen (1999)[39]	608	−47 (CI 41−53)[§]	−41 (36−48)[§]	−70 (CI 58−82)[§]

* Parentheses indicate SD unless otherwise indicated, [†]Parentheses indicate SEM, [‡]Germans on augmentation therapy, [§]Parentheses indicate 95% CI, [¶]Danes not on augmentation therapy
From: Stoller JK, Aboussouan LS. Alpha-1 antitrypsin deficiency. Lancet 2005;365:2225−36; with permission.

PROGNOSIS

On average, individuals with severe alpha-1 antitrypsin deficiency experience an accelerated yearly decline in their FEV1 which results in progressive obstructive airway disease (Table 9.3). Available studies show that the annual rate of decline of the FEV1 in PI*ZZ patients is 41–109 ml/year.[4] As with COPD in general, the degree of airflow obstruction is an important determinant of prognosis. For example in the NHLBI Registry, the three-year mortality rate of patients with a baseline value of FEV1 <15% predicted was 36% compared to only 2.6% in those subjects with values >50% predicted.[32] Registry data showed that the overall annual mortality rate of Registry participants was 3%.

As with lung disease, the course of liver disease can be quite variable. For patients who present in infancy with liver-related problems, estimates suggest that only about 10% will subsequently develop clinically significant liver disease. Nonetheless, the lack of liver problems in infancy does not assure protection from liver disease in adulthood. For example, estimates suggest that 11% to 34% of adult patients will develop cirrhosis. Also, in an 11-year follow-up study of PI*ZZ homozygotes, 37% of the individuals died (∼3%/year overall), with 59% of the deaths relating to respiratory failure and 13% due to complications of liver disease.[13] Data from the NHLBI Registry show similar results, with 10% of patients succumbing to cirrhosis.[32] Approximately 2.5% of patients with PI*ZZ die of cirrhosis or require liver transplantation by the age of 18. Although cirrhosis can be seen in children and adolescents, the incidence appears to increase beyond the age of 50, especially in nonsmokers who escape emphysema. The overall risk of liver disease is about 20-fold increased compared to the general population. As a group, survival to age 60 among individuals with severe deficiency of AAT has been shown to be significantly lower than that for the general U.S. population (16% survival vs. 85% for age-matched controls).[33]

SUMMARY

Although much is now known about the molecular and genetic basis of alpha-1 antitrypsin deficiency, many questions still remain. For example, risk factors for lung disease beyond cigarette smoking and certain occupational exposures are poorly understood and current studies are addressing the role of genetic modifiers of the PI*ZZ state for the development of lung disease. Also greater understanding of risk factors for liver disease is needed.

In summary, AAT deficiency is common but under-recognized. Enhanced suspicion by clinicians is needed to offer affected individuals the benefits of current therapy, the opportunity to partake in new and future investigational treatments, and to offer family members appropriate genetic counseling.

REFERENCES

1. Laurell, C-B, Eriksson, A. The electrophoretic alpha 1-globulin pattern of serum in alpha-1 antitrypsin deficiency. Scand J Clin Lab Invest 1963;15:132.
2. Sharp HL, Bridges RA, Krivit W, Freier ER. Cirrhosis associated with alpha-1 antitrypsin deficiency: a previously unrecognized inherited disorder. J Lab Clin Med 1969;73:934–9.
3. American Thoracic Society/European Respiratory Society: Standards for the Diagnosis and Management of Individuals with Alpha-1 Antitrypsin Deficiency Lung Disease. Am J Respir Crit Care Med 2003;168:823–49.
4. Stoller JK, Aboussouan LS. Alpha-1 antitrypsin deficiency. Lancet 2005;365:2225–36.
5. Carrell, R, Lomas, D. Alpha-1 antitrypsin deficiency- a model for conformational diseases. N Engl J Med 2002;346:45–53.
6. Turino GM, Barker AF, Brantly ML, et al. Clinical features of individuals with PI*SZ phenotype of alpha-1 antitrypsin deficiency. Am J Respir Crit Care Med 1996;154:1718–25.
7. Perlmutter DH. Alpha-1 antitrypsin deficiency: diagnosis and treatment. Clin Liver Dis 2004;8:839–59.
8. Sapienza MS, Porayko M. Alpha-1 antitrypsin deficiency and liver disease. Clinical Perspectives in Gastroenterology 2002;5:40–8.
9. Primhak RA, Tanner MS. Alpha-1 antitrypsin deficiency. Arch Dis Child. 2001;85:2–5.
10. Sveger, T. Liver disease in alpha-1 antitrypsin deficiency detected by screening of 200,000 infants. N Engl J Med 1976;294: 1316–21.
11. Lang T, Muhlbauer M, Strobelt M, Weidinger S, Hadorn HB. Alpha-1-antitrypsin deficiency in children: liver disease is not reflected by low serum levels of alpha-1 antitrypsin: a study on 48 pediatric patients. Eur J Med Res 2005;10:509–14.
12. Eriksson S. Alpha-1 antitrypsin deficiency and liver cirrhosis in adults: an analysis of 35 Swedish autopsied cases. Acta Med Scand 1987;221:461–7.
13. Campos MA, Wanner A, Zhang G, Sandhaus RA. Trends in the diagnosis of symptomatic patients with alpha-1 antitrypsin deficiency between 1968 and 2003. Chest 2005;128:1179–86.
14. Stoller JK, Sandhaus RA, Turino G, Dickson R, Rodgers K, Strange C. Delay in diagnosis of alpha-1 antitrypsin deficiency: a continuing problem. Chest 2005;128:1989–94.
15. Lieberman J, Winter B, Sastre A. Alpha-1 antitrypsin PI-types in 965 COPD patients. Chest 1986;89: 370–3.
16. The Alpha-1 Antitrypsin Deficiency Registry Study Group. Prepared by: Schluchter MD, Barker AF, Crystal RG, et al. A registry of patients with severe deficiency of alpha-1 antitrypsin: design and methods. Chest 1994;106:1223–32.

17. Silverman EK, Pierce JA, Province MA, et al. Variability of pulmonary function in alpha-1 antitrypsin deficiency: clinical correlates. Ann Intern Med 1989;111:982–991.

18. Needham M, Stockley RA. Alpha-1 antitrypsin deficiency 3: Clinical manifestations and natural history. Thorax 2004;59:441–5.

19. Pauwels RA, Buist AS, Calverley PMA, Jenkins CR, Hurd SS. Global strategy for the diagnosis, management, and prevention of chronic obstructive pulmonary disease: NHLBI/WHO Global Initiative for Chronic Obstructive Lung Disease (GOLD) Workshop summary. Am J Respir Crit Care Med 2001;163:1256–76.

20. Wewers MD, Casolaro MA, Sellers SE, Swayze S, McPhaul KM, Wittes JT, and Crystal RG. Replacement therapy for alpha-1 antitrypsin deficiency associated with emphysema. N Engl J Med 1987;316:1055–62.

21. Dirksen A, Dijkman JH, Madesen F, Stoel B, Hutchison DCS, Ulrik CS, Skovgaars LT, Kok-Jensen A, Rudolphus A, Seersholm N, Vrooman HA, Reiber JHC, Hansen NC, Hecksher T, Viskum K, Stolk J. A randomized clinical trial of alpha-1 antitrypsin augmentation therapy. Am J Respir Crit Care Med 1999;160:1468–72.

22. The Alpha-1 antitrypsin Deficiency Registry Study Group. Survival and FEV1 decline in individuals with severe deficiency of alpha-1 antitrypsin. Am J Respir Crit Care Med 1998;158:49–59.

23. Seersholm N, Wencker M, Banik N, et al. Does alpha-1 antitrypsin augmentation therapy slow the annual decline in FEV1 in patients with severe hereditary alpha-1 antitrypsin deficiency? Eur Respir J 1997;10:2260–63.

24. Wencker M, Fuhrmann B, Banik N, Konietzko N. Wissenschaftliche Arbeitsgemeinschaft zur Therapie von Lungenerkrankungen. Longitudinal follow-up of patients with alpha (1)-protease inhibitor deficiency before and during therapy with IV alpha(1)-protease inhibitor. Chest 2001;119:737–44.

25. Gildea TR, Shermock KM, Singer ME, Stoller JK. Cost-effectiveness analysis of augmentation therapy for severe alpha-1 antitrypsin deficiency. Am J Respir Crit Care Med 2003;167:1387–92.

26. Sandhaus RA. Alpha-1 antitrypsin deficiency 6: New and emerging treatments for alpha1-antitrypsin deficiency. Thorax 2004;59:904–9.

27. Lomas DA. Mahadeva R. Alpha-1 antitrypsin polymerization and the serpinopathies: pathobiology and prospects for therapy. J Clin Invest 2002;110:1585–90.

28. Flotte TR, Brantly ML, Spencer LT, et al. Phase I trial of intramuscular injection of a recombinant adeno-associated virus alpha-1 antitrypsin (rAAV2-CB-hAAT) gene vector to AAT-deficient adults. Hum Gene Ther 2004;15:93–128.

29. Kolb M, Martin G, Medina M, Ask K, Gauldie J. Gene therapy for pulmonary diseases. Chest 2006;130:879–84.

30. Burrows JA, Willis LK, Perlmutter DH. Chemical chaperones mediate increased secretion of mutant alpha-1 antitrypsin (alpha-1 AT) Z: A potential pharmacological strategy for prevention of liver injury and emphysema in alpha-1 AT deficiency. Proc Natl Acad Sci USA 2000;97:1796–1801.

31. Teckman JH. Lack of effect of oral 4-phenylbutyrate on serum alpha-1-antitrypsin in patients with alpha-1 antitrypsin deficiency: A preliminary study. J Pediatr Gastroenterol Nutr 2004;39:34–7.

32. Stoller JK, Tomashefski J, Crystal RG, Arroliga A, Strange C, Killian DN, Schluchter MD, Wiedemann HP. Mortality in individuals with severe deficiency of alpha-1 antitrypsin. Chest 2005;127:1196–1204.

33. Brantly ML, Paul LD, Miller BH, et al. Clinical features and history of the destructive lung disease associated with alpha-1 antitrypsin deficiency of adults with pulmonary symptoms. Am Rev Respir Dis 1988;138:327.

34. Janus ED, Phillips NT, Carrell RW. Smoking, lung function and alpha-1 antitrypsin deficiency. Lancet 1985;1:152–4.

35. Hutchison DC, Tobin MJ, Cooper D. Longitudinal studies in alpha-1 antitrypsin deficiency: a survey by the British Thoracic Society. In: Taylor JC, Mittman C, eds. Pulmonary emphysema and proteolysis. Orlando: Academic Press, 1987.

36. Wu MC, Eriksson S. Lung function, smoking and survival in severe alpha-1 antitrypsin deficiency, PiZZ. J Clin Epidemiol 1988;41:1157–65.

37. Seersholm N, Kok-Jensen A, Dirksen A. Decline in FEV1 among patients with severe hereditary alpha-1 antitrypsin deficiency type PiZ. Am J Respir Crit Care Med 1995;152:1922–25.

38. Seersholm N, Wencker M, Banik N, et al. Does alpha-1 antitrypsin augmentation therapy slow the annual decline in FEV1 in patients with severe hereditary alpha-1 antitrypsin deficiency? Eur Respir J 1997;10:2260–63.

39. Piitulainen E, Eriksson S. Decline in FEV1 related to smoking status in individuals with severe alpha-1 antitrypsin deficiency (PiZZ). Eur Respir J 1999;13:247–51.

Autoimmune Liver Disease

Andrea A. Gossard, MS, CNP,
and Keith D. Lindor, MD

BACKGROUND

Autoimmune liver disease encompasses several disorders. Included in this category are primary sclerosing cholangitis (PSC), primary biliary cirrhosis (PBC), and autoimmune hepatitis (AIH). There are also several "overlap syndromes" which encompass two of these diseases in combination. In this chapter, we will describe these liver conditions, including the typical clinical presentation, the diagnostic criteria, management, and potential complications. We will also discuss briefly the role of orthotopic liver transplantation.

PRIMARY SCLEROSING CHOLANGITIS

Primary sclerosing cholangitis (PSC) is a chronic, cholestatic liver disease of unknown etiology. Several potential causes have been described. These include disordered immunoregulation; which may involve altered T-cell subsets, abnormal T-cell suppressor function, circulating immune complexes, and/or abnormal complement levels; infections and bacterial products; or portal bacteremia. The disease leads to diffuse inflammation and fibrosis of the biliary tree which ultimately causes biliary cirrhosis and portal hypertension.[1,2,3]

Clinical Presentation

Clinically, patients with PSC will often present with an incidental finding of elevated liver tests in a cholestatic profile (elevated alkaline phosphatase). The majority (70%) of patients will also have inflammatory bowel disease (IBD), typically chronic ulcerative colitis. Fifteen to 44% of patients may be entirely asymptomatic. Others may present with symptoms of cholestasis such as fatigue, jaundice, hyperpigmentation, or pruritus (Table 10.1).[4] A subset may even have evidence of cholangiocarcinoma at the time of initial presentation.

Table 10.1. Clinical Presentation of PSC

Symptoms	%
Asymptomatic	15–44
Fatigue	75
Pruritus	70
Jaundice	30–69
Hepatomegaly	34–62
Abdominal pain	16–37
Weight loss	10–34
Splenomegaly	30
Ascending cholangitis	5–28
Hyperpigmentation	25
Variceal bleeding	2–14
Ascites	2–10

Table 10.2. Autoantibodies in PSC

p-ANCA	80%
Antimitochondrial antibody	< 2%
Antinuclear antibody	50–60%
Smooth muscle antibody	35%

Diagnosis

The diagnosis of PSC is typically made in the setting of liver tests elevated in a cholestatic profile and an abnormal cholangiogram. Autoantibodies may also be present (Table 10.2). Endoscopic retrograde cholangiopancreatography (ERCP) has been the preferred method of imaging the bile ducts but is rapidly being replaced by magnetic resonance (MR) cholangiography. Computed tomographic (CT) cholangiography is also being evaluated as a non-invasive alternative (Figure 10.1).

In the setting of PSC, the bile ducts demonstrate a "beaded" appearance when imaged. Approximately 5% of patients with cholestatic changes will have a normal appearing biliary tree but have changes histologically that are consistent with PSC. This condition has been termed small-duct PSC. It may be that some of these patients will eventually develop disease of the larger bile ducts as well, but this progression is unclear.[5] A liver biopsy can be helpful in confirming the diagnosis and in providing prognostic information, but is not necessary in all cases. Typical histological features include periductal fibrosis, a paucity of bile ducts, and variable degrees of fibrosis encasing the intralobular bile duct ("onion skin" fibrosis). These changes are classified into stages as seen in Table 10.3.

Complications of PSC

Biliary obstruction may develop in the setting of PSC and the etiology must be determined. Causes include dominant biliary strictures, impacted stones, or the

Table 10.3. Histological Findings in PSC

Stage 1	Portal stage: portal inflammation or bile duct inflammation, periductal fibrosis, atrophy
Stage 2	Periportal stage: portal and periportal fibrosis
Stage 3	Bridging fibrous septa
Stage 4	Cirrhosis

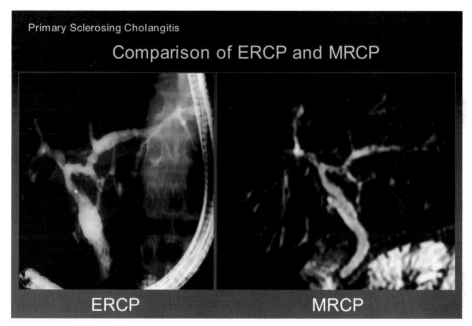

Figure 10.1. ERCP vs MRCP.

development of cholangiocarcinoma. Biopsies and cytology studies have been insensitive for detecting malignancies within strictures. Digital image analysis (DIA) and fluorescent in situ hybridization (FISH) are more sensitive but may lack specificity. Marked elevations of CA 19–9 in the setting of a dominant stricture is concerning for cholangiocarcinoma.

Cholangiocarcinoma is the most feared outcome of PSC. The lifetime risk is in the range of 7–15% and may be higher in smokers and those patients with IBD.[6] The incidence is approximately 0.5–1.0 % per year (Figure 10.2). These patients are also at an increased risk for cancers of the pancreas, liver and colon (if they have colitis). Surgery has not provided a very favorable outcome for those patients who develop a cholangiocarcinoma. Photodynamic therapy has offered some survival advantage, but is not curative. A few highly selective patients have had long-term success with liver transplantation, as well.

In advanced disease, fat-soluble vitamin deficiencies can occur (Table 10.4) and supplementation may be indicated. Metabolic bone disease can also be an issue in PSC.[7,8] as with other cholestatic liver diseases such as primary biliary cirrhosis. Bisphosphonates have been helpful in patients with cholestasis-induced osteoporosis and should be considered. In patients with evidence of esophageal varices, oral administration of bisphosphonates is contraindicated.

Table 10.4. Fat Soluble Vitamin Deficiencies in PSC

Vitamin Deficiency	
A	40%
D	14%
E	2%
K	Unknown

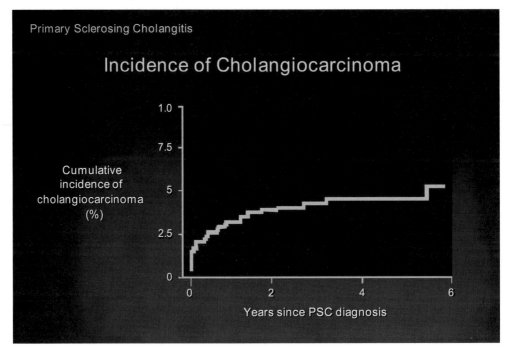

Figure 10.2. Incidence of cholangiocarcinoma in PSC.

Management

Surgical therapy for primary sclerosing cholangitis is seldom used. Endoscopic management of strictures is necessary at times and may be accomplished with balloon dilatation or stenting of the bile ducts.[9] Long-term stenting is not recommended due to stent obstruction or potential migration of the stent and the associated risk of biliary obstruction.

There is no approved medical therapy for PSC. Multiple agents have been studied with largely negative results (Table 10.5). Preliminary studies have suggested potential benefit with ursodeoxycholic acid at doses of 28–30 mg/kg/day and therefore, further investigation is currently underway.[10,11]

Liver transplantation has an excellent outcome for patients with PSC with a one-year survival rate approaching 97% and a five-year survival of 85–88%. These patients are at an increased risk of rejection and infection when compared to patients transplanted for other liver diseases. As with many other liver diseases, the disease can and does recur for a number of patients post-transplantation.[12,13]

Table 10.5. Therapies for PSC

Medical Therapies Tested to Date

Penicillamine	Colchicine	*Mycophenolate Mofetil*
Cyclosporine	Methotrexate	*Silymarin*
Pentoxifylline	Budesonide	*Tacrolimus*
Nicotine	Pirfenidone	*Ursodeoxycholic Acid*
Azathioprine	Etanercept	*(possible benefit)*

Table 10.6. Clinical Features of AMA Negative versus Positive PBC

AMA-Negative vs. AMA-Positive PBC

Clinical Picture	AMA-Negative (n = 17)	AMA-Positive (n = 17)
Female:Male	14:3	14:3
Age at diagnosis (years)	51.1	55.0
Jaundice	3	3
Fatigue	8	7
Pruritus	9	11
Hypothyroidism	3	3
Polyarthralgias	5	3
Sicca Syndrome	3	7
Raynaud's	2	4

In summary, management of the patient with PSC should include cancer surveillance with annual imaging of the liver and biliary system. This can be done with abdominal ultrasound, CT or MRI. In the setting of IBD, colon cancer screening should be done on an annual basis as the concurrent diagnosis with PSC increases the risk of colon cancer.[14] Surveillance biopsies should be obtained of the entire colon to adequately screen for early dysplastic changes. Patients with PSC should also be immunized for hepatitis A and B to decrease the risk of contracting a second liver condition. Periodic monitoring for development of osteoporosis, esophageal varices, and vitamin deficiency is important, particularly in advanced disease. In the event complications such as cholangitis or strictures develop, antibiotics and biliary dilatation should be considered.

PRIMARY BILIARY CIRRHOSIS

Primary biliary cirrhosis (PBC) is a chronic, cholestatic liver disease that affects primarily adult females. In 95% of patients, an antimitochondrial antibody is present in the serum. The demographic features and natural history of AMA negative PBC is no different than that for AMA positive PBC (Table 10.6). The histological findings in AMA negative and AMA positive PBC are also no different.[15] Histologically, the disease is characterized by chronic, nonsuppurative destruction of the interlobular bile ducts leading to fibrosis, cirrhosis, and liver failure.

Multiple case-controlled studies have attempted to ascertain a cause for PBC. Indeed, several case-control investigations have attempted to determine

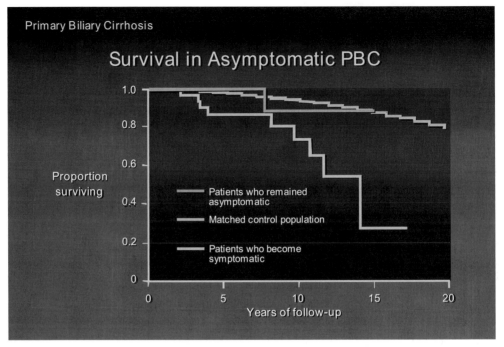

Figure 10.3. Survival in PBC

what exposures may be responsible for the development of PBC in susceptible hosts.[16] The major potential risk factors observed in patients with PBC versus unaffected controls are female sex, cigarette smoking, inflammatory diseases of the skin and thyroid, history of urinary tract infection, previous tonsillectomy, and genetic predisposition.[17]

The natural history of PBC has been reasonably well described. In a study by Springer et al.,[18] 91 asymptomatic patients were followed for a period of five years. During that time, a total of 36% of the patients became symptomatic with 11% progressing to death or liver transplantation. Median survival from the onset of disease for the entire cohort was 14 years. Patient survival was less than that predicted for age and gender matched controls ($p < 0.05$). No individual clinical, histologic, or biochemical feature at the time of presentation could distinguish those who became symptomatic from those who remained symptom free (Figure 10.3).

Clinical Presentation

Asymptomatic cholestasis as an incidental finding during blood work is the presentation for 40–60% of patients with PBC. Others may present with fatigue, pruritus, sicca syndrome, hepatosplenomegaly, jaundice, or more rarely, xanthelasma. Fatigue is the most common complaint and is present in up to 80% of symptomatic patients.[19] The etiology of fatigue is not well understood so therapeutic options are limited. There is no association between level of fatigue and histological stage or bilirubin level. Pruritus is also relatively common, reported in 25–70% of PBC patients. It may have an insidious onset and can be intractable. The etiology is unknown. There is no association between pruritus and age, sex,

Table 10.7. Extrahepatic Autoimmune Diseases

Sicca syndrome	70%
Thyroid disease	40%
Arthritis	20%
Scleroderma	15%
Raynaud's phenomenon	10%
CREST syndrome	5%

histological stage, and Mayo Risk Score.[20] Sicca syndrome is present in up to 70% of patients with PBC. Keratoconjunctivitis and xerostomia are the most common symptoms in patients with sicca syndrome. The majority of patients do not satisfy the criteria for Sjogrens syndrome, however. Xanthomata can occur in 15–50% of patients and tend to involve the extensor tendon surfaces. Xanthelasma tends to affect the eye lids. These findings are associated with elevated serum cholesterol levels.

As seen in Table 10.7, the most common extrahepatic autoimmune disease in association with PBC is keratoconjunctivitis sicca.[21] Hypothyroidism is seen in up to 40% of patients and often predates the diagnosis of PBC. Inflammatory arthritis is less well defined as degenerative joint disease is often observed. Localized or systemic scleroderma is seen in up to 20% of patients.

Diagnosis

Most patients with PBC will present with a three- to four-fold elevation of the alkaline phosphatase. The serum ALT and AST levels may also be elevated, but are typically less than 200 U/L. If they are higher than this, further investigation into a concurrent autoimmune hepatitis or drug-induced liver disease should be considered. Bilirubin elevations are more common in advanced stage disease. Cholesterol elevations are present in up to 85% of patients but are not thought to be atherogenic in this setting.

As mentioned previously, 90–95% of patients will have the anti-mitochondrial antibody (AMA) in serum. There is a subset of patients with PBC who do not have this antibody, however. There seems to be no difference in clinical presentation, natural history, and prognosis when compared to AMA positive patients. Response to therapy and outcome following liver transplantation also seems similar.[22]

The need for liver biopsy in AMA positive patients with liver tests elevated in a cholestatic profile remains unclear. In a study of 156 patients with positive AMA tests, a diagnosis was established by biopsy in 131 (85%) of the patients.[23] The histologic diagnosis was associated with a cholestatic biochemical profile (alkaline phosphatase $>1.5 \times$ upper limit of normal (ULN), AST $< 5 \times$ ULN) in 112 of the 131 patients 85.5%. The combination of alkaline phosphatase $>1.5 \times$ ULN and AST $<5 \times$ ULN yielded a 98.2% positive predictive value of PBC diagnosis on liver biopsy in AMA positive subjects. Therefore, the use of liver biopsy would be more beneficial to establish the diagnosis of PBC in only a minority of AMA positive patients with an alkaline phosphatase of $<1.5 \times$ ULN and

Table 10.8. Histologic Stages for PBC

	Ludwig, 1984	Scheuer, 1967
Stage 1	Portal inflammation	Florid duct lesion
Stage 2	Periportal inflammation	Ductular proliferation
Stage 3	Bridging fibrosis, septa or necrosis	Bridging fibrosis, loss of ducts
Stage 4	Cirrhosis	Cirrhosis

an AST of > 5 × ULN. Two histological scoring systems have been developed for the grading and staging of PBC (Table 10.8). Both the Ludwig[24] and the Scheuer[25] classification systems employ an ordinal measurement scale to describe advancing degree or stage of fibrosis. These systems remain in use today. Stage I is associated with portal tract inflammation from predominantly lymphoplasmacytic infiltrates. Focal duct obliteration with granuloma formation has been termed the "florid duct lesion" and is nearly pathognomonic for PBC when present. Stage II PBC is consistent with the descriptions of periportal hepatitis by Ludwig or ductular proliferation by Scheuer. Eosinophils may also be present within the inflammatory reaction. The histologic findings of granulomas, cholangitis, and ductular proliferation are most commonly observed in stage II disease. Stage III disease is characterized by septal or bridging fibrosis. Ductopenia, as evidenced by the loss of >50% of the interlobular bile ducts, becomes more common resulting in cholestasis with periportal and paraseptal hepatocytes. Stage IV disease in both classifications is consistent with biliary cirrhosis. Nodular regeneration in addition to the features of stage III disease are observed with a "garland" shaped appearance that is consistent with advanced PBC.

Complications of PBC

Metabolic bone disease in PBC is usually related to osteoporosis rather than osteomalacia (defective bone mineralization). Potential etiologies of osteopenia include defective osteoblast activity in pre-menopausal women, polymorphisms in vitamin D metabolism which predispose a patient to bone disease, cigarette smoking which reduces serum vitamin D levels, or malabsorption of vitamin D in advanced cholestasis. Approximately 30% of patients with PBC have osteopenia and 11% have osteoporosis. Osteoporosis is more common in late stage disease.[26]

Portal hypertension most often occurs in the setting of cirrhotic-stage PBC. Complications include variceal bleeding, ascites, and hepatic encephalopathy. In certain cases, the development of portal hypertension and ascites may occur with presinusoidal fibrosis in the absence of cirrhosis.[27] Serum platelet level, bilirubin, and platelet count are independent predictors of esophageal varices. The clinical outcome is similar to that of other parenchymal liver diseases.

In one study comparing patients with PBC and chronic hepatitis C, a total of 4% of patients developed hepatocellular carcinoma (HCC).[28] All had stage IV disease. The incidence in the 45 patients with late stages of disease (stages III–IV) was 11.1%, similar to that found in HCV-related cirrhosis (15%). The probability of developing HCC was significantly higher in patients with HCV-related cirrhosis than in PBC patients overall (p = 0.001) but was similar in patients with HCV related cirrhosis and in patients with stages III–IV PBC.

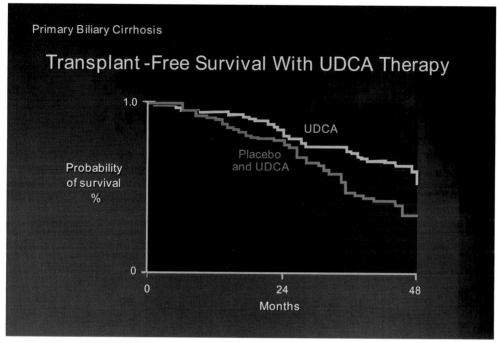

Figure 10.4. PBC – Survival with UDCA therapy

Management

The recommended long-term management of PBC includes a clinical visit once a year with laboratory assessment of cholestasis and hepatic synthetic function. Patients with advanced liver disease should have serum liver enzyme tests more frequently (every 3–6 months). In cirrhotic patients, cross sectional abdominal imaging should be performed every two to three years to screen for the development of cirrhotic changes. Cross-sectional imaging of the abdomen has been recommended every year to screen for the development of hepatocellular carcinoma. Bone mineral density testing at the time of diagnosis and after two years if therapy is initiated, or if the patient is post-menopausal is also recommended.[29] In patients with jaundice (total bilirubin > 2.5 mg/dL), serum fat-soluble vitamin levels should be obtained with oral replacement of deficient states, if found.[30] Upper endoscopy to screen for esophageal varices should be performed every two years in patients with known cirrhosis, clinical evidence of cirrhosis, or a Mayo risk score of >4.1.

A number of medical therapies to halt disease progression have been tested in PBC. The only medical therapy with proven efficacy to delay progression of disease, as well as extend transplant-free survival is ursodeoxycholic acid (UDCA).[31] The mechanism of action for UDCA therapy in PBC is multifactorial. In addition to promoting endogenous bile acid secretion, there is evidence to suggest that UDCA is associated with membrane stabilization, reduced aberrant HLA type I expression on hepatocytes, and decreased cytokine production. The inhibition of apoptosis and mitochondrial dysfunction caused by exposure to hydrophobic bile acids are also prevented by UDCA. In a large placebo-controlled study (Figure 10.4), UDCA therapy was associated with an increased transplant-free survival at four years (p = 0.04).[32] The positive effects of UDCA on disease progression and survival free of liver transplantation were questioned in a recent meta-analysis by Goulis.[33] By combining eight placebo-controlled trials involving 1,114 patients, no differences in death or the need for liver transplantation between UDCA and placebo-treated patients was reported. The majority of identified studies, however, had follow-up periods of two years or less. A number of trials also used doses of UDCA at less than 13 mg/kg/day. With the exclusion of these trials, a 32% risk reduction in death or need for liver transplantation with UDCA compared to placebo remains present.[34]

Among patients experiencing a suboptimal response to UDCA, there are a number of causes that must be excluded. In addition to medication noncompliance or inappropriate dosing, the concomitant use of cholestyramine for pruritus may result in a lack of UDCA absorption caused by resin binding. The diagnoses of uncontrolled hypothyroidism and celiac disease must be eliminated as causes of elevated serum hepatic biochemistries. Finally, a lack of complete response to UDCA may suggest the presence of true overlap syndrome with autoimmune hepatitis.

PBC is becoming a less frequent indication for liver transplantation in the United States. Patient and graft survival rates from liver transplantation are reported to approach 92% and 85% at one-year and five-year intervals, respectively. Previously considered a controversial topic, the recurrence of PBC following liver transplantation has now been demonstrated. The estimated rate of recurrent PBC may be as high as 30% at 10 years with prospective follow-up. Serum AMA status appears to be independent of recurrence risk. Recent published studies document a shorter time to recurrence with tacrolimus rather than cyclosporine as primary immunosuppression.[35] No information is available regarding the efficacy of UDCA therapy in halting disease progression from early stage recurrent PBC. Re-transplantation for recurrent PBC is uncommon.

AUTOIMMUNE HEPATITIS

Autoimmune hepatitis is an intermittently progressive liver disease characterized by hypergammaglobulinemia, autoantibodies, predominately periportal hepatitis and a usually favorable response to corticosteroid therapy. In contrast to viral hepatitis, a relatively common disease present in >1% of the population in many countries, autoimmune hepatitis has a point prevalence of <20 per 100,000 (<0.02%) in Northern Europeans. Moreover, while highly specific screening and confirmatory tests for viral hepatitis are now available, there are no pathognomonic markers for autoimmune hepatitis. Nevertheless, effective therapy for autoimmune hepatitis was reported in randomized controlled trials published in the early 1970s. However, in contrast to the large number of ongoing, large, multi-center randomized controlled trials assessing prospective new therapies for viral hepatitis, no new therapies for autoimmune hepatitis have been tested in randomized controlled trials during the past three decades.

In early clinical trials such as a study reported by Kirk et al. in *Gut* in 1980,[36] symptomatic autoimmune hepatitis patients were observed to have approximately a 50% three- to five-year mortality rate in the absence of therapy. In contrast to a >75% ten-year mortality rate among untreated, symptomatic

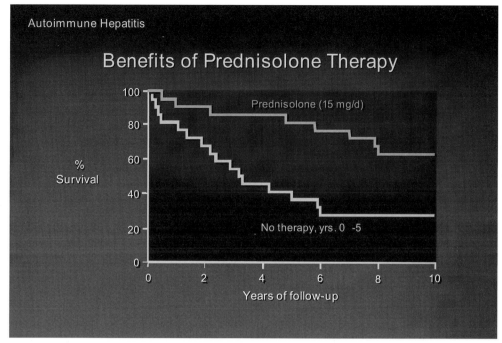

Figure 10.5. Treatment of AIH with prednisolone.

autoimmune hepatitis patients, corticosteroid therapy significantly improves both short-term and long-term survival (Figure 10.5).

Clinical Presentation

The typical patient with autoimmune hepatitis is a middle-aged or teen-aged female without environmental risk factors for liver disease who presents with insidious onset of fatigue, arthralgias, myalgias, oligomenorrhea, and then often develops jaundice. Seventy percent of patients with AIH are female, and 50% are less than 40 years of age.[37,38] Laboratory testing reveals evidence of hepatocellular injury, hypergammaglobulinemia, and usually the presence of both anti-nuclear and anti-smooth muscle antibodies. Liver histology is marked by the presence of interface hepatitis and a lymphoplasmacytic infiltrate and, when corticosteroid therapy is started, a gratifying, steady resolution of biochemical and histological abnormalities ensues. Although "typical" female patients with autoimmune hepatitis are usually readily identified, the disease also may present in men, young children, or in the elderly. Conventional autoantibodies may to be absent or only transiently present. In addition, despite use of terms such as "lupoid hepatitis" to describe this disease, there is minimal clinical overlap between ANA positive, type I autoimmune hepatitis and systemic lupus erythematosus. Although >80% of autoimmune hepatitis patients eventually exhibit complete remission on immunosuppressive therapy, complete histological remission usually requires one to three years of continuous therapy and some patients fail to respond to conventional corticosteroid based regimens. Finally, it should be noted that up to 40% of patients with autoimmune hepatitis have an acute presentation and in some cases exhibit no clinical or histological features of chronic liver disease.

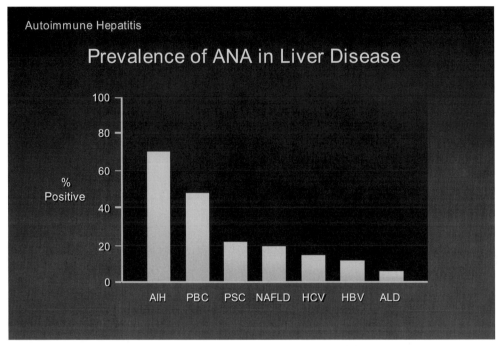

Figure 10.6. Prevalence of ANA in liver disease.

Sub-types of autoimmune hepatitis have been proposed based on differences in autoantibody markers and clinical features.[39] The most common form is type 1 autoimmune hepatitis characterized by the presence of ANA and SMA. Less common is the type 2 form characterized by the presence of LKM-1 autoantibodies but absence of ANA, SMA, or p-ANCA. Type 2 disease presents predominately in children, may be associated with low IgA levels with or without elevations of IgG and more commonly progresses to cirrhosis early in the course of the disease. A type 3 AIH, characterized by the presence of SLA autoantibodies in the absence of ANA, SMA, or LKM-1 autoantibodies, has been proposed, but this syndrome appears indistinguishable from Type 1 AIH in all other clinical and laboratory features.

Although ANA are present in 70% of AIH patients and thus are the most consistent serological marker of this disease, as a single test, ANA testing lacks specificity for AIH as ANA are also present in half of patients with primary biliary cirrhosis, at least a quarter of patients with primary sclerosing cholangitis and in 5–20% of patients with the most common causes of liver disease such as non-alcoholic liver disease, chronic hepatitis C, chronic hepatitis B, and alcoholic liver disease (Figure 10.6).

Diagnosis

The diagnosis of AIH should be considered in patients with hepatitis or cirrhosis of uncertain etiology. Because of their lack of specificity, ANA, SMA, and LKM-1 autoantibody tests should not be used as screening tests, but rather as markers supportive of the diagnosis of autoimmune liver disease in patients with the constellation of findings that define this disease. Because there are no pathognomonic markers for AIH, this diagnosis is often a "work in progress" in which the clinician must repeatedly reconsider factors that favor or argue against AIH as diagnostic evaluations and therapy progresses. The diagnosis of autoimmune hepatitis requires the presence of characteristic features and the exclusion of other diseases that may resemble AIH. Although not all cases are straightforward, typical cases of definite AIH present with prominently elevated aminotransferases and IgG levels, the presence of one or more of the conventional autoantibody markers of AIH and a liver biopsy showing interface hepatitis with no biliary lesions, granulomas, or prominent steatosis. Tests for genetic and viral liver disease are negative and there is no history of drug-, alcohol-, or toxin-induced liver injury.

An essential component in the evaluation of patients for AIH is assessment of liver histology. The International Autoimmune Hepatitis Group Scoring System assigns positive points for typical histological features such as interface hepatitis, lymphoplasmacytic infiltrates, and rosetting of liver cells. However, negative points are assigned for the absence of all of these AIH features or for the presence of biliary lesions or other changes such as granulomas or significant steatosis that are more typical of other types of inflammatory liver diseases. Following institution of corticosteroid therapy, the International Autoimmune Hepatitis Group Scoring System assigns additional positive points for two typical features of this disease: a complete remission on therapy and a remission followed by relapse after discontinuation of therapy. Following complete historical, laboratory and histological evaluation, a score of >15 indicates definite AIH whereas a score of 10–15 indicates probable AIH. After responses to therapy are considered, a score of > 17 indicates definite AIH and a score of 12–17 suggests probable AIH (Table 10.9).

Management

Based on the results of randomized controlled trials of therapy in symptomatic patients and the assessment of the natural history of disease in AIH patients with different degrees of biochemical and/or histological abnormalities, there is a general consensus that symptomatic AIH patients with AST ≥ 10-fold elevated, or AST ≥ five-fold elevated plus gamma globulins ≥ two-fold elevated or bridging necrosis on liver biopsy should be treated whereas asymptomatic patients with only inactive cirrhosis or portal hepatitis (i.e., no interface hepatitis) on liver biopsy should not. In patients with intermediate indications for therapy, clinical judgment must be used in making therapeutic decisions. In the randomized, controlled clinical trial conducted at the Mayo Clinic and reported initially by Soloway, in 1972,[40] varying combinations of prednisone and azathioprine therapy were assessed. The combination regimen using intermediate doses of prednisone and azathioprine was found to be equal in efficacy to a regimen using a higher dose or prednisone alone whereas azathioprine alone was found to have a high failure rate in preventing progression of AIH. Based on the results of this, two standard regimens for initial therapy of AIH are now recommended.[41] The first is a monotherapy regimen consisting of prednisone 60 mg/d for the first week, and then 40 mg/d during week 2, 30 mg/d for weeks 3 and 4 and then 20 mg per day until remission is achieved. The second standard regimen for

Table 10.9. AIH Classification

	Patient History	
	Favor AIH (points)	Favor Other Diagnosis (points)
Gender	Female (+2)	Male (0)
Alcohol	<25 g/d (+2)	>60 g/d (−2)
Hepatotoxic drugs	None (+1)	Present (−4)
Other autoimmune diseases	Present (+2)	None (0)
	Biochemistries	
Alkaline phosphatase elevations: ALT elevation	<1.5 (+2)	>3.0 (−2)
Serum globulins, γ globulin or IgG	>2x normal (+3) >1.5–2x normal (+2) >1–1.5x normal (+1)	Normal (0)
	Serologies	
ANA, SMA, or LKM-1	>1:80 (+3) 1:80 (+2) 1:40 (+1)	<1:40 (0)
AMA	Negative (0)	Positive (−4)
Hepatitis markers	Negative (+3)	Positive (−3)
Other autoantibodies	Present (+2)	Absent (0)
HLA-DRS or DR4	Present (+1)	Absent (0)
	Histology	
Interface Hepatitis	+3	
Lymphoplasmacytic infiltrate	+1	
Rosetting of liver cells	+1	
None of the above		−5
Biliary changes		−3
Other changes		−3
	Hepatitis Group Score	
	Score	Interpretation
Pre-therapy	>15	Definite AIH
	10–15	Probably AIH
Post-therapy	>17	Definite AIH
	12–17	Probably AIH

initial therapy of AIH is a combination approach using 50% of the dose of prednisone used in the monotherapy regimen in combination with 50 mg/d of azathioprine (Table 10.10).

Long term follow-up of patients receiving prednisone monotherapy versus prednisone and azathioprine combination therapy indicates that the two regimens achieve similar efficacy but are associated with different side effect profiles. Corticosteroid side effects are especially common in patients with AIH. For most patients and especially for patients already at risk for osteoporosis, diabetes, obesity, and/or hypertension, the combination regimen is preferred because of the steroid sparing benefits of azathioprine. However, in patients with

Table 10.10. Autoimmune Hepatitis Therapy

Interval	Monotherapy Prednisone mg/d	Combination Therapy Prednisone mg/d	Azathioprine mg/d
Week 1	60	30	50
Week 2	40	20	50
Week 3	30	15	50
Week 4	30	15	50
Daily until endpoint	20	10	50

severe cytopenias, known thiopurine methyltransferase deficiency, or azathioprine intolerance or with concerns about the teratogenic or oncogenic potential of azathioprine, prednisone monotherapy may be preferred.

Following selection of the initial therapeutic regimen, therapy should be continued until complete remission is achieved. Sixty-five percent of patients with AIH enter remission within 18 months of therapy.[37,42] Complete remission includes disappearance of symptoms, normalization of serum bilirubin and γ-globulins, decrease of AST and ALT to levels $\leq$ two-fold the upper limit of normal and resolution of interface hepatitis. It is important to understand that on average histological remission lags biochemical remission by approximately six months.

Once an in initial complete remission is achieved, corticosteroids can be tapered and eventually discontinued. Azathioprine may also be discontinued. However, patients must be monitored closely as the majority will experience a relapse of AIH requiring re-institution of therapy.

A number of studies indicate that when follow-up liver biopsies are performed following therapy of AIH, only a minority of patients with biochemical responses will exhibit normal histology and only in this sub-group is short-term risk of relapse low.[43,44] In contrast, the majority of treated AIH patients exhibit some residual interface hepatitis or the presence of cirrhosis. These histological features are associated with an approximately 75% risk of relapse within 1–3 years of follow-up. Of note, a recent study has suggested that the presence of residual portal plasma cells alone, in the presence or absence of interface hepatitis or cirrhosis is associated with a 90% risk of relapse following discontinuation of therapy.

Because of the relapsing nature of AIH, most patients require maintenance therapy. Low dose prednisone alone, prednisone in combination with 50 mg/d of azathioprine, or higher doses of azathioprine alone are effective in maintaining remission in the majority of patients. All patients receiving chronic corticosteroid therapy should be placed on supplemental calcium and vitamin D and monitored for development of hypertension, diabetes, ophthalmologic, or bone disease complications. Those on azathioprine should be monitored for myelosuppression.

In patients who fail to respond to conventional corticosteroid or corticosteroid and azathioprine regimens, higher doses of prednisone or prednisolone monotherapy, or prednis(ol)one plus azathioprine combination therapy may be tried. In patients who are either intolerant of or nonresponsive to conventional immunosuppressive regimens, mycophenolate mofetil, or calcineurin

Table 10.11. Diagnostic Criteria for Overlap Syndromes

	AIH	PBC	PSC
Symptoms	Malaise Jaundice	Fatigue Pruritus	Fatigue Pruritus
Asymptomatic	Occasionally	Often	Often
Gender	Female > Male	Female > Male	Female > Male
Biochemistry	ALT	ALP	ALP and/or GGT
Immunoglobulins	IgG	IgM	IgM/IgG
Autoantibodies	SMA/anti LKM1	AMA	None specific
ERC/MRC	Overlap PSC	Normal	Diagnostic Hallmark

inhibitor regimes as detailed have been reported to be effective in small series of patients.[45,46]

Liver transplantation is effective for AIH patients who either fail to respond to therapy or deteriorate due to complications of cirrhosis that developed before or during initial therapy. There is a modestly increased incidence of acute allograft rejection and a 30–40% disease recurrence rate in these patients, but if anticipated and treated appropriately these complications usually respond well to immunosuppressive therapy. Overall five-year survival rates after liver transplantation for AIH are 80–90%.

OVERLAP SYNDROMES

The term "overlap syndrome" encompasses patients who have two simultaneous autoimmune liver diseases, two sequential autoimmune liver diseases, or one autoimmune liver disease with features of another. In order to recognize the variants of autoimmune liver disease, the differences in symptomatology, demography, and laboratory work up of the three main autoimmune liver diseases need to be appreciated, but at the same time, it must be recognized that there are few specific diagnostic hallmarks for any of theses three disease categories (Table 10.11). The diagnostic criteria of the overlap syndromes have not been standardized nor do these variant forms have confident treatment strategies.[47]

Variants of autoimmune hepatitis include AMA positive patients with no features of PBC, bile duct lesions in otherwise overt AIH, acute AIH plus viral hepatitis, cryptogenic AIH with no autoantibodies, or cholestatic AIH with co-existent silent PSC. There is no long-term data regarding whether patients with AIH and a positive AMA will eventually develop PBC. Patients with PBC with features of AIH do seem to respond to UDCA similarly to those with only features of PBC. Survival at seven years is observed to be similar in these two groups.[48] Patients with AMA negative PBC usually have detectable high-titer ANA, sometimes with an ANA pattern that is described as multiple nuclear dot or rim. These same ANA may also be detected in AMA positive PBC patients.

There are some patients who present with a hepatitis which is not viral, not caused by drugs or toxins (including alcohol), or metabolic disorders such as Wilson's, hemochromatosis, alpha antitrypsin deficiency or NAFLD and that is not associated with any autoantibodies in serum, but hypergammaglobulinemia is present. Such individuals are described as having "cryptogenic" chronic active hepatitis and may also respond well to treatment with corticosteroids.

Autoimmune cholangitis is a term which is not well defined. Patients with absent interlobular bile ducts histologically, a normal biliary tree, and no AMA may be described as having autoimmune cholangitis, small duct PSC or even idiopathic ductopenia. There are patients who have no typical findings of PSC on endoscopic retrograde cholangiopancreatogram (ERCP) or magnetic resonance cholangiogram (MRC) who nevertheless have other features suggesting PSC. Liver histology confirms absent bile ducts. Such patients are frequently given a diagnosis of small duct PSC. It is rare for such patients subsequently to develop large duct disease but is possible. Patients with small duct PSC appear to have a significantly better survival than those with large duct PSC.[49]

Overlap syndromes are not common. The outcomes of patients with overlap syndromes are not well defined and may be dependent on the individual patient's response to empiric therapy. Continued monitoring of these patients with regular blood work and cross-sectional imaging is important.

SUMMARY

Autoimmune liver diseases are not uncommon. It is important to recognize these diseases and the differences between the various presentations. Also, it is important to appreciate the potential for overlap conditions to occur. The natural history of each of these diseases is different. In addition, the presence of overlap syndromes leads to further variability.

Progression to advanced stage liver disease in each of the diseases increases the risk of complications such as portal hypertension and esophageal varices, as well as malignancy, including hepatocellular cancer and cholangiocarcinoma. Treatment approaches for autoimmune liver disease vary, and may involve multiple therapies particularly in the setting of overlap syndromes. Regular monitoring of the autoimmune liver disease patient with blood work and imaging studies is recommended.

REFERENCES

1. Angulo P and Lindor KD. Primary sclerosing cholangitis. *Hepatol* 1999;30(1):325–32.
2. Angulo P and Lindor KD. Primary biliary cirrhosis and primary sclerosing cholangitis. *Clin Liver Dis*, 1999;3(3):529–70.
3. Mendes F and Lindor KD. Primary sclerosing cholangitis. *Clin Liver Dis*, 2004;8(1):195–211.
4. Vierling, J.M. In: Zakim & Boyer, eds. *Hepatology*, 2003;1221.
5. Broome U, Glaumann H, Lindstom E, Loof L, Almer S, Prytz H, Sandberg-Gertzen H, Lindgren S, Fork FT, Jarnerot G, and Olsson R. Natural history and outcome in 32 Swedish patients with small duct primary sclerosing cholangitis. *J Hepatol*, 2002;36:586–589.
6. Burak, K, Angulo, P, Pasha, TM, Egan, K, Petz, J, and Lindor KD. Incidence and risk factors for cholangiocarcinoma in primary sclerosing cholangitis. *Am J Gastroenterol*, 2004;99(3):523–6.
7. Hay, JE. The metabolic bone disease of primary sclerosing cholangitis. *Hepatol*, 1991;14(2):257–261.

8. Angulo P, Therneau TM, Jorgensen R, DeSotel CK, Egan KS, Dickson ER, Hay JE, and Lindor KD. Bone disease in patients with primary sclerosing cholangitis: prevalence, severity and prediction of progression. *J Hepatol*, 1998;29(5):729–735.

9. Ponsioen C, Lam K, van Milligen de Wit AW, Huibregtse K, and Tytgat GN. Four year experience with short term stenting in primary sclerosing cholangitis. *Am J Gastroenterol*, 1999;94:2403–2407.

10. Harnois D, Angulo P, Jorgensen RA, LaRusso NF, and Lindor KD. High-dose ursodeoxycholic acid as a therapy for patients with primary sclerosing cholangitis. *Am J Gastroentero*, 2001;96:1558–1562.

11. Mitchell SA, Bansi DS, Hunt N, Von Bergmann K, Fleming KA, and Chapman RW. A preliminary trial of high-dose ursodeoxycholic acid in primary sclerosing cholangitis. *Gastroenterology*, 2001;121:900–907.

12. Faust, TW. Recurrent primary biliary cirrhosis, primary sclerosing cholangitis, and autoimmune hepatitis after transplantation. *Semin Liver Dis*, 2000;20:481–495.

13. Graziadei IW, Wiesner RH, Batts KP, Marotta PJ, LaRusso NF, Porayk MK, Hay JE, Gores GJ, Charlton MR, Ludwig J, Poterucha JJ, Steers JL, and Krom RA. Recurrence of primary sclerosing cholangitis following liver transplantation. *Hepatol*, 1999;29:1050–1056.

14. Broome U, Lofberg R, Veress B, and Ericksson LS. Primary sclerosing cholangitis and ulcerative colitis: evidence for increased neoplastic potential. *Hepatol*, 1995;22:1404–1408.

15. Michieletti P, Wanless IR, Katz A, Scheuer PH, Yeaman SJ, Bassendine MF, Palmer JM, and Heathcote EJ. *Gut*, 1994;35:260.

16. Gershwin ME. The natural history of primary biliary cirrhosis: of genes and cooperation. *J Hepatol*, 2001;35:412–415.

17. Parikh-Patel A, Gold EB, Worman H, Krivy KE, and Gershwin ME. Risk factors for primary biliary cirrhosis in a cohort of patients from the United States. *Hepatol*, 2001;33:16–21.

18. Springer J, Cauch-Dudek K, O'Rourke K, Wanless IR, and Heathcote EJ. Asymptomatic primary biliary cirrhosis: a study of its natural history and prognosis. *Am J Gastroenterol*, 1999; 47–53.

19. Cauch-Dudek K, Abbey S, Stewart DE, and Heathcote EJ. Fatigue in primary biliary cirrhosis. *Gut*, 1998;43:705–710.

20. Talwalker JA, Souto E, Jorgensen RA, and Lindor KD. Natural history of pruritus in primary biliary cirrhosis. *Clin Gastro and Hepatol*, 2003;1(4):297–302.

21. Talwalkar JA, Lindor KD. in Zakim and Boyer, eds. *Hepatology*, 2005.

22. Kim WR, Poterucha JJ, Jorgensen RA, Batts KP, Homburger HA, Dickson ER, Krom RA, and Wiesner RH. Does antimitochondrial antibody status affect response to treatment in patients with primary biliary cirrhosis? Outcomes of ursodeoxycholic acid therapy and liver transplantation. *Hepatology*, 1997;26(1):22–6.

23. Zein CO, Angulo P, and Lindor KD. When is liver biopsy needed in the diagnosis of primary biliary cirrhosis? *Clin Gastroenterol Hepatol*, 2003;1(2):89–95.

24. Ludwig J, Czaja A, Dickson ER, La Russo NF, Wiesner RH. Manifestations of nonsuppurative cholangitis in chronic hepatobiliary diseases: morphologic spectrum, clinical correlations and terminology. *Liver*, 1984;4:105.

25. Scheuer PJ. Primary biliary cirrhosis. *Proc R Soc Med*, 1967;60:1257–1260.

26. Menon KVN, Angulo P, Weston S, Dickson ER, and Lindor KD. Bone disease in primary biliary cirrhosis: independent indicators and rate of progression. *J Hepatol*, 2001;35:316–323.

27. Leuschner U. Primary biliary cirrhosis–presentation and diagnosis. *Clin Liver Dis*, 2003;7:741–58.

28. Caballeria L, Pares A, Castells A, Gines A, Bru C, and Rodes J. Hepatocellular carcinoma in primary biliary cirrhosis: similar incidence to that in hepatitis C virus-related cirrhosis. *Am J Gastroenterol*, 2001;96(4):1160–3.

29. Lindor, KD. Management of osteopenia of liver disease with special emphasis on primary biliary cirrhosis. *Semin Liver Dis*, 1993;13(4);367–373.

30. Jorgensen RA, Lindor KD, Sartin JS, LaRusso NF, and Wiesner RH. Serum lipid and fat-soluble vitamin levels in primary sclerosing cholangitis. *J Clin Gastroenterol*, 1995;20(3)215–9.

31. Angulo P, Batts KP, Therneau TM, Jorgensen RA, Dickson ER, and Lindor KD. Long-term ursodeoxycholic acid delays histological progression in primary biliary cirrhosis. *Hepatol*, 1999;29(3):644–647.

32. Lindor KD, Therneau TM, Jorgensen RA, Malinchoc M, Dickson ER. Effects of ursodeoxycholic acid on survival in patients with primary biliary cirrhosis. *Gastroenterology*, 1996;110(5):1515–8.

33. Goulis J, Leandro G, and Burroughs AK. Randomised controlled trials of urso-deoxycholic-acid therapy for primary biliary cirrhosis: a meta-analysis. *Lancet 25*, 1999;354(9184):1053–60.

34. Poupon RE. Ursodeoxycholic acid for primary biliary cirrhosis: lessons from the past-issues for the future. *J Hepatol*, 2000;32:689.

35. Neuberger J. Recurrent primary biliary cirrhosis. *Liver Transplantation*, 2003;9(6):539–46.

36. Kirk AP, Jain S, Pocock S, Thomas HC and Sherlock S. Late results of the Royal Free Hospital prospective controlled trial of prednisolone therapy in hepatitis B surface antigen negative chronic active hepatitis. *Gut*, 1980; 21:78.

37. Cjaza AJ and Freese DK. Diagnosis and treatment of autoimmune hepatitis. *Hepatology*, 2002;36:479–497.

38. Ben-Ari Z. and Cjaza AJ. Autoimmune hepatitis and its variant syndromes. *Gut*, 2001;49:589–594.

39. Czaja AJ and Manns MP. The validity and importance of subtypes in autoimmune hepatitis – a point of view. *Am J Gastroenterol*, 1995;90:1206–11.

40. Soloway RD, Summerskill WH, Baggenstoss AH, GEall MG, Gitnick GL, Elveback IR and Schoenfield LJ. *Gastroenterology*, 1972;63:828.

41. AASLD Practice Guidelines, *Hepatology* 2002;36:479.

42. Czaja AJ. Treatment of autoimmune hepatitis. *Semin Liver Dis*, 2002;22,365–377.

43. Czaja AJ, Davis GL, Ludwig J, Taswell HF. Complete resolution of inflammatory activity following corticosteroid treatment of HBsAG-negative chronic active hepatitis. *Hepatology*, 1984;4:622–7.

44. Czaja AJ, Carpenter HA. Histological features associated with relapse after corticosteroid withdrawal in type 1 autoimmune hepatitis. *Liver International*, 2003;23:116.

45. Heneghan MA, and McFarlane Ig. Current and novel immunosuppressive therapy for autoimmne hepatitis. *Hepatology*, 2002;35:7–13.

46. Czaja A. Treatment of autoimmune hepatitis. *Semin Liver Dis*, 2002;22:365–78.

47. Czaja A. The variant forms of autoimmune hepatitis. *Ann Intern Med*, 1996;125:588–598.

48. Joshi S, Cauch-Dudek K, Wanless IR, Lindor KD, Jorgensen R., and Heathcote, EJ. Primary biliary cirrhosis with additional features of autoimmune hepatitis: response to therapy with ursodeoxycholic acid. *Hepatology*, 2002;35(2):409–413.

49. Bjornsson E, Boberg KM, Cullen S, Fleming K, Clausen O, Fausa O, Schrumpf E, and Chapman R. Patients with small duct primary sclerosing cholangitis have a favourable long term prognosis. *Gut*, 2002;51:731–735.

Drug-Induced Liver Disease (DILI)

Julie Polson, MD, and Naga Chalasani, MD

BACKGROUND

Hepatotoxicity is among the most common and feared adverse drug reactions. Television commercials advertising pharmaceuticals warn patients to beware of taking various medications if they have liver disease. Lawyers publicly recruit business from patients or loved ones of patients who may have had a hepatotoxic drug reaction; there were several newspaper ads placed by law firms after troglitazone was removed from the market, for example. Clinicians are wary of prescribing medications described to have potential adverse effects on the liver without frequent monitoring of liver tests or referral to a hepatologist. In fact, hepatotoxicity is the most common single adverse drug reaction leading to drug withdrawal and refusal for FDA approval.[1] For hepatologists and primary care physicians alike, drug hepatotoxicity is a tough clinical problem because it is a diagnosis of exclusion, may be difficult to diagnose, and there is no clear treatment other than drug withdrawal in many cases. From a public health standpoint, the difficulty in studying and predicting hepatotoxic drug reactions in a few patients may prevent thousands from receiving medications that would be beneficial to them. In short, drug-induced liver injury (DILI) is a complicated and often confusing entity that can pose problems for patients and the practitioners who care for them. In this article, we will provide an overview of idiosyncratic DILI with relatively minor focus on acetaminophen hepatotoxicity.

EPIDEMIOLOGY

The true incidence of idiosyncratic DILI is unknown. The difficulty of correctly establishing the diagnosis[2,3] as well as underreporting to regulatory agencies[4,5] makes determining disease frequency problematic. Despite these issues, several recent studies give us a picture of the occurrence of drug hepatotoxicity. Analysis of a Spanish registry over a ten year period beginning in the mid 1990's put population estimates around 3.4 episodes of drug induced liver injury per 100,000 per year, with 1.6 per 100,000 cases per year designated as serious

Table 11.1. Historically Reported Frequency of Idiosyncratic DILI in the United States

	Patient Population Studied	Study Design	Sample Size	Study Period	Proportion with Idiosyncratic DILI
ALF Study Group, unpublished data	Acute liver failure, (adults)	Multiple referral centers	1033	1998–2006	12%
Ostapowicz et al, Hepatology 2001[8]	Severe liver injury	Multiple referral centers	307	Not reported	20%
Galan, et al, J Clin Gastroenterol 2005[10]	Referrals for evaluation of acute and chronic liver disease	Tertiary care referral center	4039	1993–2002	0.8%
Vuppalanchi et al, Am J Gastroenterol 2007[9]	Total bilirubin > 3mg/dL	Community health-care system	732	1999–2003	0.7%
Squires et al, J Pediatr 2006 [12]	Acute liver failure (children)	Multiple referral centers	348	2000–2004	5%

Adapted from Vuppalanchi R, et al, Am J Gastroenterol 2007, with permission (ref 9).

(requiring hospitalization at least).[6] A Swiss study reported an incidence of drug hepatotoxicity of just over 1% in inpatients studied at two major hospitals from 1996–2000.[3] A population-based case control study from the United Kingdom General Practice Research Database placed drug induced liver injury incidence at 2.4 per 100,000 per year,[7] while in France a well-done general population based cohort study found a global crude annual incidence of nearly 14 per 100,000 inhabitants. 12% of the studied cases resulted in hospitalization, and 6% died.[4] A Swedish study published in 2006 reported 77 of 1164 (6.6%) new consults seen in a university hospital outpatient hepatology clinic between 1995 and 2005 were for drug induced liver injury. Half of these were outpatient referrals for evaluation of abnormal liver tests, while half were initial follow-up appointments after inpatient hospitalizations. A population incidence of approximately 2.3 per 100,000 per year was extrapolated from this data.[5]

While there are no population based estimates for incidence of DILI in the U.S., there are several studies illustrating the impact of DILI (Table 11.1). A United States study of an academic hospital and its affiliated outpatient primary care clinics in inner city Indianapolis found that of 732 patients seen with new-onset jaundice from 1999–2003, 29 were due to medications. Of these, most were due to acetaminophen, with only 5 (0.7% of the overall group) as the result of idiosyncratic drug hepatotoxicity. All five of these patients were alive at 6 week follow-up.[9] A Michigan study found that 32 of 4039 (0.8%) outpatients referred for hepatology evaluation over a ten year period had acute self-limited drug-induced liver injury.[10]

While majority episodes of drug hepatotoxicity are indeed self-limited, at the other end of the spectrum is drug induced acute liver failure. More than half of the cases of acute liver failure in the United States are caused by drug hepatotoxicity according to the most updated information from the United States Acute Liver Failure Study Group (unpublished data), which shows at least 45%

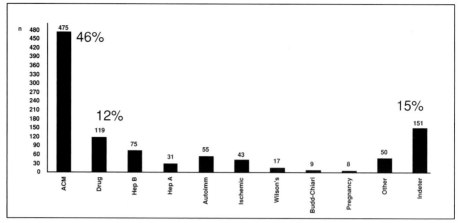

(Data from the United States ALF Study Group)

Figure 11.1. Etiology of ALF in the USA. *Source:* Adult Registry (n = 1033).

of cases due to acetaminophen and 12% due to more idiosyncratic types of drug reactions (Figure 11.1). The true impact may be higher than these numbers indicate, as some of the large group of indeterminate cases of acute liver failure are being found to be potentially related to acetaminophen,[11] and it is possible that still others in the indeterminate group may have been due to another drug not identified during the workup of these patients. In contrast to the mild, self-limited cases described above, idiosyncratic drug-induced liver injury that progresses to acute liver failure is particularly ominous, as only 22% of these patients survive without undergoing liver transplantation. In the Pediatric US Acute Liver Failure Study, 14% of all acute liver failure cases are due to acetaminophen, while 5% are due to idiosyncratic drug hepatotoxicity. Fortunately, the outcomes in children are somewhat better than in adults, with 94% of acetaminophen and 41% of idiosyncratic cases resulting in spontaneous (without transplant) survival.[12] The United Network of Organ Sharing (UNOS) data from 1990–2002 indicate that 15% of liver transplants done for acute liver failure were in cases of drug hepatotoxicity.[13]

Commonly Implicated Agents

Hundreds of drugs have been implicated in causing liver injury.[14] In addition to removal of several drugs from the market, the FDA has placed restrictions or serious warnings on a number of other medications because of hepatotoxicity (Table 11.2). The problem of drug induced liver injury is growing, partly because more medications are available than ever before and because numerous medications are often taken simultaneously, raising the risk of drug-drug interactions which in certain cases could magnify potential toxicity and in other cases makes identification of the specific 'culprit' drug nearly impossible. Another area of concern is the growing popularity of complementary and alternative medicines, several of which have been associated with hepatotoxicity. Unlike standard pharmaceuticals, these agents are not regulated by the FDA, and not considered as true

Table 11.2. FDA Regulatory Actions due to Hepatotoxicity (Partial List)

Drug	Regulatory Action
Benoxaprofen	Withdrawal (1982)
Bromfenac	Withdrawal (1998)
Troglitazone	Withdrawal (2000)
Perhexiline	Non-approval (1980's)
Dilevalol	Non-approval (1990)
Tasosartan	Non-approval (1998)
Ximelagatran	Non-approval (2006)
Pemoline	Restricted use
Tolcapone	Restricted use
Trovafloxacin	Restricted use
Felbamate	Restricted use
Telethromycin	Restricted use
Valproic acid	Warning
Ketoconazole	Warning
Nicotinic acid	Warning
Acetaminophen	Warning
Chlorzoxazone	Warning
Isoniazid	Warning
Rifampin	Warning
Pyrazinamide	Warning
Dantrolene	Warning
Nefazodone	Warning
Nevirapine	Warning
Terbinafine	Warning
Tacrine	Warning
Labetalol	Warning
Diclofenac	Warning

Adapted from presentation by Robert Temple, MD, accessed April 9, 2007 at: http://www.fda.gov/cder/livertox/ Presentations/im1389/sld002.htm.

"medicines" by many patients, who may neglect to mention them to physicians or may assume them to be harmless because they bear the label "natural."

While nearly any medication has the potential to induce idiosyncratic drug induced liver injury, certain medications or classes of medications have been more frequently associated with hepatotoxicity than others. The group of medications most commonly associated with drug induced liver injury is the antimicrobial category. French, Swedish, and Spanish studies found 25%, 30%, and 32%, respectively, of their drug induced liver injury cases were due to antibiotic agents,[4–6] and early data from the NIH-supported Drug Induced Liver Injury Network (DILIN) shows antimicrobials responsible for 43% of their prospectively collected cases.[17] Within this category, antituberculous agents are well-recognized offenders (INH and rifampin are known to cause hepatotoxicity alone or in combination with each other and/or pyrazinamide.) Antibacterial agents such as Augmentin, Bactrim, certain floroquinolones, and erythromycin are among the more frequent causative agents, but antifungal drugs have also

---

Table 11.3. Common Groups of Agents to Cause DILI

*Antimicrobials**	*NSAIDs*
Isoniazid	Diclofenac
Rifampin	Sulindac
Amox/Clavulanate	Naproxen
Erythromycin	Ibuprofen
TMP/SMX	Rofecoxib (no longer available)
Nitrofurantoin	Bromfenac (no longer available)
Ciprofloxacin	
Flucloxacillin	*Other notables*
Ketoconazole	Halothane
Nevirapine and other HAART	Isoflurane
	Disulfiram
Psychiatric agents/Anti-epileptics	Propylthiouracil
Chlorpromazine	Azathioprine
Paroxetine	Ticlopidine
Phenytoin	Enalapril
Carbamazepine	Captopril
Valproic acid	
Atomoxetine	

*Antimicrobials are the most common group of agents to cause DILI

Table 11.4. Some Herbal Medications Associated with Liver Toxicity

Atractylis gummifera	Impala
Black cohosh	Jin Bu Huan
Camphor	Kava
Cascara	Ma Huang
Chapparal	Mistletoe (skullcap, valeria)
Chaso	Pennyroyal
Greater celandine	Pyrrolizodine (comfrey, bush tea)
Germander	Sho saiko-to

Adapted with permission from reference 67

---

been implicated. Some antiviral medications, particularly HAART drugs such as nevirapine are now recognized as causes of drug induced liver injury as well.[4,8] Nonsteroidal anti-inflammatory drugs (primarily diclofenac and sulindac) and anticonvulsants are the more common hepatotoxic medications; psychiatric and anesthetic agents have been implicated as well. Some of the medications associated with drug induced liver injury are listed in Table 11.3. Increasingly, the category of complementary and alternative (CAM), or herbal medications are identified as causing liver injury (Table 11.4). The number of acute liver failure cases due to herbal medications has increased in the later compared to earlier years of the US ALF Study (US ALFSG, unpublished data). The DILIN has already identified cases of CAM hepatotoxicity, and 5% of the Swedish study cases were caused by herbal medications.[5,17]

Drug-Induced Liver Injury and Drug Development

One reason drug-induced liver injury remains such a tough problem is that the rarity of an adverse reaction to a specific drug makes study difficult. With the exception of intrinsic, largely dose-dependent toxins such as acetaminophen, most drugs that cause hepatotoxicity do so at a rate of 1 in 1,000 (as with INH) to 1 in 100,000 or more patients exposed (as with Augmentin). Added to this infrequency is a lack of a suitable animal model in which to research the disease. In part because of these hindrances, pathogenesis and risk factors for drug induced liver injury are not well understood, making it nearly impossible to predict which patients are likely to have adverse liver events with a given medication. Confounding the matter further is the fact that the signs and symptoms of drug induced liver injury are nonspecific and can mimic almost all types of liver disease. While certain patterns and presentations tend to predominate for certain drugs or drug classes, this does not always hold true, and one agent may cause more than one clinical picture. The diagnosis, therefore, is one of exclusion and difficult to make at that. Assessment of causality remains subjective, circumstantial, and of questionable accuracy.

Evaluating potential drug hepatotoxicity has clearly proven difficult not only for clinicians but for the FDA and pharmaceutical companies as well – as mentioned, hepatotoxicity is the most common reason for drug non-approval or post-marketing withdrawal.[1] The example of troglitazone (rezulin) provides an illustration of this situation. Troglitazone, the first PPAR-gamma agonist approved by the FDA for treatment of type II diabetes, was greeted with enthusiasm by patients and physicians when it was originally marketed in 1997. In less than one year of its release, however, cases of acute liver failure linked to troglitazone began to be reported. Recommendations were made for routine monitoring of liver chemistries in patients taking troglitazone, and when other PPAR-gamma agonist compounds with apparently better liver safety profiles became available, troglitazone was removed from the market in March of 2000. In the final analysis, 94 people developed acute liver failure while taking troglitazone, which was used by close to two million patients overall.[18] With the troglitazone experience came not only a wave of litigation against pharmaceutical companies but also increased scrutiny on the drug development and approval process particularly with regard to detecting potential hepatotoxicity. How can preclinical and clinical studies fail to identify drug compounds with such potentially toxic effects? Preclinical animal studies with troglitazone did not discover its potential for liver injury; this is not surprising since studies in animals are more helpful for evaluating predictable, dose-dependent hepatotoxic agents than for identifying more idiosyncratic types of hepatotoxicity in humans. Even in clinical studies when human patients are exposed to a drug compound, the low occurrence of significant drug induced liver injury with most idiosyncratic hepatotoxins makes detecting the potential for serious liver damage quite difficult. Statistically speaking, if the true incidence of an event is 1 in 1,000 per year it would require observation of nearly 3,000 patients for that amount of time to have 95%

confidence of seeing one case.[19] Given that most drugs known to be associated with idiosyncratic drug induced liver injury do so even less often than 1 in 1000 exposures, and that most pre-approval clinical drug trials contain typically less than 10,000 subjects, the likelihood of detecting serious adverse liver effects in pre-approval trials is uncertain at best.

During pre-approval clinical trials of troglitazone, elevations of serum alanine aminotransferase (ALT) levels above the normal range actually developed in more patients taking placebo than in those taking troglitazone,[20] an observation which could be related to potential beneficial effects of PPAR-gamma agonists on fatty liver disease.[21] Elevations of ALT above 3 times the upper limit of normal were seen in 2% of subjects receiving troglitazone as compared to 0.5% of those receiving placebo, however. Of the 2510 patients given troglitazone, 12 developed ALT levels more than 10 times the upper limit of normal and 5 had levels at least 20 times greater than the upper limit of normal. Two patients did develop jaundice in the setting of significantly elevated ALT, but as ALT continued to rise several days following drug discontinuation, it was thought that troglitazone was unlikely to be the cause of the liver injury in these cases. Ultimately, this biochemical pattern was seen to be consistent with troglitazone induced liver injury and in retrospect these pre-approval occurrences were seen as predictive of the adverse events that took place post-marketing.[22]

More than three decades ago Hyman Zimmerman noted that the development of jaundice in the setting of drug-induced hepatocellular injury is particularly ominous and carries a 10% mortality risk.[23] 'Hepatocellular jaundice' is a signal of potentially serious drug hepatotoxicity, indicating true dysfunction of the liver in terms of its ability to remove bilirubin from the serum, conjugate it and secrete it into bile. The observation that drug-induced hepatitis accompanied by elevated bilirubin is associated with approximately a 1 in 10 likelihood of death or at least acute liver failure has been termed "Hy's Rule." Hy's Rule defined as drug-induced elevation of ALT over 3 times the upper limit of normal plus a serum total bilirubin greater than 2 times the upper limit of normal in the absence of biliary obstruction or Gilbert's syndrome has been adopted by the FDA as an indicator of potential serious liver injury in the evaluation of new drug compounds.[24] The experience with troglitazone has been seen as validating Hy's Rule. 2 of 2510 patients, just under 0.1%, of patients who received the medication during the pre-approval trial developed hepatocellular jaundice. Hy's Rule would thus predict development of acute liver failure and possibly death in approximately 1 in 10,000 patients treated with troglitazone, which is fairly close to the numbers that were seen with the drug after its release on the market.[18] Recent studies from Sweden and Spain have validated Hy's Rule as well.[6,25] The occurrence of hepatocellular jaundice in pre-approval drug trials is indeed a signal of likely hepatotoxic potential, but its absence does not guarantee the drug is safe since trial subject numbers may be too small to catch rare events and since there are other presentations of drug-induced liver injury (cholestatic patterns for example). Given the lack of certainty in determining a drug's liver safety profile during development and testing, the time following release of a medication is important in terms of continuing to evaluate its safety. Once a drug is released on the market, it is crucial for suspected adverse events to be reported.

Table 11.5. Risk Factors Associated with DILI

Variable	Comment
Older age	May reflect increased underlying medication use and polypharmacy. Valproate and other anti-seizure medicines cause DILI in children.
Female gender	Various series of DILI and ALF show female preponderance. Underlying mechanism is not known.
Polypharmacy	May reflect drug-drug interactions
Pregnancy	Traditionally considered a risk factor but no definitive data
Obesity	Traditionally considered a risk factor but no definitive data
Alcoholism	Increases the risk of hepatotoxicity from acetaminophen, INH, duloxetine, etc
Malnutrition	Increases the risk of hepatotoxicity from acetaminophen and possibly INH
Underlying liver disease	May increase the risk of hepatotoxicity from INH, Antiretroviral agents
Genetic polymorphism	Suspected to play a significant role in most cases of idiosyncratic DILI. Recent studies have reported genetic basis for INH and diclofenac hepatotoxicity.

Risk Factors

The fact that many drugs known to cause liver injury do so in only a small fraction of patients exposed to them highlights the role of individual variability in patient-drug interactions. Determining which patients are more likely to develop hepatotoxicity with certain medications would potentially help to avoid some cases of drug-induced liver injury (Table 11.5). Unfortunately the individual risk factors for developing drug hepatotoxicity have been difficult to pinpoint and data are in most cases not clear-cut. It has generally been accepted that older patients are more susceptible to drug induced liver injury. Adults develop hepatotoxicity more often than children (though there are exceptions with medications such as valproic acid and other anti-epileptics as well as anti-neoplastic medications and aspirin).[14,28,29] Drug-induced liver injury is generally seen more commonly in patients over the age of 50 or 60,[4–6,30] but this has not been found by all studies[3] and may be at least partly due to the increased exposure to medications in older age groups. Certain medications do appear more clearly associated with older age.[31,32] Hepatotoxicity with INH, for example, is seen in approximately 2% of patients over the age of 45–50 years, and is only very rarely seen in patients under 20 years old. There is some evidence that in patients who do develop drug-induced liver injury may have worse prognosis than younger patients,[25] but this is not borne out in all studies.[33]

Drug-induced liver injury has generally been reported to be more frequent in women than in men[5,17,25] but this has not been seen with all drugs or in all studies, some of which have found equal preponderance among males and females or even higher occurrence in males.[3,6,8,9,34] This apparent effect, as with that of older age, may be partially related to increased exposure to drugs in women (who may be more likely to take medications or seek medical advice). Another possibility is the increased likelihood of autoimmune propensity in females, which could in theory increase likelihood of more autoimmune-type drug reactions. There is some evidence that women might fare worse than men when they do develop drug-induced liver injury, but this is not definitive. The United States ALF Study Group reports a female preponderance of 68% in their drug-induced cases (unpublished data), and 76% of UNOS transplants for drug-induced liver damage between 1990 and 2002 were performed in female patients.[13] The recent Swedish study of risk factors and outcome in drug-induced liver injury, however, did not show any difference in outcome between men and women.[25]

A past history of drug-induced liver injury is likely a predictor of future episodes, and this is definitely true for a specific medication which has caused hepatotoxicity in a patient previously. Pregnancy and obesity may also increase risk of drug-induced liver injury, and the use of multiple medications at the same time may in certain cases predispose patients to hepatotoxicity as well.[35] Malnutrition and chronic alcohol use seem to increase the likelihood of developing acetaminophen-induced hepatotoxicity,[36,37] but the role of alcohol and nutritional status is less understood with more idiosyncratic hepatotoxins. Genetic variability is probably the most important risk factor for drug hepatotoxicity but specifics here remain elusive[31] Genetic polymorphisms can alter metabolism of drug compounds and may make certain individuals more or less at risk for toxicity. N-acetyltransferase 2 gene polymorphisms, for example, have been found to affect susceptibility to isoniazid.[38] Preexisting liver disease is likely much more important in determining a patient's capacity to tolerate and recover from drug-induced liver injury than on whether or not the reaction occurs.

Pathogenesis

The liver plays a vital role in the metabolism of drugs and other toxins. Located between the absorptive surface of the gastrointestinal tract and the systemic circulation, it is central to the metabolism of most foreign substances. Most drugs are lipophilic and because of this are able to diffuse across stomach or intestinal cells. These substances are then transported to the liver, where they must be transformed into more hydrophilic compounds in order to be ultimately excreted in urine or bile. This process of biotransformation is accomplished within hepatocytes by a series of steps involving a vast array of enzymes and metabolic pathways. Most xenobiotics including drug compounds are biotransformed via one or both of two basic processes known as phase I and phase II metabolic reactions. Phase I pathways include oxidation, reduction, and hydrolytic reactions whose products are either readily excretable or must undergo further modification. Phase II reactions are known as conjugation reactions and involve esterification of either the parent compound or a metabolite formed via phase I reactions. Most drug compounds go through phase I metabolism within hepatocytes by enzymes of the cytochrome P450 (CYP) system, located in the smooth endoplasmic reticulum of the cells. The P450 family contains many different enzymes which metabolize specific drugs and xenobiotics. There are more than twenty known different CYPs within the human liver.[39] Parent drug compounds are generally metabolized by the P450 system into either non-toxic metabolites or toxic metabolites which must undergo further metabolism by either P450 or other enzymes in order to be rendered nontoxic. There is marked genetic variability in the CYP family, so a given CYP may generate slightly different metabolites in different people. Thus, toxic metabolites may be generated in some but not other people exposed to a single drug compound. In some cases, CYPs may produce a metabolite which is recognized by the host's particular immune system and may lead to immune attack on the hepatocytes producing this "allergenic" metabolite.

The known CYPs have been grouped into types and subtypes, and specific subtypes metabolize specific drugs. Drugs which are metabolized by the same CYP subtype may interact to either increase or decrease rate of metabolism of one or both of the compounds. Some medications such as quinidine, erythromycin, and ketoconazole are powerful inhibitors of specific CYPs and can thus significantly reduce the metabolism of drugs metabolized by those CYPs. Other compounds may induce or cause increased production of certain CYPs and thus increase the metabolism of any drugs metabolized by those CYPs. In some cases this increased metabolic rate results in decreased plasma levels of the drugs. In cases where a toxic metabolite is generated, however, such enhancement of the process will result in increased toxicity of certain drugs. This mechanism is the primary way in which drug-drug interactions may produce or contribute to drug induced liver injury. There are numerous inducers of CYPs, including ethanol, isoniazid, rifampin, phenytoin, and even cigarette smoke.

Hepatotoxins are generally classified as either intrinsic or idiosyncratic types. Intrinsic toxins produce liver damage in a fairly predictable, dose-dependent manner and are usually reproducible in animal models. These reactions occur in most people who are exposed to one of these medications or environmental toxins when certain levels of the parent compound, or more often, a toxic metabolite, accumulate within the liver. Examples of intrinsic hepatotoxins include carbon tetrachloride, phosphorous, and acetaminophen. In acetaminophen metabolism, phase II reactions usually predominate, but when the quantity of the drug exceeds the capacity of these pathways, the excess is metabolized by cytochrome P450, particularly CYP2E1. This process generates the toxic intermediate, N-acetyl-p-benzoquinoneamine (NAPQI), which damages hepatocytes at least in part by covalently binding to cell proteins which causes disruption of cellular membranes and derangement of normal cellular activities.[37] NAPQI can be detoxified by conjugation via glutathione-S-transferase to form the harmless, water-soluble mercapturic acid, but when larger doses of acetaminophen are ingested this safety mechanism is overwhelmed (Figure 11.2). Supplying glutathione by administration of N-acetylcysteine thus protects against acetaminophen-induced liver injury.[40,41] Starvation depletes glutathione stores and thus enhances acetaminophen-induced liver damage and increases susceptibility of individuals to lower doses of the drug. Ethanol intake has varying effects on acetaminophen metabolism, depending on whether ingestion is chronic or acute, but in some cases may increase toxicity.[37] Doses of up to 4g per day of acetaminophen have been considered very safe in generally healthy, nutritionally replete individuals, but recent work indicates that daily intake of this dose for several days causes nontrivial ALT elevations in some healthy adults.[42] The long-term significance of this effect is as yet unknown.

In contrast to acetaminophen, the vast majority of drugs that cause liver injury do so in an unpredictable and (for the most part) dose-independent manner. They are tolerated by most people exposed to them and cause hepatotoxicity only in rare cases, as discussed in a previous section of this chapter. These idiosyncratic reactions are not reproducible in animal species and may occur at varying intervals after beginning a medication. Much remains unknown regarding the pathogenesis of idiosyncratic drug induced liver injury but it is likely that several

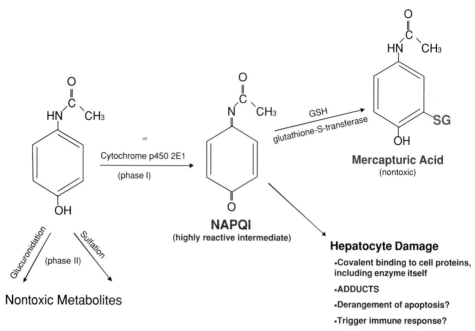

Figure 11.2. Mechanism of Acetaminophen Hepatotoxicity. NAPQI is a highly reactive metabolic intermediary of acetaminophen metabolism. When therapeutic doses of acetaminophen are given, the NAPQI that is produced is rapidly detoxified through conjugation into non-toxic mercapturic acid. However, in acetaminophen overdose, massive amounts of NAPQI that are produced overwhelm conjugation process. Sometimes, therapeutic doses of acetaminophen could lead to toxicity if there is co-existing depletion of conjugating enzymes (GSH) due to alcoholism or malnutrition.

"hits" are required for the development of significant hepatotoxicity. Genetic variations in CYPs may lead to development of toxic intermediates in some but not other individuals. Intermediate drug products may directly injure and/or trigger immune attack against hepatocytes. Genetic variability and other factors such as differences in HLA binding, nutritional state, coexistent diseases, age and gender may modulate immune responses and thus help determine whether a given individual will develop hepatotoxicity to a given medication as well as how severe a given reaction may be.

Whether direct or idiosyncratic in nature, drug induced liver injury occurs via many different mechanisms. Detailed discussions of these mechanisms are beyond the scope of this chapter but can be found in recent well-written review articles.[37,43]

Clinical Presentation

Drug-induced liver injury mimics essentially all forms of acute and chronic liver diseases. Different biochemical patterns are seen and correlate with different mechanisms or sites of injury. Most commonly, drug-induced liver injury involves damage and destruction of hepatocytes with resulting elevation of serum aminotransferase levels which may or may not be followed by milder increase in serum alkaline phosphatase and/or bilirubin. As previously discussed, the development of jaundice in the setting of this hepatocellular or hepatitic pattern of drug-induced liver injury is an indicator of severity and potentially poor outcome. Isoniazid, diclofenac, troglitazone, and acetaminophen are examples of drugs typically producing this type of injury. With acetaminophen hepatotoxicity in particular, patients may have extremely high aminotransferases and only mildly elevated bilirubin, especially early in the course.[44] This biochemical profile should be a signal to the clinician to consider acetaminophen overdose (either suicidal or a 'therapeutic misadventure') as highly likely in the differential diagnosis. Other drugs principally injure canalicular membranes and bile ducts. This cholestatic injury is characterized by alkaline phosphatase elevation that is out of proportion to and generally precedent to any increase in levels of aminotransferases. Erythromycin, Augmentin, estrogens, and chlorpromazine are examples of medications which tend to cause this type of injury pattern. Elevation of bilirubin may or may not occur in these cases and is less concerning in conjunction with cholestatic as opposed to hepatocellular liver injury. Some drug compounds cause both types of injury and biochemical abnormalities concurrently and this is known as a "mixed" pattern. Immunoallergic drug-induced liver injury such as with halothane, phenytoin, methyldopa, and nitrofurantoin is often more severe with repeated exposure and though typically associated with hepatocellular injury may also cause cholestatic or mixed patterns of biochemical abnormalities. In some of these cases peripheral eosinophilia and/or even positive anti-nuclear antibodies may be present. Other drugs may react to damage hepatic sinusoidal cells or mitochondria. A single drug may cause different patterns of injury in different instances, and patterns of injury may overlap to further confuse the picture. Whatever the pattern of injury in a particular case of drug hepatotoxicity, the development of coagulopathy (elevation in prothrombin time / international normalized ratio) and decline in serum levels of albumin are biochemical signs of worsening synthetic function and overall clinical picture.

Overt, systemic signs and symptoms of drug-induced liver injury are variable and nonspecific. Outward clinical evidence of liver injury may be minimal or absent even in cases where biochemical or histologic evaluation would reveal significant insult. Symptoms are protean and may include malaise, anorexia, nausea with or without vomiting, vague abdominal discomfort or right upper quadrant pain, and headache. Jaundice, as previously discussed, may or may not be present depending in part upon the type and severity of the hepatotoxic reaction. Immunoallergic reactions may produce the systemic signs and symptoms of hypersensitivity or autoimmune disease, including fever, rash, lymphadenopathy, and eosinophilia. Development of altered mental status is an ominous symptom, especially in conjunction with coagulopathy, when it signifies the development of liver failure with its dismal prognosis.

Many histologic abnormalities may be caused by drug hepatotoxicity. As with biochemical abnormalities, a drug may have different histopathologic effects in different people, but most hepatotoxins are more commonly associated with one or another type of histologic effect. While liver biopsy is rarely diagnostic in cases of drug-induced liver injury, the categorization of drug reactions according to the histologic changes involved (Table 11.6) is helpful in understanding the spectrum of drug-induced liver injury.

Table 11.6. Clinical and Histological Patterns of DILI*

HC Necrosis/ Acute Hepatitis		*Acute Cholestasis*	
Isoniazid	Diclofenac	Erythromycin	Sulindac
Methyldopa	Phenytoin	Bactrim	Captopril
Ketoconazole	Halothane	Allopurinol	Naproxen
Disulfiram	Nitrofurantoin	Carbamazepine	Amox/Clavu
Ma Huang	Carbamazepine	Chlorpromazine	Azathioprine
Kava	Propylthioruacil	Propylthiouracil	Estrogens
Nefazodone	Acetaminophen		
		Chronic Hepatitis or Cholestasis	
Acute Liver Failure		Diclofenac	TMP/SMX
Isoniazid	Augmentin	Chlorpromazine	Minocycline
Rifampin	Ciprofloxacin	Nitrofurantoin	Methyldopa
Halothane	Propylthiouracil		
Itraconazole	Bactrim	*Immuno-allergic or Autoimmune*	
Phenytoin	Valproic acid	Halothane	Bactrim
Nitrofurantoin	Kava	Phenytoin	Methyldopa
Disulfiram	Ma Huang	Nitrofurantoin	Minocycline
Granulomas		*Steatosis/ steatohepatitis*	
Allopurinol	Bactrim	Valproic acid	Amiodarone
Hydralazine	Carbamazepine	Stavudine	Tamoxifen
Methyldopa	Chaparral	Intravenous tetracycline	
Amox/Clavu	Phenytoin		
Quinidine			

*Note there is much overlap.

HEPATOCELLULAR NECROSIS

Many hepatotoxins cause hepatocyte death in the form of necrosis and probably also apoptosis.[37,45] Loss of hepatocytes due to drug toxicity tends to be most pronounced in the centrilobular area, which is the region of the lobule most sensitive to drug-induced injury. Several idiosyncratic toxins such as isoniazid and diclofenac cause this type of liver injury, but intrinsic hepatotoxins such as acetaminophen are the most classic examples of this direct hepatocyte damage.

HEPATITIS

Hepatocellular necrosis occurs in this type of reaction, but inflammation in the form of infiltrates composed of plasma cells, mononuclear cells, and occasionally eosinophils, also characterizes this type of drug toxicity, which may histologically resemble viral or autoimmune hepatitis and can be either acute or, in rarer cases, chronic. Such pathologic changes usually correlate with the biochemical pattern of predominant serum aminotransferase elevation. Immunoallergic type hepatotoxic reactions are among those that will cause this kind of histologic picture. Examples of drugs causing hepatitic histologic changes include nitrofurantoin, halothane, phenytoin, and methyldopa.

CHOLESTASIS

Injury to hepatocyte canalicular membranes or less frequently to bile ducts by certain toxins can disrupt bile flow, leading to cholestasis. In some cases this occurs without accompanying hepatitis; estrogens tend to cause this picture.[46] Cholestasis accompanied by hepatocellular necrosis and inflammatory infiltrates occurs with many drugs including chlorpromazine, erythromycin, TMP/SMX, and amox/clavu. Most of the drugs which cause cholestatic hepatitis can also cause cholestasis without hepatitis. Bile duct injury may sometimes be observed with chlorpromazine, carbamazepine, and flucloxacillin. In some cases cholestasis can become chronic and/or lead to vanishing bile duct syndrome.[47]

FIBROSIS

Chronic, large total-dose exposure to methotrexate or excess vitamin A can cause development of fibrosis without inflammation.[47]

GRANULOMAS

Granulomatous reactions may occur with a number of hepatotoxic agents and across a wide spectrum of injury types. Evidence of inflammation and systemic hypersensitivity may or may not be present. Carbamazepine, phenytoin, allopurinol, augmentin, methyldopa and hydralazine are among the medications which have been associated with hepatic granuloma formation.[48]

STEATOSIS AND STEATOHEPATITIS

Microvesicular steatosis may be seen in cases of hepatotoxicity due to certain nucleoside analogs, valproic acid and intravenous tetracycline. The mechanism in this case is mitochondrial injury, and acute liver failure may result. Young children appear to be particularly susceptible to valproate-induced hepatotoxicity.[49] Steatosis and steatohepatitis may also occur in association with amiodarone and tamoxifen, both of which can cause acute or chronic liver injury. Amiodarone may also cause phospholipidosis, cholestasis, and acute liver failure.[50] An unusual characteristic of amiodarone hepatotoxicity is that damage may continue for many months due to gradual release of accumulated drug stores.[51]

VASCULAR LESIONS

Drug-induced vascular injury may lead to several types of liver disease. Peliosis hepatis has been associated with oral contraceptives, anabolic steroids, and azathioprine. This lesion is characterized histologically by development of large sinusoidal cavities filled with blood and may present clinically as hepatomegaly with or without discomfort, may be asymptomatic, or may in rare cases lead to hepatic rupture or liver failure. Sinusoidal dilation without peliosis also may be seen with use of oral contraceptives. Hepatic venous obstruction has been related to oral contraceptives as well, and may produce mild venous congestion or in severe cases can produce centrilobular hemorrhage. When chronic and subacute, cirrhosis can be a consequence. Sinusoidal obstruction syndrome or veno-occlusive disease results from damage to sinusoidal endothelial cells. This has been seen with pyrrolizodine alkaloids (common in Jamaican herbal teas where it was first described, and in comfrey) and with certain chemotherapeutic agents especially after bone marrow transplantation. The injury results in nonthrombotic occlusion of sinusoids, terminal hepatic venules and small intrahepatic veins, and may present clinically as tender hepatomegaly with ascites and sometimes liver failure. Occasionally chronic liver disease with portal

---

Table 11.7. Keys Elements in the Diagnosis of DILI

■ High index of suspicion
■ Thorough history of prescription and OTC medications and herbal agents
■ Establish a plausible temporal association
■ Exclusion of competing etiologies
■ Some drugs may have characteristic "signature"
■ Available causality instruments are not user-friendly

---

hypertension and cirrhosis may develop. Nodular regenerative hyperplasia has also been described.[52]

NEOPLASMS

Development of several hepatic tumors has been linked to drugs and toxins. Hepatic adenoma may develop in women taking oral contraceptives; anabolic steroids have also been associated with this lesion. Though regression generally occurs with medication withdrawal, lesions which are large or symptomatic should be resected. There is a small risk of transformation to hepatocellular carcinoma. Angiosarcoma has been associated with arsenic, vinyl chloride, and thorotrast. Association of this lesion with anabolic steroids has rarely been reported. Connection between drugs and several other hepatic tumors are less certain and rarely reported.[47]

Since drug-induced liver injury is generally indistinguishable from many other liver diseases on the basis of clinical symptoms, biochemical abnormalities, and even histopathology, its diagnosis is often challenging. Detection of drug hepatotoxicity thus depends on the awareness, index of suspicion, and careful history-taking of the clinician.

Diagnosis

As DILI can masquerade a variety of acute and chronic forms of liver disease and as there is no single test to establish the diagnosis, it is largely a diagnosis of exclusion and requires high index of suspicion and careful history taking. As a matter of practice, DILI should be considered in the differential diagnosis of every patient with new onset liver disease. One should keep in mind about the hepatotoxic potential of herbal and over-the counter medications. Prompt diagnosis is essential for recovery because continued consumption of a suspected medication after the clinical onset of DILI carries high mortality (Table 11.7).

There is almost always a temporal relationship between starting the implicated medication and onset of DILI or temporal relationship between stopping the implicated medication and improvement in DILI. Although most cases of DILI occur within days to weeks after starting a new medication, there are exceptions (e.g., nitrofurantoin, diclofenac, troglitazone) where DILI may develop months to years after starting a medication. The rapid clinical improvement upon the discontinuation of an implicated agent (dechallenge) can also be helpful in confirming the diagnosis. Although dechallenge is one of the key components of the causality instruments (see below), its utility in day to day clinical practice is limited due to its retrospective nature. Furthermore, even after stopping the implicated agent, liver injury may initially worsen for days or weeks before exhibiting stability and subsequent improvement. Traditionally, rechallenge is considered a gold standard in the diagnosis of DILI, but it is very rarely attempted and it may have false negative results if adaptive tolerance has developed. Some drug exhibit a characteristic "signature" of liver injury and this may facilitate the diagnosis. However, medications with a known signature pattern of liver injury may sometimes present with non-signature pattern of liver injury. For example, although amox/clavulanate typically causes a cholestatic pattern of liver injury, it has been reported to cause hepatocellular DILI as well.

The role of liver biopsy in establishing the diagnosis of DILI is not clear. In selected cases, liver biopsy may provide appropriate diagnostic and/or prognostic information. Extensive portal infiltration with eosinophils is suggestive of DILI whereas lobular hepatitis with plasma cell infiltration is more indicative of autoimmune liver disease. Some transplant centers routinely obtain liver biopsy by transjugular approach in patients with presenting with acute liver failure caused by acetaminophen and other etiologies to assess the degree of hepatic necrosis. In patients with cholestatic DILI, a liver biopsy can identify whether there is simple cholestasis (excellent prognosis) or significant bile duct loss (vanishing bile duct syndrome) which may subsequently lead to biliary cirrhosis.

The United States Acute Liver Failure Study Group has recently reported that measurement of acetaminophen cysteine protein adducts reliably identifies acetaminophen toxicity and may be a useful diagnostic test in patients with acute liver failure from indeterminate causes.[53,54] This test is commercially unavailable and further studies are needed to establish its clinical utility.

There are several published instruments that assess the causal association between an episode of liver injury and suspected agent(s).[55–57] A scoring system termed "the Roussel Uclaf Causality Assessment Method" (RUCAM) is commonly used by the pharmaceutical industry and the regulators. Based on the numerical score, the causality is classified as highly probable, probable, possible, unlikely, or excluded. This and other scoring systems are fraught with problems and are rarely used in clinical practice.[58,59]

Management

The successful management of a patient with potential DILI includes (a) consideration of DILI as a potential etiology, (b) assessment of severity of liver damage, (c) prompt discontinuation of all suspected medications, (d) administration of N-acetyl cysteine in cases of acetaminophen hepatotoxicity, (e) hospitalization of patients with symptomatic or significant injury (jaundice with coagulopathy), and (f) referral to a liver transplant center if patients have acute liver failure (Table 11.8).

An international consensus meeting (1989) on drug induced liver disease defined DILI as ALT or direct bilirubin > 2 times ULN or a combined increase of AST, alkaline phosphatase (AP) or bilirubin provided one of them is two fold above ULN.[60] Unfortunately this definition is far too inclusive and does not distinguish clinically significant DILI from asymptomatic and largely inconsequential increases in aminotransferases. For practical purposes, one may define clinically significant drug induced liver injury as one that is associated with symptoms (e.g. nausea, vomiting, right upper quadrant abdominal pain) or elevated

Table 11.8. Key Guidelines in Managing Patients with Clinically Significant DILI[a,b]

Explain symptoms to patients	When a drug with potential for hepatotoxicity is prescribed, patients should be explicitly explained that they should report vague symptoms such as nausea, anorexia, abdominal discomfort as well as liver specific symptoms such as dark urine, itching, and jaundice
Careful history is crucial	It is essential to obtain detailed history of all prescription, over-the counter, and herbal remedies. Continued use of implicated medication after the onset of DILI carries significant morbidity and mortality
Removal of suspected agent(s)	Stop the suspected agent immediately. If a specific agent cannot be pinpointed, all agents started within last 6 months should be stopped
Prognosis	Prognosis depends on the level of initial injury and also whether the offending agent has been withdrawn in a timely fashion. As a general rule, if a patient has jaundice along with increased aminotransferases, the mortality can be 10% or more. If the causality is certain, rechallenge should be avoided as much as possible.
Chronic DILI	Improvement is quite common but some patients may evolve into chronic liver disease. Therefore, even in those with improvement, liver biochemistries should be checked at 6 months to document that they returned to normal or their baseline.
Timely referral to a specialist or liver transplant center	Patients with clinically significant should be seen by a gastroenterologist and referral to a transplant center should be considered for patients with progressive acute liver failure

[a]Clinically significant DILI can be defined as elevated liver biochemistries with jaundice and/or attributable symptoms.
[b]Modified with permission from Navarro VJ, Senior JR (Ref 111).

direct fraction of serum bilirubin in addition to increased aminotransferases or alkaline phosphatase.

As a general rule, when a patient with clinically significant DILI is encountered, suspected agents should be discontinued and the patient should be monitored closely with periodic clinical and laboratory assessment. In this era of polypharmacy, it is not uncommon to have multiple suspected agents, and in such situations authors recommend that all medications which have been started within the previous six months should be stopped. If patients have significant symptoms and/or jaundice with evidence of coagulopathy, patients may need to be hospitalized for further evaluation, management of symptoms, and close monitoring. In patients with clinically significant DILI, if a decision is made for outpatient follow-up, patients and their family members should be explicitly explained to watch for symptoms of worsening liver function and liver biochemistries should be followed closely. In patients with signs and symptoms of acute liver failure, referral to a liver transplant center should be considered.

Improvement occurs in majority of cases but at variable rates, depending on the type and nature of liver injury. The improvement can be dramatic in cases of acetaminophen induced acute liver injury, whereas it can be quite protracted in patients with cholestatic forms of liver injury. Largely ignored is the fact that some patients with acute DILI may evolved into chronic DILI.[61-63] A recent study from Spain has shown that the incidence of chronic DILI is 5.7% and patients with cholestatic/mixed pattern of DILI are significantly more prone to develop chronic DILI than those with hepatocellular DILI.[62]

In patients with clinically significant DILI, the implicated agent (and possibly same class of agents) should be avoided in future as rechallenge may lead to more severe liver disease, especially if the initial injury was immune-mediated. However, if the DILI is asymptomatic and consists of isolated elevations in aminotransferases without accompanying hyperbilirubinemia, it may be appropriate to continue the implicated medication. An example of this situation is patients received statins frequently exhibit asymptomatic elevations in aminotransferases. These elevations are largely inconsequential, and many authors have recommended that routine monitoring of liver biochemistries in patients receiving statins is not required and should be abandoned.[64–66]

Although the role of steroids in the treatment of DILI is controversial, their use by practicing clinicians is not too uncommon. The preliminary results from the DILIN prospective study show that nearly 15% of patients with suspected DILI received systemic steroids.[62] Anecdotes and small case series report successful use of steroids in patients with DILI with marked hypersensitivity or autoimmune features. Some scenarios where steroids may be justified include if DILI is associated with Stevens-Johnson Syndrome (e.g., phenytoin) or autoimmune features (nitrofurantoin, diclofenac, minocycline, halothane, etc). One noted expert recently recommended a short trial of steroids (prednisone 40–60 mg for one week followed by a rapid taper) for severe DILI if there are features of hypersensitivity (rash, eosinophilia) and if there is no rapid improvement within 3–4 days after stopping the offending agent.[66]

Summary

Although Idiosyncratic DILI is rare, it is a highly significant health condition because it can cause significant impediment to medication development and availability. As idiosyncratic DILI can masquerade a variety of acute and chronic liver diseases, it is one condition that should always kept in the differential when evaluating a patients with new onset liver disease. Its diagnosis hinges on careful history taking and establishing temporal association, and by excluding competing etiologies. In majority of the instances, patients with DILI improve if the offending agent is withdrawn in a timely fashion. Depending on the nature and severity of initial injury, some patients with idiosyncratic DILI may evolve into chronic liver disease and may develop cirrhosis.

ACKNOWLEDGMENTS

Supported in part by K24 DK 069290 (NC). Dr. Chalasani has received consulting fees from Merck, Ortho-McNeil, Advanced Life Sciences, Metabasis, Atherogenesis, and Abbott Pharmaceuticals. Dr. Polson has no conflicts to declare.

REFERENCES

1.   Temple RJ, Himmel MH. Safety of newly approved drugs: implications for prescribing. JAMA 2002;287:2273–5.

2. Aithal GP, Rawlins MD, Day CP. Accuracy of hepatic adverse drug reaction reporting in one English health region. BMJ 1999;319:1541–4.

3. Meier Y, Cavallaro M, Roos M, et al. Incidence of drug-induced liver injury in medical inpatients. Eur J Clin Pharmacol 2005;61:135–43.

4. Sgro C, Clinard F, Ouazir K, et al. Incidence of drug-induced hepatic injuries: a French population-based study. Hepatology 2002;36:451–5.

5. De Valle MB, Klinteberg VA, Alem N, et al. Drug-induced liver injury in a Swedish University hospital outpatient hepatology clinic. Aliment Pharmacol Ther 2006; 1187–95.

6. Andrade RJ, Lucena MI, Fernandez MC, et al. Drug-induced liver injury: an analysis of 461 incidences submitted to the Spanish registry over a 10-year period. Gastroenterology 2005;129:512–21.

7. de Abajo FJ, Montero D, Madurga M, Garcia Rodriguez LA. Acute and clinically relevant drug-induced liver injury: a population based case-control study. Br J Clin Pharmacol 2004;58:71–80.

8. Ostapowicz G, Samuel G, Larson AM et al. Identification of drug-induced liver innury among 307 cases of severe liver injury: a retrospective multi-center study. Hepatology 2001;34:454A 1127 Part 2 Suppl.

9. Vuppalanchi R, Liangpunsakul S, Chalasani N. Etiology of new-onset jaundice: how often is it caused by idiosyncratic drug-induced liver injury in the United States? Am J Gastroenterol 2007;102:558–62.

10. Galan MV, Potts JA, Silverman AL, et al. The burden of acute nonfulminant drug-induced hepatitis in a United Status tertiary referral center (corrected). J Clin Gastroenterol 2005;39:64–7.

11. Davern TJ, James LP, Hinson JA, et al. Measurement of serum acetaminophen-protein adducts in patients with acute liver failure. Gastroenterology 2006;130:687–94.

12. Squires RH, Shneider BL, Bucuvalas J, et al. Acute liver failure in children: the first 348 patients in the Pediatric Acute Liver Failure Study Group. J Pediatr 2006;148:652–8.

13. Russo MW, Galanko JA, Shrestha R, et al. Liver transplantation for acute liver failure from drug-induced liver injury in the United States. Liver Transplantation 2004;10:1018–23.

14. Zimmerman HJ. Hepatotoxicity: the adverse effects of drugs and other chemicals on the liver. 2nd ed. Philadelphia: Lippincott Williams & Wilkins, 1999.

15. Temple RJ. Hepatotoxicity through the years: impact on the FDA. (Accessed April 9, 2007 at htttp://www.fda.gov/cder/livertox/Presentations/im1389/ sld002.htm).

16. Kaplowitz N. Idiosyncratic drug hepatotoxicity. Nat Rev Drug Discov 2005;4:489–99.

17. Chalasani N, Fontana R, Watkins PB, et al. Drug Induced Liver Injury Network (DILIN) prospective study: initial results (abstracted). Am J Gastroenterol 2006;101 (9 Suppl):S169.

18. Graham DJ, Green L, Senior JR, Nourjah P. Troglitazone-induced liver failure: a case study. Am J Med 2003;114:299–306.

19. Rosner B. The binomial distribution. In Fundamentals of Biostatistics. B Rosner, ed. 4th ed. Duxbury Press, Boston: 82–7.

20. Watkins PB. Idiosyncratic liver injury: challenges and approaches. Toxicol Pathol 2005;33:1–5.

21. Liangpunsakul S, Chalasani N. Treatment of nonalcoholic fatty liver disease. Curr Treat Options Gastroenterol 2003;6:455–63.

22. Watkins PB, Whitcomb RW. Hepatic dysfunction associated with troglitazone. N Engl J Med 1998;338:916–7.

23. Black M, Mitchell JR, Zimmerman HJ, et al. Isoniazid-associated hepatitis in 114 patients. Gastroenterology 1975;69:289–302.

24. Senior JR. Regulatory perspectives. In: Drug Induced Liver Disease. Kaplowitz N, DeLeve L, eds. New York: Marcel Dekker 2003: 739–754.

25. Bjornsson E, Olsson R. Outcome and prognostic markers in severs drug-induced liver disease. Hepatology 2005;42:481–9.

26. Kessler DA. Introducing MEDWatch: a new approach to reporting medication and device adverse effects and product problems. JAMA 1993;269:2765–8.

27. Arnaiz JA, Carne X, Riba N, et al. The use of evidence in pharmacovigilance: case reports as the referente source for drug withdrawals. Eur J Clin Pharmacol 2001;57:89–91.

28. Clarkson A, Choonara I. Surveillance for fatal suspected adverse drug reactions in the UK. Arch Dis Child 2002;87:462–6.

29. Schwabe MJ, Dobyns WM, Burke B, Armstrong DL. Valproate-induced liver failure in one of two siblings with Alpers disease. Pediatr Neurol 1997;16:337–43.

30. James OF. Drugs and the ageing liver. J Hepatol 1985;1:431–5.

31. Larrey D. Epidemiology and individual susceptibility to adverse drug reactions affecting the liver. Semin Liver Dis 2002;22:145–55.

32. Olsson R, Wiholm BE, Sand C, et al. Liver damage from flucloxacillin, cloxacillin, and dicloxacillin. J Hepatol 1992;15:154–61.

33. Ohmori S, Shiraki K, Inoue H, et al. Clinical characteristics and prognostic indicators of drug-induced fulminant hepatic failure. Hepato-Gastroenterology 2003;50: 1531–4.

34. Ibanez L, Perez E, Vidal X, et al. Prospective surveillance of acute serious liver disease unrelated to infectious, obstructive, or metabolic diseases: epidemiological and clinical features, and exposure to drugs. J Hepatol 2002;37:592–600.

35. Navarro VJ, Senior JR. Drug-related hepatotoxicity. N Engl J Med 2006;354:731–9.

36. Whitcomb DC, Block GD. Association of acetaminophen hepatotoxicity with fasting and ethanol use. JAMA 1994;272:1845–50.

37. Lee WM. Drug-induced hepatotoxicity. N Engl J Med 2003;349:474–85.

38. Huang Y-S, Chern H-D, Su W-J, et al. Polymorphism of the N-acetyltransferase 2 gene as a susceptibility risk factor for anti-tuberculous drug-induced hepatitis. Hepatology 2002;35:883–9.

39. Hasler JA, Estrabrook R, Murray M, et al. Human cytochromes P450. Molec Aspects Med 1999;20:5–137.

40. Smilkstein MJ, Knapp GL, Kulig KW, Rumack BH. Efficacy of oral N-acetylcysteine in the treatment of acetaminophen overdose. N Engl J Med 1988;319:1557–62.

41. Keays R, Harrison PM, Wendon JA, et al. A prospective controlled trial of intravenous N-acetylcysteine in paracetamol-induced fulminant hepatic failure. BMJ 1991;303:1024–9.

42. Watkins PB, Kaplowitz N, Slattery JT, et al. Aminotransferase levels in healthy adults receiving 4 grams of acetaminophen daily. JAMA 2006;296:87–93.

43. Kaplowitz N. Biochemical and cellular mechanisms of toxic liver injury. Semin Liver Dis 2002;22:137–44.

44. Larson AM, Polson J, Fontana RJ, et al. Acetaminophen-induced acute liver failure: results of a United States multi-center, prospective study. Hepatology 2005;42: 1364–72.

45. Reed JC. Apoptosis-regulating proteins as targets for drug discovery. Trends Molec Med 2001;7:314–9.

46. Kreek MJ. Female sex steroids and cholestasis. Semin Liver Dis 1987;7:8–23.

47. Farrell GC. Liver disease caused by drugs, anesthetics, and toxins. In: Gastrointestinal and Liver Disease. Feldman, Friedman, Sleisenger eds. 7th ed. 2002; 1426–8, 1431–3, 1435–7.

48. Maddrey WC. Granulomas of the liver. In: Schiff's Diseases of the Liver. Schiff EF, Sorrell M, Maddrey WC, eds. 8th ed. Philadelphia: Lippincott-Raven 1999: 1571–85.

49. Bryant AE, Dreifuss FE. Valprioc acid hepatic fatalities. III. US Experience since 1986. Neurology 1996;46:465–9.

50. Snir Y, Pick N, Riesenberg K, et al. Fatal hepatic failure due to prolonged amiodarone treatment. J Clin Gastroenterol 1995;20:265–6.

51. Chang CC, Petrelli M, Tomashefski JF, McCullough AJ. Severe intrahepatic cholestasis caused by amiodarone toxicity after withdrawal of the drug: a case report and review of the literature. Arch Pathol Lab Med 1999;123:251–6.

52. DeLeve L. Cancer chemotherapy. In: Drug Induced Liver Disease. Kaplowitz N, DeLeve L eds. New York: Marcel Dekker 2003: 601–7.

53. Davern TJ 2nd, James LP, Hinson JA, Polson J, Larson AM, Fontana RJ, et al. Measurement of serum acetaminophen-protein adducts in patients with acute liver failure. Gastroenterology 2006;130:687–694.

54. James LP, Alonso EM, Hynan LS, Hinson JA, Davern TJ, Lee WM, et al. Detection of acetaminophen protein adducts in children with acute failure of indeterminate cause. Pediatrics 2006;118: 676–681.

55. Danan G, Benichou C. Causality assessment of adverse reactions to drugs – I. A novel method based on the conclusions of international consensus meeting. J Clin Epidemiol 1993;46:1323–1330.

56. Maria VAJ, Victorino RMM. Development and validation of a clnical scale for the diagnosis of drug induced hepatitis. Hepatology 1996;26:664–669.

57. Aithal GP, Rawlins MD, ay CP. Clinical diagnostic scale: a useful tool in the evaluation of suspected hepatotoxic adverse reactions. J Hepatol 2000;33: 949–952.

58. Kaplowiitz N. Causality assessment versus guilt by association in drug hepatotoxicity. Hepatology 2001;33: 308–310.

59. Rockey DC, Seeff LB, Freston JW, Chalasani NP, Bonacini M, Fontana RJ, Russo MW, Drug Induced Liver Injury Network. Comparison between expert opinion and RUCAM for assignment of causality in drug induced liver injury. Gastroenterology 2007;132: A773 (Abstract).

60. Criteria of drug induced liver disorders: Report of an international consensus meeting. J Hepatol 1990;11:272–276.

61. Aithal PG, Day CP. The natural history of histologically proved drug induced liver disease. Gut 1999;44:731–735.

62. Chalasani N, Fontana R, Watkins PB, et al. Drug Induced Liver Injury Network (DILIN) prospective study: initial results (abstracted). Am J Gastroenterol 2006;101 (9 Suppl):S169.

63. Andrade RJ, Lucena MI, Kaplowitz N, Garcia-Munoz B, Borraz Y, Pachkoria K, Garcia-Cortes M, et al. Outcome of acute idiosyncratic drug-induced liver injury: long-term follow-up in a hepatotoxicity registry. Hepatology 2006;44:1581–1588.

64. Chalasani N. Statin hepatotoxicity: focus on statin usage in nonalcoholic fatty liver disease. Hepatology 2005;41:690–695.

65. Cohen D, Anania F, Chalasani N. Report of the liver expert panel. Statin Safety Task Force, National Lipid Association. Am J Cardiology 2006;97(Supplement):77C–81C

66. Nathwani RA, Kaplowitz N. Drug Hepatotoxicity. Clinics in Liver Disease 2006;10:207–217.

67. Strader DB, Seeff LB. Hepatotoxicity of Herbal preparations. In Boyer TD, Wright TL, Manns MP (Eds): Zakim and Boyer's Hepatology: A text book of liver disease (5th edition). Elseviar Health, Philadelphia, PA, Pages 551–560.

Benign and Malignant Tumors of the Liver

Morris Sherman, MD, PhD

BACKGROUND

There are a large number of tumors that may grow in the liver. Most are rare, and do not merit more than a passing mention. This discussion will therefore be limited to the three benign tumors or tumor-like lesions, hemangioma, focal nodular hyperplasia, and hepatic adenoma, and to the two most common malignant tumors of the liver, hepatocellular carcinoma (HCC) and intrahepatic cholangiocarcinoma (CC). These five entities account for the vast majority of nodular lesions found on radiological examination of the liver.

HEMANGIOMA

Hemangioma is the most common liver tumor. It is found in up to 20% of autopsy series.[1] Hemangiomas tend to occur more frequently in women than men. They may be single or multiple and may vary in size from a few millimeters to 10 cm or more, although most are smaller than 5 cm in diameter. They consist of vascular channels lined by a single endothelial layer, supported by fibrous tissue. The vascular spaces may contain thrombi that may calcify. In some hemangiomas, the calcified thrombus might be large enough to be seen radiologically. Hemangioma may be associated with focal nodular hyperplasia.[2]

Hemangioma is a benign lesion, and never develops malignancy. Whether the lesion is hormone sensitive is controversial.[3,4] There are reports of enlargement of hemangiomas with pregnancy or exogenous estrogen administration.[5,6,7] However, hemangiomas may enlarge in the absence of these stimuli. Furthermore, the vast majority of hemangiomas are not hormone sensitive and do not grow significantly over the reported observation periods, whether in the presence of sex hormones or not.

Diagnosis

The diagnosis of hemangioma can almost always be made radiologically, so that there is no need for biopsy. This is fortunate, because biopsy can be associated with significant risk of bleeding. Because the majority of hemangiomas are clinically silent, they most commonly present as an incidental finding on an ultrasound done for unrelated purposes. Typically, hemangiomas are described as brightly echogenic on ultrasound. The nature of the lesion can be confirmed by one of several methods. A labeled red-blood cell scan with delayed images (late portal phase) shows pooling of the label in the lesion that persists into the delayed phases.[8] However, the sensitivity of this nuclear medicine study is dependent on the size of the lesion. Hemangiomas that are smaller than about 2 cm may not be detected by labeled red blood cell scanning. All forms of dynamic imaging, i.e., contrast ultrasound, tri- or four-phase CT scanning or MRI are quite sensitive for the detection of hemangioma.[9–13] Again, there are size limitations, but all three modalities can detect and identify lesions not seen labeled red blood cell scanning. The characteristic features are centripetal filling of the lesion with contrast agent, and peripheral nodularity in the venous or late phases.

Clinical Presentation

Hemangiomas of the liver rarely cause symptoms. Thrombosis of very large lesions may present as pain. The diagnosis is made radiologically, using a dynamic contrast enhanced study. Usually analgesia is the only treatment required, because once the thrombus has formed and is stable the pain will subside. Occasionally giant hemangiomas may bleed, either into the liver, or into the peritoneal cavity.[14] Rupture has been reported in associated with enlargement during pregnancy.[15] These are exceptionally rare events, and are the only indications for resection of these lesions.

Large hemangiomas may rarely be associated with thrombocytopenia (Kasabach-Merritt Syndrome)[16] particularly in children. Fibrin deposition within the lesion has been reported to cause hypofibrinogenemia.

TREATMENT

No treatment is required, except for the occasional resection as discussed above.

Focal Nodular Hyperplasia

This is a tumor-like lesion that consists mainly of normal hepatocytes. Like hemangioma, it has no malignant potential. Focal nodular hyperplasia (FNH) occurs more frequently in women than in men.[17] The etiology is unknown. Some believe that the FNH is a hypertrophic lesion that grows in response to the development of a spider-like arterial vascular abnormality.[18] The cause of the initial vascular abnormality is unknown. In most instances, the lesion presents as an incidental finding on an imaging study ordered for other reasons. Although there are reports of apparent enlargement of FNH in response to estrogen exposure[19] it is difficult to know whether the association is real or due to selective reporting.

There are few prospective series that included sufficient subjects to completely exclude the possibility that some FNH's do develop in relation to sex hormone exposure[20] but the vast majority of FNH are not hormone sensitive.[21]

Clinical Presentation

FNH may vary in size from smaller than 2 cm to many cm in diameter. The larger lesions may infarct, or may bleed into the lesion. In this situation the lesions presents with pain. External rupture into the peritoneum is rare. Occasionally FNH may shrink in size or even regress completely.[22,23]

Pathologically, FNH consists of normal hepatocytes in plates 2–3 cells thick (compared to the single or double cell plates in normal liver. The vascular supply is usually by unpaired arteries (without accompanying vein or duct) within a fibrous band. The arteries appear to drain directly into the sinusoids between adjacent plates. In the center of the lesion there is usually a fibrous stellate scar, carrying the vascular supply, which, if present, is characteristic of FNH.

Diagnosis

FNH can usually be diagnosed radiologically without having to resort to biopsy. Perhaps the most sensitive and specific imaging technique is contrast-enhanced ultrasound (CEUS).[13,24] In this technique microbubbles are injected peripherally and scanned as they flow through the liver. The microbubbles provide multiple surfaces for the incoming sounds waves to reflect off, giving a very bright pattern and outlining the blood vessels. CEUS can often clearly demonstrate the central stellate scar that fills centripetally, and the feeding artery, which if present is a diagnostic finding. Dynamic MRI and three-phase CT scan can also often show the central scar[25–27]. However, even in the absence of the scar pattern the enhancement characteristics can distinguish FNH from HCC.

Treatment

Because FNH does not undergo malignant transformation the need to treat the lesion is limited to symptomatic lesions. Occasionally very large lesions, causing pressure symptoms may need to be resected. Other treatments that have been applied include arterial embolization.[29–31] Large FNH lesions are at risk for rupture, and may require prophylactic resection. Lesions that do rupture also require surgical intervention, although embolization has also been used to treat these lesions.[32]

HEPATIC ADENOMA

This is a rare benign liver tumor. That adenomas are frequently hormone dependent is now well established. The evidence of a causal association rests on small case series and the temporal relationship between the introduction of the oral contraceptive pill and a sudden significant increase in the number of case reports of hepatic adenoma appearing in the literature.[33–36] However, there are no large-scale epidemiological studies confirming the association. The association was enforced by the finding that hepatic adenoma may enlarge during pregnancy, and may regress after delivery, or on withdrawal of the oral contraceptives.[37,38] Similarly, adenoma associated with androgen use may regress once the androgen therapy is withdrawn. Today's oral contraceptives have much lower estrogen concentrations that those that were in use when the association was first recognized, and some do not even contain the C17-alkyl substituted estrogens that are thought to be incriminated.[39] Although development of hepatic adenoma is usually associated with longer-term oral contraceptive use, the development of adenoma has been described after as little as six months of use. Hepatic adenomas in men are seen in association with use of anabolic steroids, initially reported with therapeutic use of anabolic steroids for Fanconi's anemia or aplastic anemia, and more recently following illicit use of androgens in athletes.[40–43] Glycogen storage disease type 1A is associated with the development of multiple hepatic adenomas.[44] Multiple hepatic adenomatosis is a rare condition, in which the liver may contain 10 or more lesions of various sizes. This may occur in the setting of exogenous hormone administration, although there may be no such history.[46] Hepatic adenomas tend to enlarge over time and have the potential to become malignant.[47,48] The development of HCC in a pre-existing hepatic adenoma has been well described, but is a rare event.

Clinical Presentation

As with other liver masses, hepatic adenomas are often incidental findings in patients undergoing radiological imaging, usually ultrasound, for other reasons. Symptomatic presentation is seen with large lesions, that may cause pressure symptoms, a palpable right upper quadrant mass, or rarely may present with pain due to bleeding into the tumor, or rupture into the peritoneum.

Diagnosis

Radiological diagnosis is moderately specific. Technecium-labelled liver spleen scans may show a cold area, because the adenoma contains relatively few Kuppfer cells. However, this is not a highly sensitive or specific test. The ultrasound appearances are not specific. The lesion may be hyper- or hypoechoic, or of mixed echogenicity.[49] Contrast-enhanced ultrasonography is useful to exclude the differential diagnoses of HCC and focal nodular hyperplasia[49,] but the appearances are not highly specific for adenoma. CT and MRI may also show rapid arterial enhancement.[50,51] Other features that may be detected radiologically include the presence of fat in the lesion, abnormal vessels, or intra-tumoral hemorrhage. Because the radiologic features are not sufficiently specific needle biopsy of the lesion is required for definitive diagnosis.

Pathologically, the hallmark of the hepatic adenoma is that it consists solely of hepatocytes, arranged in chords that are seldom more than three cells wide, separated by very narrow sinusoids. The hepatocytes are often larger than normal hepatocytes and may contain fat. Kupffer cells are variably present, although usually in reduced numbers. Bile ducts are absent and mitoses are rare. The differential diagnosis is primarily with HCC, in which the chords are usually more than three cells wide, and the overall architecture is more disorganized.

Treatment

Hepatic adenomas diagnosed in the setting of exogenous hormone administration often regress when the offending drug is withdrawn, and this constitutes the treatment of choice. However, lesions that do not regress need to be treated, because of the risk of growth and complications related to bleeding or rupture, or to malignant transformation. The usual therapy in the past has been resection, but today local ablation with radiofrequency probes is more commonly used for smaller lesions.[52,53]

HEPATOCELLULAR CARCINOMA

Hepatocellular carcinoma (HCC), also known as hepatoma, is among the 10 most common tumors in the world, accounting for about 300,000 deaths each year.[54] Unlike many other cancers, there are close epidemiological links with a several diseases that predispose to the development of HCC. In most countries and in most patients HCC arises in the setting of chronic liver disease, usually cirrhosis. HCC arising in a previously normal liver accounts for less than 10% of all HCCs in regions of the world where the underlying liver diseases are common, and for about 10% of cases where those diseases are less common. Numerically, the most frequent underlying cause of HCC is chronic hepatitis B, given that there are about 300 million people infected with this virus in the world. The next most common cause is hepatitis C, which infects about 170 million people. Other causes of cirrhosis that predispose to HCC include alcoholic cirrhosis, cirrhosis associated with genetic hemochromatosis[55] and alpha 1-antitrypsin deficiency,[56] primary biliary cirrhosis[57] and more recently it has been recognized that cirrhosis following steatohepatitis is also a risk factor for HCC.[58] Thus, those parts of the world where there is a high prevalence of chronic viral hepatitis are also those parts of the world where the incidence of HCC is highest.[59] Hepatitis B is common in South East Asia and sub-Saharan Africa. In those parts of the world the incidence of HCC is more than 5/100,000/ year,[59] and may be as high as more than 50/100,000/year in parts of China. In contrast, in parts of the world where chronic viral hepatitis is not common, e.g., northern Europe and North America, the incidence of HCC is closer to 1–5/100,000/year.[59]

In patients with hepatitis B HCC can occur in non-cirrhotic liver, but for hepatitis C and other causes of liver disease cirrhosis seems to be a prerequisite condition. This may not be true in Japan, where HCC in hepatitis C occurs with appreciable frequency in the absence of cirrhosis. The explanation for these differences is not clear.

The incidence of HCC is rising in many countries in the West.[60–63] This is as a result of a number of factors. In some countries, e.g., Italy, there was a silent epidemic of hepatitis C infection in the period between about 1945 and 1970. Those who were infected during that era are now of an age where HCC is more common, i.e., in their sixties and seventies. In other countries epidemics of hepatitis C occurred as a result of injection drug use, a practice that became widespread during the 1960s and 1970s. Those infected during that period are now 30–40 years older, and are also now at risk for the development of HCC.

Finally, immigration from parts of the world where hepatitis B and hepatitis C are common is also contributing to the pool of infected individuals in many countries, and also to the rising incidence of HCC.

Screening for HCC

Until recently there was no evidence that screening at-risk individuals for HCC had any effect on the mortality from the disease. Recently, however, a randomized controlled trial in hepatitis B carriers in China has shown that six monthly screening with ultrasound and alphafetoprotein resulted in a reduction in mortality of 37%.[64] It is not certain that these results can be generalized to other populations or to other diseases. Nonetheless these results and others have led to the recommendation by many different groups that patients at risk for HCC should be screened. The study referred to above was initiated a number of years ago. Since then it has become apparent that alphafetoprotein was not a very good screening test.[65] Overall, AFP screening is insufficiently sensitive and insufficiently specific for general use as a screening test. There are too many false-positives and too many false negatives. Therefore screening should be with ultrasound alone. The screening interval should be between six and 12 months, preferably six months. This is based on the anticipated tumor doubling time, which on average is about three to five months. Patients deemed at higher than average risk do not need to be screened more frequently, because the screening interval depends on tumor growth rate, not degree of risk.

With good ultrasound it is possible to detect lesions smaller than 1 cm. With appropriate follow-up and intervention, it is at least theoretically possible to cure the majority of these small lesions (see later). Thus we are entering an era where a disease that was once considered a death sentence can be cured with appreciable frequency, even in the majority of patients, provided that good ultrasound is followed by appropriate intervention.

Diagnosis

The diagnosis of HCC depends on the clinical circumstances. Screening of at-risk individuals has become common in many parts of the world. Patients whose tumors are diagnosed through screening present with small lesions. Unfortunately, even in parts of the world where screening is common, the majority of patients do not undergo screening, and present with late-stage disease. The diagnostic criteria for HCC are different at different stages of disease.

Diagnosis of Small HCC

Small HCC is defined as a lesion smaller than 2 cm in diameter. These are either found incidentally, or on routine screening of patients at risk for HCC. The recommended screening test is ultrasound,[66] so the diagnostic algorithms have been developed on the assumption that an ultrasound examination has identified a lesion smaller than 2 cm. Recommended algorithms are shown in Figures 12.1, 12.2, and 12.3. In summary, if the lesion is smaller than 1 cm, it should be monitored by repeat ultrasonography at more frequent intervals, e.g., every three to four months. If it grows to larger than 2 cm the diagnostic algorithm is as for

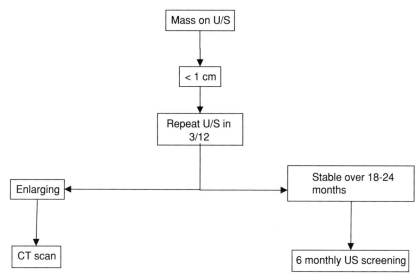

Figure 12.1. Assessment of liver mass less than 1 cm in size.

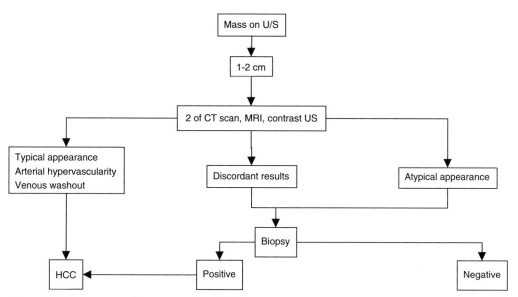

Figure 12.2. Assessment of liver mass 1–2 cm in size.

lesions first presenting at that size. If the lesion does not change in size the more frequent ultrasounds should be continued for up to two years. If the lesion is stable in size over two years it is not likely to be HCC, and the patient can resume the regular six monthly screening. If the lesion is between 1–2 cm in diameter the recommendation is that it should be investigated further using two dynamic imaging studies, such as four-phase CT scan, gadolinium-enhanced MRI, or contrast enhanced ultrasound.[65] If two such studies show typical features of HCC, namely enhancement in the arterial phase, with decreased signal intensity compared to the liver in the portal venous or delayed phases, this is sufficient for the diagnosis and no biopsy is required. If however, one or both studies show features that are not typical of HCC a biopsy is required. A positive biopsy

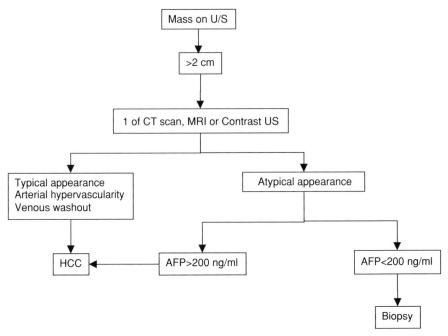

Figure 12.3. Assessment of liver mass more than 2 cm in size.

obviously confirms the diagnosis, but a negative biopsy can never exclude the possibility that HCC is present. This is because there is a significant false-negative diagnosis rate on biopsy. The placement of the needle may be inaccurate in such small lesions, and pathological interpretation of the very earliest HCC lesions is also difficult.

Lesions larger than 2 cm that present without symptoms can also be diagnosed radiologically, without resort to biopsy.[66] In these larger lesions the diagnostic radiology is more frequently present, so that only a single typical radiological examination result is necessary.

Serum alphafetoprotein concentration has long been used as a diagnostic test for HCC. Large tumors may be associated with AFP concentrations that exceed 1 mg/ml. However, in smaller tumors the AFP is less often elevated in the diagnostic range.[65] It is common for AFP to be elevated in cirrhosis due either to hepatitis B or C infection, in the absence of HCC. However, in those situations the AFP is seldom higher than 200 ng/ml. In a cirrhotic liver with a small mass if the AFP is greater than 200 ng/ml the specificity of these findings for HCC is in excess of 90%.[65] However, it is also important to note that AFP is normal in up to 40% of all HCCs. Thus, AFP concentration is neither sensitive nor specific.

Pathologically, the earliest lesions of HCC consist of well-differentiated cells in plates that may not be more than three cells wide. There may still be portal tracts present, and there may be some arterialization, but portal veins may also still be present. These lesions often contain fat, and seldom show any invasion of vessels. These small lesions are often unencapsulated. At the lesion progresses the cellular differentiation changes, more typical nuclear/cytoplasmic ratio changes are seen and there is nuclear pleiomorphism. These lesions may be encapsulated, and there may be microvascular vessel invasion. More advanced lesions no longer have portal tracts and there are no portal veins. All the blood supply is arterial.

Clinical Presentation

HCC that causes symptoms is late-stage disease, and at that point is seldom curable, and often is to far advanced for any form of therapy, including liver transplantation. Late-stage disease usually presents as deterioration in clinical status in a patient known to have liver disease, or as new onset ascites in patients not previously known to have liver disease. Ascites is usually the first clinical manifestation, followed or accompanied by weight loss and jaundice. Occasionally, an HCC may present with abdominal pain due to rupture into the peritoneum or intra-hepatic bleeding. The diagnosis is confirmed radiologically in these patients.

Treatment

Treatment of HCC can be divided into three broad categories.[67] Curative therapy includes local ablation with either injection of alcohol, or radiofrequency ablation, resection or transplantation. Palliative therapy includes chemoembolization or experimental therapies, and finally, the latest stages of disease require only supportive care. A schematic representation of the types of patients who are suitable for the different types of treatment is shown in Figure 12.4.

LIVER TRANSPLANTATION

Liver transplantation is reserved for relatively early-stage disease. The original criteria within which transplant was effective were first propounded in 1996, by a group in Milan, Italy, and have become known as the "Milan Criteria."[68] These are that there should be s single tumor smaller than 5 cm in diameter, or up to three tumors, none larger than 3 cm in diameter. Within these criteria other predictive features such as vascular invasion or poor cellular differentiation are not operative. Others have expanded the criteria to a maximum single tumor diameter of 6.5 cm, no more than three lesions, with a maximal combined tumor diameter of 8 cm.[69] It has been suggested that the survival in patients selected using these criteria is the same as for the Milan criteria. The Milan criteria have been externally well validated. The expanded criteria are less well validated, and are less well accepted.

For patients transplanted within the Milan Criteria the five-year survival is about 70%, with a tumor recurrence rate that is less than 20%. However, in an intention to treat analysis of all patients listed for transplant overall survival is only 65% at five years, i.e., similar to survival following resection.[70] However, the recurrence rate is much better than surgery, i.e., about 20%. Thus, liver transplantation has become the treatment of choice for HCC in the West. However, a lack of donor organs has meant that many patients on the waiting list for liver transplant are removed from the list because their tumors exceed listing criteria over time.

SURGICAL RESECTION

Resection for HCC has been used for many years. Improvements in patient selection and post-operative management has resulted in better survival – up to 70% at five years, but with a recurrence rate of about 50%.[71] Patients with cirrhosis and poor liver function cannot tolerate resection. Thus resection is

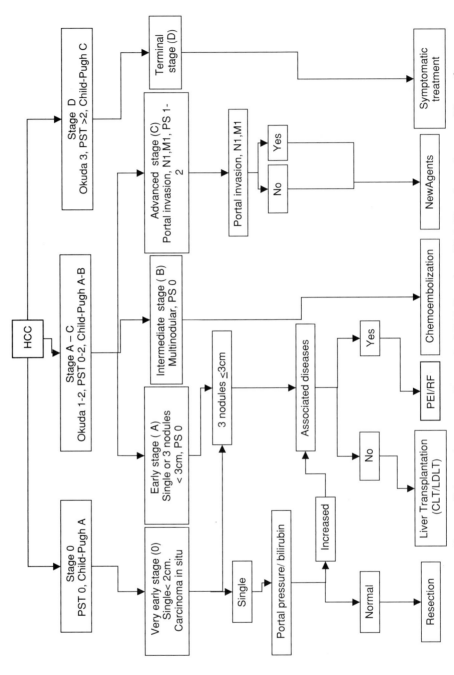

Figure 12.4. Staging of hepatocellular carcinoma according to the BCLC (Barcelona Clinic Liver Cancer) system. PS – performance status according to the Eastern Cooperative Oncology Group. CP – Child-Pugh score. OLT – orthotopic liver transplantation. PEI – percutaneous ethanol injection. RFA – radiofrequency ablation.

limited to patients with Child's A cirrhosis and normal liver function. The presence of significant portal hypertension (esophageal varices, splenomegaly, portal-venous pressure gradient of more than 10 mmHg) or elevated bilirubin are contraindications to resection.[72] Extensive resections, such a tri-segmentectomy, are also usually not possible in cirrhotic patients. Thus, in patients with chronic hepatitis C, almost all of whom have cirrhosis resection is seldom possible. However, in patients with HCC due to chronic hepatitis B, in whom up to 40% have fibrosis but not cirrhosis, resection is more often possible.

LOCAL ABLATION

This term refers to the local application of a noxious stimulus directly to the tumor. The initial studies were performed by injections of absolute alcohol directly into the lesion.[73] More recently application of heat using radiofrequency waves generated at the tip of the needle has replaced alcohol injection.[74] Radiofrequency ablation will produce complete ablation of a HCC in fewer sessions than alcohol injection, although each session takes more time.[75] Radiofrequency ablation provides more complete ablation than alcohol for lesions that are smaller than about 3–4 cm. Indeed radiofrequency ablation is usually restricted to tumors smaller than 4.5 cm, in order to achieve necrosis of the visible tumor and a margin of 0.5–1 cm around the lesion. Lesions smaller than 2 cm can be ablated completely in more than 95% of cases.[76] Lesions larger than 3 cm can be completely ablated in about 58% of cases. Because survival is related to the ability to achieve complete ablation, the smaller the tumor at diagnosis the more likely it is to be completely ablated, and the more likely is survival to be enhanced.

CHEMOEMBOLIZATION

In this technique a chemotherapeutic agent, usually doxorubicin or cisplatin, is injected directly into an artery feeding the tumor. The drug is mixed with lipiodol to create an emulsion. Lipiodol is a viscous oily radiographic contrast agent. Following injection into HCC the lesion takes up lipiodol, so that the lesion is intensely white on CT scan. The lipiodol probably has its effect by slowing down the flow of blood, or even stopping the flow of blood completely, creating some local ischemia. Following the injection of the lipiodol-drug mix the artery feeding the tumor is embolized with gelfoam, polyvinyl alcohol, or other embolic agent. The induction of ischemia in the tumor cells appears to enhance the killing effect of the chemotherapeutic agent.

Two randomized controlled trials and a meta-analysis confirm that chemoembolization does prolong survival.[77–79] Chemoembolization can only be given to patients with reasonably good liver function, i.e., child's A cirrhosis. It is associated with some destruction of viable liver tissue, and is often associated with some degree of worsening of liver function. On average the two-year survival after chemoembolization is about 60%, compared to about 30% in untreated controls.[77–79]

OTHER THERAPY FOR HCC

There are a large number of different forms of therapy that have been applied to patients with HCC. Unfortunately, none have been tested in randomized controlled trials. Combination of chemoembolization and local ablation seems a logical approach, but this has never been shown to be superior to either alone. Although the liver is radiosensitive external beam conformal radiotherapy has been used to limit the exposure of uninvolved liver to radiation. Enhanced survival has not been demonstrated. Internal radiotherapy using [99] Yttrium-labelled glass beads injected into the feeding artery is a promising therapy,[80] but this has also not been shown to enhance survival. Intra-arterial chemotherapy or systemic chemotherapy has been shown in controlled trials to enhance survival only by a matter of a few weeks, but at the cost of a significant decrease in quality of life. A number of small molecule inhibitors of tumor cell biology and monoclonal antibodies are currently being tested. These include sorafenib, a raf-kinase inhibitor, and bevacizimab (an angiogenesis inhibitor), among others.

INTRAHEPATIC CHOLANGIOCARCINOMA

This is a disease of the fifth and sixth decades, and occurs equally in males and females. Intrahepatic cholangiocarcinoma (ICC) is a tumor arising in the bile duct radicles in within the liver (at and above the hilum of the liver). This is a relatively common tumor all over the world, and often has recognized predisposing causes. These include infestations with liver flukes, such as clonorchis sinensus or opisthorchis viverrini, hepatolithiasis, Caroli's disease, a diet high in nitrosamines, or exposure to Thorotrast. Opisthorchis viverini infection is a major cause of disease in parts of Thailand, where this tumor is very common. Hilar cholangiocarcinoma has a slightly different demographic distribution, and is more common in males, and more often associated with inflammatory bowel disease and sclerosing cholangitis.

The incidence of intrahepatic cholangiocarcinoma is rising, whereas the incidence of extrahepatic cholangiocarcinoma is falling.[81,82] This may be related to the modern high rate of cholecystectomy, and a significant decrease of gall bladder carcinoma. The causes of the increased incidence of intrahepatic cholangiocarcinoma are not known.[83] It has been suggested that it may be related to the increased incidence of HCC, related to hepatitis C and hepatitis B. However, the demographics of the populations that have HCC and cholangiocarcinoma are different,[84] suggesting that they do not really have a common etiology.

Diagnosis

Intrahepatic cholangiocarcinoma presents as a mass-like lesion, and because it is usually clinically silent until late, often presents with cancer symptoms of weight loss, malaise, abdominal pain, and decreased performance status, rather than symptoms that bring attention to the liver. Lesions that obstruct the bifurcation of the hepatic duct present with jaundice.[85,86] Intrahepatic cholangiocarcinoma spreads to local lymph nodes early in the course of the disease.

Diagnosis

The diagnosis is primarily radiological.[87] Ultrasound will show a peripheral mass lesion in the liver, and will show dilated intrahepatic bile ducts in the hilar carcinoma. Thickening of the bile duct wall may also be identified. For hilar cholangiocarcinoma MRI has become the investigation of choice because of its superior ability to identify the level of bile duct obstruction,[88,89] and ability to delineate tumor anatomy and to determine resectability. It does not require injection of contrast, and thus there is no need to leave a drain in situ to prevent cholangitis in the obstructed duct. MRI however, does understage disease in about 20% of cases. Endoscopic ultrasound allows fine needle biopsy of the lesion.[90] This is much more accurate than obtaining brushings at ERCP. It also allows identification of local involved lymph nodes. PET scanning has also been used to assist with the staging and planning of therapy of cholangiocarcinoma. It is less specific than CT scanning for the primary lesion, but is better at detecting regional and distant lymphadenopathy.[91–94] Although both CEA and CA 19–9 either alone or in combination have been described as tumor markers of cholangiocarcinoma, neither is sufficiently sensitive or specific for routine use as diagnostic tumor markers.[95,96]

Pathologically, the lesion is an adenocarcinoma and may demonstrate a tubular appearance set in fibrous stroma, occasionally the cells may be very pleiomorphic. In tumors arising in the larger ducts the tumor is usually surrounded by a wide zone of biliary epithelial cell dysplasia.

Treatment

Despite advances in treatment, the prognosis of intrahepatic cholangiocarcinoma remains poor, with most patients dying within five years, and 90% dying with the first two years.[84] Although reports from single centers suggest that resection improves survival,[97–104] mortality data do not support this conclusion. Nonetheless, surgical resection remains the only chance of curative therapy. Unfortunately early spread of the disease results in a high recurrence rate. The location of the tumor may also limit the ability to resect the lesion. Lesions involving the hilum may not be resectable, particularly if the tumor extends into the second order branches of the right and left hepatic ducts. Radiotherapy and chemotherapy have not been shown to extend life.[105–108] For tumors that obstruct the hepatic duct and cause biliary dilatation insertion of a stent to drain the duct may be required. This can be placed by endoscopy at ERCP, or percutaneously under ultrasound guidance.[109] Liver transplantation is usually associated with a 90% recurrence rate.[110] Recently an aggressive management protocol developed at the Mayo Clinic has allowed post transplant survival of 85% at five years.[111] However, few patients are suitable for this protocol.

Other Liver Tumors

There are about 20 other mass-like lesions that may develop in the liver. Benign lesions include bile duct adenomas, and cystadenomas, hemangioendothelioma, lymphangioma, angiomyolipoma, and other rare benign soft tissue tumors. Of the malignant lesions not discussed that occur in the liver metastatic cancer is the most common, and the colon is the most common primary site. The radiological appearances of metastases are similar, wherever the source, but in the setting of a previous known carcinoma elsewhere, the diagnosis is not difficult. Metastases from neuroendocrine tumors merit special mention. These are often slow growing, and may present with symptoms of the carcinoid syndrome, or phaeochromocytoma. However, the majority of the tumors are non-secreting, and present commonly during surveillance for metastatic disease after treatment of a primary neuroendocrine tumor, or in patients in whom a primary has not been diagnosed, as an incidental finding on an ultrasound. These are usually very vascular tumors that may be mistaken for hepatocellular carcinoma. However, they do not usually display the typical "washout" that characterizes HCC. Tissue from a needle biopsy may be difficult to interpret, and often special stains for either hepatocyte markers or neuroendocrine markers, such as synaptophysin or chromaogranin may be necessary.

In addition, malignancies can arise from any component of liver tissue. Endothelium can give rise to angiosarcoma or malignant hemangioendothelioma, muscle can give rise to rhabdomyosarcoma. Other, other primary sarcomas and primary lymphoma of the liver have also been reported. These are all exceptionally rare and all require tissue diagnosis.

SUMMARY

The vast majority of liver masses can be accounted for by a limited number of benign or malignant diagnoses. Differentiating benign from malignant is obviously important and can be easily accomplished in most cases by radiology alone. Suspected adenoma and atypical (often early) HCC may require biopsy diagnosis, which is usually quite specific. Most benign lesions, what ever their nature need treatment only if they cause symptoms. Adenoma that does not resolve on withdrawal of an inciting estrogen or androgen might also require resection. HCC is the most common malignancy of the liver and usually arises in patients with pre-existing liver disease. Early diagnosis and effective treatment will cure the majority of HCC's although second primaries often occur. Cholangiocarcinoma has a bad prognosis, and the only treatment that is offered to patients is surgery.

REFERENCES

1. Karhunen PJ. Benign hepatic tumours and tumour like conditions in men. J Clin Pathol. 1986;39:183–8.
2. Di Carlo I, Urrico GS, Ursino V, Russello D, Puleo S, Latteri F. Simultaneous occurrence of adenoma, focal nodular hyperplasia, and hemangioma of the liver: are they derived from a common origin? J Gastroenterol Hepatol. 2003;18:227–30.
3. Gemer O, Moscovici O, Ben-Horin CL, Linov L, Peled R, Segal S. Oral contraceptives and liver hemangioma: a case-control study. Acta Obstet Gynecol Scand. 2004;83:1199–201.
4. Glinkova V, Shevah O, Boaz M, Levine A, Shirin H. Hepatic haemangiomas: possible association with female sex hormones. Gut. 2004;53:1352–5.
5. Au WY, Liu CL. Growth of giant hepatic hemangioma after triplet pregnancy. J Hepatol. 2005;42:781.
6. Saegusa T, Ito K, Oba N, Matsuda M, Kojima K, Tohyama K, Matsumoto M, Miura K, Suzuki H. Enlargement of multiple cavernous hemangioma of the liver in association with pregnancy. Intern Med. 1995;34:207–11.
7. Ozakyol A, Kebapci M. Enhanced growth of hepatic hemangiomatosis in two adults after postmenopausal estrogen replacement therapy. Tohoku J Exp Med. 2006;210:257–61.

8. Piga M, Satta L, Corrias M, Montaldo C, Loi GL, Madeddu G. Simultaneous 99mTc double labelling of the hepatic reticuloendothelial system and of the red blood cells: a simplified method for the detection of liver hemangiomas. J Nucl Med Allied Sci. 1990;34:77–80.

9. Numminen K, Halavaara J, Isoniemi H, Tervahartiala P, Kivisaari L, Numminen J, Hockerstedt K. Magnetic resonance imaging of the liver: true fast imaging with steady state free precession sequence facilitates rapid and reliable distinction between hepatic hemangiomas and liver malignancies. J Comput Assist Tomogr. 2003;27:571–6.

10. Peterson MS, Murakami T, Baron RL. MR imaging patterns of gadolinium retention within liver neoplasms. Abdom Imaging. 1998;23:592–9.

11. Johnson CM, Sheedy PF 2nd, Stanson AW, Stephens DH, Hattery RR, Adson MA. Computed tomography and angiography of cavernous hemangiomas of the liver. Radiology. 1981;138:115–21.

12. Birnbaum BA, Weinreb JC, Megibow AJ, Sanger JJ, Lubat E, Kanamuller H, Noz ME, Bosniak MA. Definitive diagnosis of hepatic hemangiomas: MR imaging versus Tc-99m-labeled red blood cell SPECT. Radiology. 1990;176:95–101.

13. Kim TK, Jang HJ, Wilson SR. Benign liver masses: imaging with microbubble contrast agents. Ultrasound Q. 2006;22:31–9.

14. Shimoji K, Shiraishi R, Kuwatsuru A, Maehara T, Matsumoto T, Kurosaki Y. Spontaneous subacute intratumoral hemorrhage of hepatic cavernous hemangioma. Abdom Imaging. 2004;29:443–5.

15. Krasuski P, Poniecka A, Gal E, Wali A. Intrapartum spontaneous rupture of liver hemangioma. J Matern Fetal Med. 2001;10:290–2.

16. Ontachi Y, Asakura H, Omote M, Yoshida T, Matsui O, Nakao S. Kasabach-Merritt syndrome associated with giant liver hemangioma: the effect of combined therapy with danaparoid sodium and tranexamic acid. Haematologica. 2005 Nov;90.

17. Reddy KR, Kligerman S, Levi J, Livingstone A, Molina E, Franceschi D, Badalamenti S, Jeffers L, Tzakis A, Schiff ER. Benign and solid tumors of the liver: relationship to sex, age, size of tumors, and outcome. Am Surg. 2001;67:173–8.

18. Wanless IR, Mawdsley C, Adams R. On the pathogenesis of focal nodular hyperplasia of the liver. Hepatology. 1985;5:1194–200.

19. Byrnes V, Cardenas A, Afdhal N, Hanto D. Symptomatic focal nodular hyperplasia during pregnancy: a case report. Ann Hepatol. 2004;3:35–7.

20. Scalori A, Tavani A, Gallus S, La Vecchia C, Colombo M. Oral contraceptives and the risk of focal nodular hyperplasia of the liver: a case-control study. Am J Obstet Gynecol. 2002;186:195–7.

21. Mathieu D, Kobeiter H, Maison P, Rahmouni A, Cherqui D, Zafrani ES, Dhumeaux D. Oral contraceptive use and focal nodular hyperplasia of the liver. Gastroenterology. 2000;118:560–4.

22. Ohmoto K, Honda T, Hirokawa M, Mitsui Y, Iguchi Y, Kuboki M, Yamamoto S. Spontaneous regression of focal nodular hyperplasia of the liver. J Gastroenterol. 2002;37:849–53.

23. Di Stasi M, Caturelli E, De Sio I, Salmi A, Buscarini E, Buscarini L. Natural history of focal nodular hyperplasia of the liver: an ultrasound study. J Clin Ultrasound. 1996;24:345–50.

24. Yen YH, Wang JH, Lu SN, Chen TY, Changchien CS, Chen CH, Hung CH, Lee CM. Contrast-enhanced ultrasonographic spoke-wheel sign in hepatic focal nodular hyperplasia. Eur J Radiol. 2006;14.

25. Terkivatan T, van den Bos IC, Hussain SM, Wielopolski PA, de Man RA, IJzermans JN. Focal nodular hyperplasia: lesion characteristics on state-of-the-art MRI including dynamic gadolinium-enhanced and superparamagnetic iron-oxide-uptake sequences in a prospective study. J Magn Reson Imaging. 2006;24:864–72.

26. Nicolau C, Vilana R, Catala V, Bianchi L, Gilabert R, Garcia A, Bru C. Importance of evaluating all vascular phases on contrast-enhanced sonography in the differentiation of benign from malignant focal liver lesions. AJR Am J Roentgenol. 2006;186:158–67.

27. Lee MJ, Saini S, Hamm B, Taupitz M, Hahn PF, Seneterre E, Ferrucci JT. Focal nodular hyperplasia of the liver: MR findings in 35 proved cases. AJR Am J Roentgenol. 1991;156:317–20.

28. Nicolau C, Vilana R, Catala V, Bianchi L, Gilabert R, Garcia A, Bru C. Importance of evaluating all vascular phases on contrast-enhanced sonography in the differentiation of benign from malignant focal liver lesions. AJR Am J Roentgenol. 2006;186:158–67.

29. Vogl TJ, Own A, Hammerstingl R, Reichel P, Balzer JO. Transarterial embolization as a therapeutic option for focal nodular hyperplasia in four patients. Eur Radiol. 2006;16:670–5.

30. Geschwind JF, Degli MS, Morris JM, Choti MA. Treatment of focal nodular hyperplasia with selective transcatheter arterial embolization using iodized oil and polyvinyl alcohol. Cardiovasc Intervent Radiol. 2002;25:340–1.

31. Terkivatan T, Hussain SM, Lameris JS, IJzermans JN. Transcatheter arterial embolization as a safe and effective treatment for focal nodular hyperplasia of the liver. Cardiovasc Intervent Radiol. 2002;25:450–3.

32. Erdogan D, Busch OR, van Delden OM, Ten Kate FJ, Gouma DJ, van Gulik TM. Management of spontaneous haemorrhage and rupture of hepatocellular adenomas. A single centre experience. Liver Int. 2006;26:433–8.

33. Baum JK, Bookstein JJ, Holtz F, Klein EW. Possible association between benign hepatomas and oral contraceptives. Lancet. 1973;2(7835):926–9.

34. Ammentorp PA, Carson RP. Hepatocellular adenoma and oral contraceptives. Ohio State Med J. 1976;72:283–6.

35. Rooks JB, Ory HW, Ishak KG, Strauss LT, Greenspan JR, Hill AP, Tyler CW Jr. Epidemiology of hepatocellular adenoma. The role of oral contraceptive use. JAMA. 1979;242:644–8.

36. Nissen ED, Kent DR, Nissen SE. Role of oral contraceptive agents in the pathogenesis of liver tumors. J Toxicol Environ Health. 1979;5:231–54.

37. Aseni P, Sansalone CV, Sammartino C, Benedetto FD, Carrafiello G, Giacomoni A, Osio C, Vertemati M, Forti D. Rapid disappearance of hepatic adenoma after contraceptive withdrawal. J Clin Gastroenterol. 2001;33:234–6.

38. Steinbrecher UP, Lisbona R, Huang SN, Mishkin S. Complete regression of hepatocellular adenoma after withdrawal of oral contraceptives. Dig Dis Sci. 1981;26:1045–50.

39. Heinemann LA, Weimann A, Gerken G, Thiel C, Schlaud M, DoMinh T. Modern oral contraceptive use and benign liver tumors: the German Benign Liver Tumor Case-Control Study. Eur J Contracept Reprod Health Care. 1998;3:194–200.

40. Grange JD, Guechot J, Legendre C, Giboudeau J, Darnis F, Poupon R. Liver adenoma and focal nodular hyperplasia in a man with high endogenous sex steroids. Gastroenterology. 1987;93:1409–13.

41. Nakao A, Sakagami K, Nakata Y, Komazawa K, Amimoto T, Nakashima K, Isozaki H, Takakura N, Tanaka N. Multiple hepatic adenomas caused by long-term administration of androgenic steroids for aplastic anemia in association with familial adenomatous polyposis. J Gastroenterol. 2000;35:557–62.

42. de Menis E, Tramontin P, Conte N. Danazol and multiple hepatic adenomas: peculiar clinical findings in an acromegalic patient. Horm Metab Res. 1999;31:476–7.

43. Socas L, Zumbado M, Perez-Luzardo O, Ramos A, Perez C, Hernandez JR, Boada LD. Hepatocellular adenomas associated with anabolic androgenic steroid abuse in bodybuilders: a report of two cases and a review of the literature. Br J Sports Med. 2005;39.

44. Franco LM, Krishnamurthy V, Bali D, Weinstein DA, Arn P, Clary B, Boney A, Sullivan J, Frush DP, Chen YT, Kishnani PS. Hepatocellular carcinoma in glycogen storage disease type Ia: a case series. J Inherit Metab Dis. 2005;28:153–62.

45. Hagiwara S, Takagi H, Kanda D, Sohara N, Kakizaki S, Katakai K, Yoshinaga T, Higuchi T, Nomoto K, Kuwano H, Mori M. Hepatic adenomatosis associated with hormone replacement therapy and hemosiderosis: a case report. World J Gastroenterol. 2006;12:652–5.

46. Grazioli L, Federle MP, Brancatelli G, Ichikawa T, Olivetti L, Blachar A. Hepatic adenomas: imaging and pathologic findings. Radiographics. 2001;21:877–92.

47. Ito M, Sasaki M, Wen CY, Nakashima M, Ueki T, Ishibashi H, Yano M, Kage M, Kojiro M. Liver cell adenoma with malignant transformation: a case report. World J Gastroenterol. 2003;9:2379–81.

48. Gyorffy EJ, Bredfeldt JE, Black WC. Transformation of hepatic cell adenoma to hepatocellular carcinoma due to oral contraceptive use. Ann Intern Med. 1989;15;110: 489–90.

49. Dietrich CF, Schuessler G, Trojan J, Fellbaum C, Ignee A. Differentiation of focal nodular hyperplasia and hepatocellular adenoma by contrast-enhanced ultrasound. Br J Radiol. 2005;78:704–7.

50. Brancatelli G, Federle MP, Vullierme MP, Lagalla R, Midiri M, Vilgrain V. CT and MR imaging evaluation of hepatic adenoma. J Comput Assist Tomogr. 2006;30:745–50.

51. Kebapci M, Kaya T, Aslan O, Bor O, Entok E. Hepatic adenomatosis: gadolinium-enhanced dynamic MR findings. Abdom Imaging. 2001;26:264–8.

52. Fujita S, Kushihata F, Herrmann GE, Mergo PJ, Liu C, Nelson D, Fujikawa T, Hemming AW. Combined hepatic resection and radiofrequency ablation for multiple hepatic adenomas. J Gastroenterol Hepatol. 2006;21:1351–4.

53. Rocourt DV, Shiels WE, Hammond S, Besner GE. Contemporary management of benign hepatic adenoma using percutaneous radiofrequency ablation. J Pediatr Surg. 2006;41:1149–52.

54. Parkin DM, Bray F, Ferlay J, Pisani P. Estimating the world cancer burden: Globocan 2000. Int J Cancer 2001;94:153–156.

55. Elmberg M, Hultcrantz R, Ekbom A, Brandt L, Olsson S, Olsson R et al. Cancer risk in patients with hereditary hemochromatosis and in their first-degree relatives. Gastroenterology 2003;125:1733–41.

56. Eriksson S, Carlson J, Velez R. Risk of cirrhosis and primary liver cancer in alpha 1-antitrypsin deficiency. N Engl J Med 1986;314:736–9.

57. Caballeria L, Pares A, Castells A, Gines A, Bru C, Rodes J. Hepatocellular carcinoma in primary biliary cirrhosis: similar incidence to that in hepatitis C virus-related cirrhosis. Am J Gastroenterol 2001; 96(4):1160–3.

58. Shimada M, Hashimoto E, Taniai M, Hasegawa K, Okuda H, Hayashi N et al. Hepatocellular carcinoma in patients with non-alcoholic steatohepatitis. J Hepatol 2002; 37:154–160.

59. Bosch FX, Ribes J, Diaz M, Cleries R. Primary liver cancer: worldwide incidence and trends. Gastroenterology 2004; 127(5 Suppl 1):S5–S16.

60. El Serag HB, Mason AC. Rising incidence of hepatocellular carcinoma in the United States. N Engl J Med 1999; 340:745–50.

61. Deuffic S, Poynard T, Buffat L, Valleron AJ. Trends in primary liver cancer. Lancet 1998; 351(9097):214–15.

62. Stroffolini T, Andreone P, Andriulli A, Ascione A, Craxi A, Chiaramonte M et al. Characteristics of hepatocellular carcinoma in Italy. J Hepatol 1998; 29:944–52.

63. Taylor-Robinson SD, Foster GR, Arora S, Hargreaves S, Thomas HC. Increase in primary liver cancer in the UK, 1979–94. Lancet 1997; 350(9085):1142–3.

64. Zhang BH, Yang BH, Tang ZY. Randomized controlled trial of screening for hepatocellular carcinoma. J Cancer Res Clin Oncol 2004; 130:417–22.

65. Trevisani F, D'Intino PE, Morselli-Labate AM, Mazzella G, Accogli E, Caraceni P et al. Serum alpha-fetoprotein for diagnosis of hepatocellular carcinoma in patients with chronic liver disease: influence of HBsAg and anti-HCV status. J Hepatol 2001; 34:570–5.

66. Bruix J, Sherman M; Practice Guidelines Committee, American Association for the Study of Liver Diseases. Management of hepatocellular carcinoma. Hepatology. 2005;42:1208–36.

67. Bruix J, Llovet JM. Prognostic prediction and treatment strategy in HCC. Hepatology 2002; 35:519–24

68. Mazzaferro V, Regalia E, Doci R, Andreola S, Pulvirenti A, Bozzetti F et al. Liver transplantation for the treatment of small hepatocellular carcinomas in patients with cirrhosis. N Engl J Med 1996; 334:693–9.

69. Yao FY, Ferrell L, Bass NM, Watson JJ, Bacchetti P, Venook A et al. Liver transplantation for hepatocellular carcinoma: expansion of the tumor size limits does not adversely impact survival. Hepatology 2001; 33:1394–1403.

70. Llovet JM, Fuster J, Bruix J. Intention-to-Treat Analysis of Surgical Treatment for Early Hepatocellular Carcinoma: Resection Versus Transplantation. Hepatology 1999; 30:1434–440.

71. Grazi GL, Ercolani G, Pierangeli F, Del Gaudio M, Cescon M, Cavallari A et al. Improved results of liver resection for hepatocellular carcinoma on cirrhosis give the procedure added value. Ann Surg 2001; 234:71–8.

72. Bruix J, Castells A, Bosch J, Feu F, Fuster J, Garcia-Pagan JC et al. Surgical resection of hepatocellular carcinoma in cirrhotic patients: prognostic value of preoperative portal pressure. Gastroenterology 1996; 111:1018–22.

73. Andriulli A, De Sio I, Brunello F, Salmi A, Solmi L, Facciorusso D, Caturelli E, Perri F. Survival of patients with early hepatocellular carcinoma treated by percutaneous alcohol injection. Aliment Pharmacol Ther. 2006;23:1329–35.

74. Livraghi T, Solbiati L, Meloni MF, Gazelle GS, Halpern EF, Goldberg SN. Treatment of focal liver tumors with percutaneous radio-frequency ablation: complications encountered in a multicenter study. Radiology 2003; 226:441–451.

75. Chen MS, Li JQ, Zheng Y, Guo RP, Liang HH, Zhang YQ, Lin XJ, Lau WY. A prospective randomized trial comparing percutaneous local ablative therapy and partial hepatectomy for small hepatocellular carcinoma. Ann Surg. 2006 Mar;243(3):321–8.

76. Sala M, Llovet JM, Vilana R, Bianchi L, Sole M, Ayuso C, Bru C, Bruix J; Barcelona Clinic Liver Cancer Group. Initial response to percutaneous ablation predicts survival in patients with hepatocellular carcinoma. Hepatology. 2004 Dec;40(6):1352–60.

77. Llovet JM, Real MI, Montanya X, Planas R, Coll S, Aponte AJ et al. Arterial embolization, chemoembolization versus symptomatic treatment in patients with unresectable hepatocellular carcinoma: a randomized controlled trial. The Lancet 2002; 359:1734–9.

78. Lo CM, Ngan H, Tso WK, Liu CL, Lam CM, Poon RT et al. Randomized controlled trial of transarterial lipiodol chemoembolization for unresectable hepatocellular carcinoma. Hepatology 2002; 35:1164–71.

79. Llovet JM, Bruix J. Systematic review of randomized trials for unresectable hepatocellular carcinoma: Chemoembolization improves survival. Hepatology. 2003;37:429–42.

80. Salem R, Lewandowski RJ, Atassi B, Gordon SC, Gates VL, Barakat O, Sergie Z, Wong CY, Thurston KG. Treatment of unresectable hepatocellular carcinoma with use of 90Y microspheres (TheraSphere): safety, tumor response, and survival. J Vasc Interv Radiol. 2005;16:1627–39.

81. Shaib YH, Davila JA, McGlynn K, El-Serag HB. Rising incidence of intrahepatic cholangiocarcinoma in the United States: a true increase? J Hepatol. 2004;40:472–7.

82. Khan SA, Thomas HC, Davidson BR, Taylor-Robinson SD. Cholangiocarcinoma. Lancet. 2005;366(9493):1303–14.

83. Shaib YH, El-Serag HB, Davila JA, Morgan R, McGlynn KA. Risk factors of intrahepatic cholangiocarcinoma in the United States: a case-control study. Gastroenterology. 2005;128:620–6.

84. McGlynn KA, Tarone RE, El-Serag HB. A comparison of trends in the incidence of hepatocellular carcinoma and intrahepatic cholangiocarcinoma in the United States. Cancer Epidemiol Biomarkers Prev. 2006;15:1198–203.

85. Anderson CD, Pinson CW, Berlin J, Chari RS. Diagnosis and treatment of cholangiocarcinoma. Oncologist. 2004;9:43–57.86. Khan SA, Davidson BR, Goldin R, Pereira SP, Rosenberg WM, Taylor-Robinson SD, Thillainayagam AV, Thomas HC, Thursz MR, Wasan H; British Society of Gastroenterology. Guidelines for the diagnosis and treatment of cholangiocarcinoma: consensus document. Gut. 2002;51 Suppl 6: VI1–9.

86. Saini S. Imaging of the hepatobiliary tract. N Engl J Med. 1997;336:1889–94.

87. Zhang Y, Uchida M, Abe T, Nishimura H, Hayabuchi N, Nakashima Y. Intrahepatic peripheral cholangiocarcinoma: comparison of dynamic CT and dynamic MRI. J Comput Assist Tomogr. 1999;23:670–7.

88. Yeh TS, Jan YY, Tseng JH, Chiu CT, Chen TC, Hwang TL, Chen MF. Malignant perihilar biliary obstruction: magnetic resonance cholangiopancreatographic findings. Am J Gastroenterol. 2000;95:432–40.

89. Abu-Hamda EM, Baron TH. Endoscopic management of cholangiocarcinoma. Semin Liver Dis. 2004;24:165–75.

90. Kim SK, Kang KW, Lee JS, Kim HK, Chang HJ, Choi JY, Lee JH, Ryu KW, Kim YW, Bae JM. Assessment of lymph node metastases using 18F-FDG PET in patients with advanced gastric cancer. Eur J Nucl Med Mol Imaging. 2006;33:148–55.

91. Fritscher-Ravens A, Bohuslavizki KH, Broering DC, Jenicke L, Schafer H, Buchert R, Rogiers X, Clausen M. FDG PET in the diagnosis of hilar cholangiocarcinoma. Nucl Med Commun. 2001;22:1277–85.

92. Anderson CD, Rice MH, Pinson CW, Chapman WC, Chari RS, Delbeke D. Fluo-rodeoxyglucose PET imaging in the evaluation of gallbladder carcinoma and cholan-giocarcinoma. J Gastrointest Surg. 2004;8:90–7.

93. Kato T, Tsukamoto E, Kuge Y, Katoh C, Nambu T, Nobuta A, Kondo S, Asaka M, Tamaki N. Clinical role of (18)F-FDG PET for initial staging of patients with extrahepatic bile duct cancer. Eur J Nucl Med Mol Imaging. 2002;29:1047–54.

94. Nehls O, Gregor M, Klump B. Serum and bile markers for cholangiocarcinoma. Semin Liver Dis. 2004;24:139–54.

95. Patel AH, Harnois DM, Klee GG, LaRusso NF Gores GJ The utility of CA 19–9 in the diagnoses of cholangiocarcinoma in patients without primary sclerosing cholangitis Am J Gastroenterol. 2000;95:204–7.

96. Jarnagin WR, Shoup M Surgical management of cholangiocarcinoma Semin Liver Dis. 2004;24:189–99.

97. Su CH, Tsay SH, Wu CC, Shyr YM, King KL, Lee CH, Lui WY, Liu TJ, P'eng FK. Factors influencing postoperative morbidity, mortality, and survival after resection for hilar cholangiocarcinoma. Ann Surg. 1996;223:384–94.

98. Nimura Y, Hayakawa N, Kamiya J, Kondo S, Shionoya S. Hepatic segmentectomy with caudate lobe resection for bile duct carcinoma of the hepatic hilus. World J Surg. 1990;14:535–43.

99. Nakeeb A, Tran KQ, Black MJ, Erickson BA, Ritch PS, Quebbeman EJ, Wilson SD, Demeure MJ, Rilling WS, Dua KS, Pitt HA. Improved survival in resected biliary malignancies. Surgery. 2002;132:555–63.

100. Hadjis NS, Blenkharn JI, Alexander N, Benjamin IS, Blumgart LH.Outcome of radical surgery in hilar cholangiocarcinoma. Surgery. 1990 Jun;107(6):597–604.

101. Pichlmayr R, Weimann A, Klempnauer J, Oldhafer KJ, Maschek H, Tusch G, Ringe B. Surgical treatment in proximal bile duct cancer. A single-center experience. Ann Surg. 1996;224:628–38.

102. Jarnagin WR, Fong Y, DeMatteo RP, Gonen M, Burke EC, Bodniewicz BS J, Youssef BA M, Klimstra D, Blumgart LH. Staging, resectability, and outcome in 225 patients with hilar cholangiocarcinoma. Ann Surg. 2001;234:507–17.

103. Wade TP, Prasad CN, Virgo KS, Johnson FE. Experience with distal bile duct cancers in U.S. Veterans Affairs hospitals: 1987–1991. Surg Oncol. 1997;64:242–5.

104. Cameron JL, Pitt HA, Zinner MJ, Kaufman SL, Coleman J. Management of proximal cholangiocarcinomas by surgical resection and radiotherapy. Am J Surg. 1990;159:91–98.

105. Todoroki T. Chemotherapy for bile duct carcinoma in the light of adjuvant chemother-apy to surgery. Hepatogastroenterology. 2000;47:644–9.

106. Todoroki T, Ohara K, Kawamoto T, Koike N, Yoshida S, Kashiwagi H, Otsuka M, Fukao K. Benefits of adjuvant radiotherapy after radical resection of locally advanced main hepatic duct carcinoma. Int J Radiat Oncol Biol Phys. 2000;46:581–7.

107. Ohnishi H, Asada M, Shichijo Y, Iijima N, Itobayashi E, Shimura K, Suzuki T, Yoshida S, Mine T. External radiotherapy for biliary decompression of hilar cholangiocarcinoma Hepatogastroenterology. 1995;42:265–8.

108. Pitt HA, Gomes AS, Lois JF, Mann LL, Deutsch LS, Longmire WP Jr. Does preoperative percutaneous biliary drainage reduce operative risk or increase hospital cost? Ann Surg. 1985;201:545–53.

109. Meyer CG, Penn I, James L. Liver transplantation for cholangiocarcinoma: results in 207 patients. Transplantation. 2000;69:1633–7.

110. Rea DJ, Heimbach JK, Rosen CB, Haddock MG, Alberts SR, Kremers WK, Gores GJ, Nagorney DM. Liver transplantation with neoadjuvant chemoradiation is more effective than resection for hilar cholangiocarcinoma. Ann Surg. 2005;242:451–8.

Complications of Cirrhosis

Jorge L. Herrera, MD

BACKGROUND

Chronic liver disease is one of the leading causes of death in the United States.[1] As a result of the hepatitis C virus (HCV) epidemic 20–30 years ago, it is expected that by 2020 the proportion of chronic HCV patients with cirrhosis will double from 16% to 32%, and there will be a 180% increase in liver-related deaths.[2] Although only liver transplantation is able to reverse the complications of advanced liver disease, the number of patients awaiting orthotopic liver transplantation has grown to 17,562 as of November 2006.[3] Many patients with cirrhosis are not eligible for liver transplantation or may not receive an organ transplant during their lifetime.

Most patients with chronic liver disease receive their medical care from primary care physicians or gastroenterologists. A clear understanding of the pathophysiology of chronic liver disease, its possible complications, and management are important to deliver state of the art care to patients with chronic liver disease.

PROGNOSIS OF CIRRHOSIS

Most chronic liver diseases generally run a steady course with gradual deterioration over time. The natural history of cirrhosis is characterized by an asymptomatic phase, also known as "compensated cirrhosis," followed by a rapidly progressive phase marked by the development of complications of portal hypertension and/or liver dysfunction, termed "decompensated cirrhosis." Transition from a compensated to a decompensated stage occurs at a rate of approximately 5–7% per year.[4] The development of decompensation is an important milestone in the natural history of cirrhosis. Patients with compensated cirrhosis have a median survival of 12 years, compared with a two-year median survival among patients with decompensated cirrhosis.

Table 13.1. Modified Child-Turcotte Criteria: Points Assigned to Laboratory Values and Signs

Parameter	1	2	3
Total serum bilirubin (mg/dL)	<2	2–3	>3
Serum albumin (g/dL)	>3.5	2.8–3.5	<2.8
INR	<1.70	1.71–2.20	>2.20
Ascites	None	Controlled medically	Poorly controlled
Encephalopathy	None	Controlled medically	Poorly controlled

Based on total points: Class A = 5 to 6 points; Class B = 7 to 9 points, Class C = 10 to 15 points.

The etiology of the liver disease also plays an important etiology in determining its natural history. Alcoholic cirrhosis usually portends a worse prognosis in those patients who continue to drink alcohol after the diagnosis. Among patients with chronic hepatitis C, a retrospective five-year study of 384 patients showed that 91% were still alive at five years and the 10-year survival probability was calculated at 70%.[5] Other investigators have assessed the five-year risk of hepatocellular carcinoma at 10% and decompensation at 15–20%.[6]

Although a liver biopsy is often required to establish the diagnosis of cirrhosis in asymptomatic patients, the biopsy provides little information regarding the severity or prognosis of the liver disease. Several prognostic models have been developed to predict the course and outcome of chronic liver disease.[7] Despite its multiple shortcomings, the Pugh modification of the Child-Turcotte criteria (CTP)[8] (Table 13.1) is the most frequently used model to establish the severity of liver disease in cirrhotic patients. Progression to a CTP score of 8 or higher signals early decompensation and should prompt consideration for referral to a liver transplant center. The model for end-stage liver disease (MELD)[9] is a recently developed prognostic model that utilizes the prothrombin time, serum bilirubin, serum creatinine level, and the need for dialysis to asses severity of liver disease. The MELD score is most useful in predicting short-term mortality in the setting of advanced liver disease among patients awaiting liver transplantation. Those patients with a score of 15 or higher have a three-month mortality that equals or exceed that of liver transplantation and should be considered for transplant. In contrast with the CTP score, which can be calculated at the bedside, the MELD score is calculated based on a complex equation. A web-based calculator can be found at http://www.unos.org/resources/. Longitudinal monitoring of patients with compensated cirrhosis using the CTP score is recommended to detect evidence of early hepatic decompensation. Once the CTP score rises to 8 or higher, computation of the MELD score is recommended to determine the ideal timing for liver transplantation.

Portal hypertension is an almost unavoidable complication of cirrhosis and is responsible for the more lethal complications of this syndrome: variceal bleeding, ascites, hepatorenal syndrome, bacterial infections, and hepatic encephalopathy. Timely recognition of these complications allows for prophylactic and therapeutic measures that may result in decreased morbidity and improved survival of patients with advanced liver disease.

VARICEAL HEMORRHAGE

Primary Prophylaxis

Among the portosystemic collaterals, gastroesophageal varices are the most clinically important because of their propensity to rupture and cause life-threatening hemorrhage. The presence of gastroesophageal varices is not universal among patients with cirrhosis, only one-third of patients with cirrhosis have varices on cross-sectional studies.[10] The prevalence of varices increases with advancing severity of liver disease. Among patients with decompensated cirrhosis and ascites, varices are found in up to 60%.[11] About one-third of patients with documented varices will bleed within two years from diagnosis with an associated mortality of 20–40% per episode.[12]

Prophylactic treatment with non-selective beta blockers in patients with cirrhosis and documented varices decreases the risk of the initial hemorrhage from esophageal varices by approximately 40% in individuals at increased risk for variceal bleeding.[13,14] In contrast, treatment with non-selective beta-blockers of all patients with cirrhosis regardless of the presence or absence of varices has failed to show any benefit, probably because of the low bleeding rates in patients without varices.[15] Nonselective beta blockers have also been found to be ineffective in preventing formation of varices among patients with portal hypertension but without varices on initial endoscopy[16] Thus, it is important to screen for varices and select patients at increased risk for bleeding, with the risk being highest for those patients with moderate to large varices on screening endoscopy.[17] The presence of red signs (red wale markings, cherry red spots, and hematocystic spots) further increase the risk of bleeding.[12] Attempts have been made at improving selection of patients for screening endoscopy based on clinical, laboratory, and radiologic parameters predicting increased risk for variceal hemorrhage. Unfortunately, most non-invasive markers of severe portal hypertension lack sensitivity or specificity in selecting patients at high risk for variceal bleeding.[18] The American College of Gastroenterology practice guidelines[19] and the American Society of Gastrointestinal Endoscopy[20] recommend endoscopic screening to detect varices in all patients with cirrhosis and no previous episodes of variceal hemorrhage.

Patients at low risk for bleeding do not require specific therapy. Those with no varices on index endoscopy should undergo repeat endoscopy in two to three years, or sooner if decompensation develops. Patients with small varices with no high risk stigmata should undergo repeat surveillance endoscopy in one year.[21] Patients with medium or large varices are at high risk for bleeding should be treated with non-selective beta blockers. Propranolol is generally used as a long-acting preparation with a starting dose of 60 mg/day. The dose is titrated to decrease resting heart rate by 25% but not less than 55 beats/minute. The mean maintenance dose of propranolol required to reach this goal is 160 mg/day. Evening administration is recommended to minimize some of the adverse events. About 30% of patients are unable to tolerate propranolol. Nadolol, also a non-selective beta blocker does not cross the blood brain barrier and is generally better tolerated. The starting dose for nadolol is 20 to 40 mg/day, and the usual daily effective dose ranges from 20 to 240 mg/day.[22] Once initiated, therapy with non-selective beta blockers should be maintained indefinitely as when they are withdrawn the risk of variceal hemorrhage rises to pre-treatment levels.[23] Those

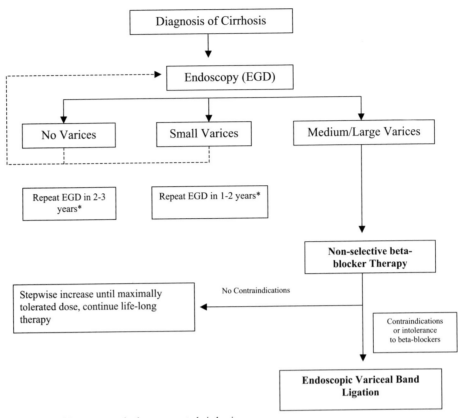

* Repeat EGD every year in decompensated cirrhosis

Figure 13.1. Prophylaxis of variceal hemorrhage.

who are unable to tolerate nonselective beta blockers and are at high risk for bleeding should be considered for prophylactic endoscopic banding of varices.[24] The recommendations for prophylaxis of variceal hemorrhage are summarized in Figure 13.1.

Treatment of Acute Variceal Hemorrhage

Acute variceal hemorrhage is a life-threatening complication of cirrhosis, with current mortality rates of 15–20% per bleeding episode.[25] The general management of variceal hemorrhage is directed at correcting hypovolemia and preventing complications associated with gastrointestinal hemorrhage such as renal failure, bacterial infections, and hepatic encephalopathy. Hypovolemia should be corrected judiciously as overcorrection may cause an increase in portal pressure and promote further bleeding. Blood volume replacement should aim at a hemoglobin level of approximately 8 g/L (equivalent to a hematocrit of approximately 25%). Platelet and fresh frozen plasma transfusions to correct coagulopathy contribute further to volume overload and re-bleeding risk. The use of recombinant activated factor VII is under evaluation for correcting the prothrombin time in cirrhotics avoiding volume overload in the acute setting.[26]

Bacterial infections are associated with an increased risk for early rebleeding from varices. The incidence of bacterial infections in cirrhotic patients hospitalized with gastrointestinal hemorrhage is 45%. Prophylaxis of bacterial infections in bleeding patients with cirrhosis results in a significant decrease in the incidence of infections, and is associated with a significant improvement in survival.[27] The use of short-term antibiotic prophylaxis should be considered standard of care in cirrhotic patients admitted with gastrointestinal hemorrhage. The simplest and most studied approach is norfloxacin administered orally at a dose of 400 mg twice a day for seven days. In patients in who cannot tolerate oral administration, systemic ciprofloxacin or ceftriaxone may be used.[28]

Pharmacologic agents to control variceal bleeding are important adjuncts to the management of actively bleeding patients. Octreotide, a somatostatin analog with a longer half-life decreases portal pressure and collateral blood flow. The efficacy of octreotide as single therapy for variceal bleeding is controversial, but its use in conjunction with endoscopic variceal ligation has shown a significant benefit in reducing early rebleeding.[29] The optimal dose of octreotide is not known, but it is usually given as a bolus of 50 micrograms intravenously, followed by an infusion of 50 micrograms per hour. The infusion is maintained for five days to prevent early rebleeding. Vasopressin has been found to be less effective and with more side effects than octreotide and should not be used as first line therapy for variceal bleeding. Terlipressin, a long-acting derivative of vasopressin is associated with good clinical efficacy and less frequent and severe side effects compared with vasopressin.[30] Currently terlipressin is not available for use in the United States, however, clinical trials are in progress.

Endoscopic therapy in the form of variceal sclerotherapy or ligation is highly effective in controlling active hemorrhage and preventing early rebleeding. Endoscopic variceal ligation is more effective than sclerotherapy in achieving bleeding control and is associated with a lower complication rate.[31]

The recommended approach to the patient with acute variceal hemorrhage is to initiate pharmacologic therapy with octreotide while providing adequate resuscitation. Once the patient is stable, endoscopic intervention with band ligation will control the bleeding and prevent early recurrence. Initial stabilization and patient resuscitation with the use of vasoactive drugs also allows for a safer and more complete endoscopic exam after most of the blood has been cleared from the stomach.

In 10–20% of patients, endoscopic and pharmacologic interventions fail to control bleeding. Balloon tamponade achieves hemostasis in 60–90% of these patients[32] but should only be used by experienced individuals and for a short period of time (less than 24 hours), as a bridge to definitive therapy. Transjugular intrahepatic protosystemic shunts (TIPS) or surgical shunts can then be used as definitive therapy in these patients depending on hepatic reserve.[32] The recommended approach to the management of acute variceal bleeding is shown in Figure 13.2.

Prevention of Recurrent Variceal Bleeding

Variceal hemorrhage has a two-year recurrence rate of approximately 80%.[33] Patients who survive the initial episode of variceal bleeding should be started

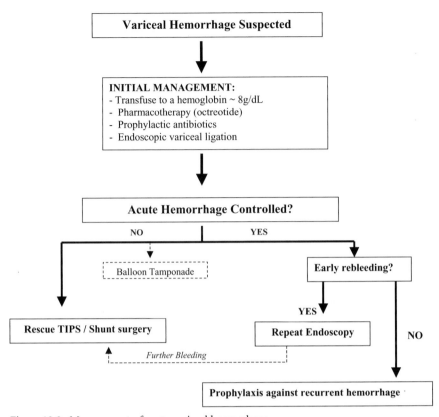

Figure 13.2. Management of acute variceal hemorrhage.

on therapy to decrease the risk of rebleeding. In addition, liver transplantation should be considered for those who have poor liver function or other recurrent complications of portal hypertension.

Non-selective beta blockers have been to be effective in decreasing the risk of rebleeding and mortality.[34] Endoscopic variceal band ligation has been found to be as effective as pharmacologic therapy in preventing rebleeding,[35] and the combination of endoscopic therapy and the use of nonselective beta-blockers appear to be synergistic and is the preferred approach to prevention of rebleeding.[36] Repeat endoscopy with ligation of varices should be done at two- to four-week intervals until variceal eradication is achieved. Thereafter, patients should be maintained on non-selective beta blockers and surveillance endoscopies repeated every six months to detect recurrence of varices. A recommended approach to prevent rebleeding from esophageal varices is shown in Figure 13.3.

Gastric Varices

Gastric varices develop in approximately 20% of patients with portal hypertension and are the source of bleeding in 5–10% of upper GI bleeding episodes in patients with cirrhosis. The optimal treatment of gastric varices has not been determined. Although there is a lack of randomized data, it seems reasonable to use nonselective beta blockers to prevent the first bleeding episode in patient who have gastric varices.[37]

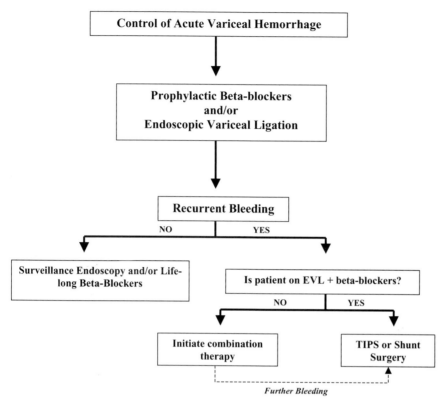

Figure 13.3 Prophylaxis of recurrent variceal hemorrhage.

The management of acute bleeding from gastric varices is controversial. The initial approach is similar to esophageal variceal bleeding, including the use of vasoactive drugs such as octreotide. Endoscopic variceal sclerotherapy and ligation are not as effective as in esophageal varices and is only recommended for the treatment of actively bleeding gastric varices that are contiguous with the esophageal varices or as a bridge to more definitive therapy. TIPS is effective for treating bleeding gastric varices and should be considered as the treatment of choice after the first episode of bleeding from gastric varices. If surgical expertise is available, a distal splenorenal shunt is an option for patients with well-compensated Child's-Pugh class A cirrhosis. Promising endoscopic interventions such as the use of cyanoacrylate endoscopic glue[38] are being investigated but are currently not available for general use in the United States.

ASCITES

Ascites is a common manifestation of portal hypertension. Approximately 50% of patients with compensated cirrhosis will develop ascites over 10 years.[39] Development of ascites is an important manifestation of advanced liver disease, with 50% mortality two years after onset of ascites.[39] Development of ascites leads to a decreased quality of life and risk of complications such as spontaneous bacterial peritonitis and renal failure.

The pathophysiology of ascites in cirrhosis is not completely understood but ascites is believed to develop as a direct consequence of sinusoidal portal hypertension in association with a state of systemic vascular vasodilation mediated by increased nitric oxide (NO) activity. The systemic vasodilation is most prominent in the splanchnic arterial bed resulting in redistribution of the circulating blood volume to the dilated vascular beds. These changes result in a decreased effective circulating blood volume and leads to increased cardiac output, renal sodium retention, and a hyperdynamic circulatory state.[40]

The development of ascites should prompt rapid investigation to establish its cause and exclude complications. Although the most common cause of ascites in the United States is cirrhosis, up to 15% of patients may have a nonhepatic cause for the ascites. Abdominal paracentesis with analysis of the ascitic fluid is the most rapid and cost-effective method to investigate the cause of the ascites and exclude complications.[41] Because of the high prevalence of unsuspected ascitic fluid infection in patients with ascites admitted to the hospital, a paracentesis should be performed in all patients with ascites at the time of admission.[42]

Diagnostic paracentesis is a safe procedure with minor complications reported in <1% of patients,[43] it is performed at the bedside using a 22- or 25-gauge needle and requires no pre-procedure laboratory testing to evaluate hemostasis.[44] Ultrasound localization of ascites may be helpful but is not necessary in most cases. Common sites for needle insertion include a point 2 cm below the umbilicus in the midline or in the left lower quadrant, 2–4 cm medial and cephalad to the anterior superior iliac spine. The midline approach avoids major blood vessels; the left lower quadrant approach is preferred in obese patients where the abdominal wall may be thinner in this area. Surgical scars should be avoided.[45]

Analysis of the Ascitic Fluid

Analysis of the ascitic fluid should answer four important questions[46]: (1) Is the fluid infected? (2) Is portal hypertension present? (3) Is the fluid at risk of infection? and (4) If portal hypertension is not present, what is the cause of the ascites? Most of these questions can be answered by routinely obtaining a cell count and differential, albumin, total protein and cultures on the ascitic fluid. To maximize the yield of bacterial cultures, 10 cc of ascitic fluid should be inoculated directly into aerobic and anaerobic blood culture bottles at the bedside. An extra aliquot of fluid should be sent to the laboratory in case additional testing is necessary after initial evaluation of the fluid. A serum albumin level should be determined simultaneously at the time of paracentesis to aid in the evaluation of the ascitic fluid results. The recommended tests that should be ordered when performing a diagnostic paracentesis are listed on Table 13.2.

Cell count and differential is used to detect the presence of infection. An absolute polymorphonuclear (PMN) count >250 cells/mm^3 in the appropriate setting strongly suggests the presence of infection and indicates the need for empiric antibiotics regardless of the culture results. The presence of portal hypertension is determined by calculating the serum-ascites albumin gradient (SAAG). The SAAG is calculated by subtracting the ascitic fluid albumin level from a simultaneously measured serum albumin level. If the difference is ≥1.1 g/dL,

Table 13.2. Ascitic Fluid Analysis – Recommended Tests

Test	Purpose
Routine Tests	
Cell count and differential	Detect infection
Albumin	Calculate the serum-ascites albumin gradient (SAAG)
Total Protein	Determine the susceptibility of the fluid to infection
Cultures	Narrowing spectrum of antibiotic coverage
Optional Tests*	
Amylase	Pancreatic ascites
Triglycerides	Chylous ascites
LDH, glucose	Secondary peritonitis
Cytology	Peritoneal carcinomatosis
Acid-fast bacilli smears and cultures	Mycobacterial peritonitis
Red blood cell count / hematocrit	Evaluation of hemoperitoneum
Bilirubin	Suspected bile leak

*Optional tests are ordered only when the clinical presentation or the initial ascites fluid analysis suggests a cause for ascites other than cirrhosis

portal hypertension is present with a 97% accuracy rate.[47] It should be noted that a high SAAG indicates the presence of portal hypertension, but not necessarily cirrhosis. Conditions such as cardiac ascites, Budd-Chiari syndrome and myxedema may cause high SAAG ascites in the absence of cirrhosis. Likewise, patients who have portal hypertension plus a second cause for ascites formation, such as malignant ascites, will also have a SAAG greater than 1.1 g/dL.

The ascites fluid total protein level indicates the susceptibility of the fluid to become spontaneously infected. Bactericidal fluid activity parallels the total protein concentration of the ascitic fluid. Prospective studies have shown that during hospitalization, spontaneous bacterial peritonitis develops 10 times more commonly in patients with ascites fluid protein concentration of <1 g/dL, compared to those with total protein ≥2 g/dL.[48] Patients with non-infected, low total protein ascites who are admitted to the hospital should be placed on oral antibiotic prophylaxis to decrease the risk of spontaneous bacterial peritonitis. Norfloxacin, 400 mg once a day eliminates aerobic gram-negative bacilli from the intestinal flora without interfering with other microorganisms and substantially reduces the risk of spontaneous bacterial peritonitis.[49] Using the SAAG and ascites total protein values, a differential diagnosis for the cause of the ascites can be formulated as shown in Figure 13.4.

Additional tests in the ascitic fluid are necessary when the initial evaluation reveals no evidence of portal hypertension or if additional diagnosis are being considered. Ascitic fluid cytology is positive only in the setting of peritoneal carcinomatosis, and should be ordered only when this diagnosis is suspected.[50] Acid-fast bacilli stain and culture, amylase and triglycerides may help in diagnosing tuberculous peritonitis, pancreatic ascites, or chylous ascites respectively. These tests should be ordered only when the clinical presentation suggest the diagnosis.

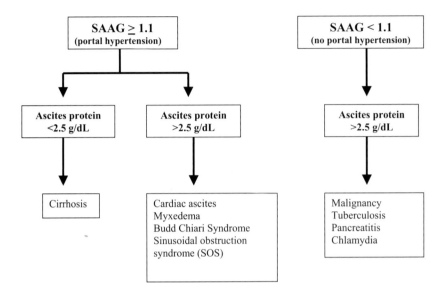

SAAG: Serum Ascites Albumin Gradient

Figure 13.4. Differential diagnosis of the cause of ascites based on the total protein and saag saag: serum ascites albumin gradient.

Treatment of Ascites

Cirrhotic patients with high SAAG ascites respond to salt restriction and diuretics. The most important aspect of treatment is patient education. A maximum of 2,000 mg (88 mEq) of sodium per day should be recommended, fluid restriction is not necessary in the absence of significant hyponatremia (Na < 120–125 mEq/L). Determining the sodium and potassium content in a random urine sample can be helpful. A random urine sodium concentration that is greater than the potassium concentration correlates with a 24-hour sodium excretion greater than 78 mEq per day with approximately a 90% accuracy.[51] Patients with a spot urine Na/K ratio >1 who are not responding to therapy are likely not compliant with a sodium restricted diet.

The usual diuretic regimen consists of a single morning dose of an oral loop diuretic (furosemide, 40 mg) and a distal tubule acting agent (spironolactone, 100 mg). Single-agent therapy with furosemide is rarely effective in the treatment of ascites.[52] In contrast, single agent diuresis with spironolactone may be effective in the treatment of moderate ascites,[53] and may be considered in patients with no peripheral edema.

In the absence of a clinical response, the dose of both diuretics can be increased simultaneously every three to five days. Usual maximum doses are 400 mg per day of spironolactone and 160 mg per day of furosemide.[54] This diuretic regimen is effective in more than 90% of patients and lack of response should raise suspicion for non-compliance or complicated ascites. For patients presenting with tense ascites, a single large volume paracentesis followed by sodium restriction and diuretic therapy results in a faster therapeutic response. Repeated large volume paracentesis is not recommended for patients who are responsive to diuretics and sodium restriction.

Refractory Ascites

Lack of response to maximum doses of diuretics and a sodium restricted diet characterize patients with diuretic-resistant ascites. A subset of patients with refractory ascites is unable to tolerate maximum doses of diuretics due to clinically significant complications such as azotemia, hyperkalemia, or encephalopathy, and cannot achieve adequate diuresis with lower doses; these patients are labeled as "diuretic-intractable." Prior to labeling a patient as having refractory ascites, it is important to exclude use of non-steroidal anti-inflammatory drugs (NSAIDs). NSAIDs reduce urinary sodium excretion and can induce azotemia, rendering patients diuretic resistant. Selective COX-2 inhibitors also have detrimental effects on renal sodium handling by the kidney in noncirrhotic individuals[55] and chronic use should be avoided in cirrhotics with ascites, although short term use may be tolerated by some.[56]

Options for patients with refractory ascites include large volume paracentesis (LVP), liver transplantation, TIPS, or peritoneovenous shunts. Liver transplantation is rarely an option for patients with otherwise preserved liver function, as the presence of refractory ascites is not factored into the computation of the MELD score currently used to determine eligibility for liver transplantation. Repeated LVP with or without albumin infusion is usually the first line therapy for refractory ascites. Infusion of albumin at a dose of 6–8 grams per liter of fluid removed appears to be associated with fewer post-paracentesis complications and better results,[57] particularly when removing more than 5 liters of ascites. Albumin infusion is usually not necessary when removing less than 5 liters of fluid.[54] Diuretics and sodium restriction should be continued while performing LVPs. Unfortunately, ascites recurs in most subjects, necessitating repeated paracentesis.

TIPS is an attractive option for patients who require frequent (more often than every 3–4 weeks) LVP. The North American Study of Treatment of Refractory Ascites showed that while TIPS was more effective than LVP in controlling ascites, it did not improve survival, quality of life or reduced the number of emergency room visits or hospitalizations.[58] TIPS should be reserved for subjects who repeatedly fail LVP and have relatively preserved liver function. The frequent need for TIPS revisions and the higher incidence of hepatic encephalopathy after TIPS make this a second line therapeutic option compared to LVP.

Peritoneovenous shunts (PVS) have been used to control refractory ascites. Although response is noted in some, poor long-term patency rates, excessive complications, and no survival advantage compared to medical therapy make this a rarely used option in the management of refractory ascites.[59] Shunt-related adhesions can make subsequent liver transplantation more difficult, and PVS should only be considered in patients who are otherwise not eligible for liver transplant.

Spontaneous Bacterial Peritonitis

Spontaneous bacterial peritonitis (SBP) has a prevalence of 10% to 30% among hospitalized individuals with ascites[33] and is defined as a monomicrobial infection of ascites in the absence of a contiguous source of infection.[60] Early diagnosis is crucial in improving survival. With early recognition and prompt therapy, mortality of an episode of SBP is approximately 20%.

A diagnostic paracentesis should be done in any patient with cirrhosis and ascites admitted to the hospital for any reason, regardless of the presence or absence of symptoms suggestive of SBP. A paracentesis should also be performed in any cirrhotic who develops signs or symptoms of peritoneal infection, worsening of liver or renal function, or worsening ascites control. The diagnosis of SBP is established if the absolute PMN count in the ascitic fluid is $\geq$250 cells/mm^3.

Gram negative bacilli (primarily *Escherichia coli*) are the most frequent organisms implicated in SBP, although the incidence of gram positive cocci infection is rapidly rising. A landmark study comparing the combination of ampicllin-tobramycin with cefotaxime for the treatment of serious infections in cirrhosis showed that cefotaxime was superior with cure rates in the order of 84–94%.[61] In uncontrolled studies, other third-generation cephalosporins such as ceftriaxone and more recently the combination of amoxicillin and clavulanic acid have been shown to be as effective as cefotaxime.[28] Although quinolones may be effective in the treatment of SBP, they have not been rigorously studied and the increasingly common emergence of quinolone-resistant organisms in patients with cirrhosis may limit their use. Aminoglycosides should be avoided in cirrhotics as they are particularly prone to develop nephrotoxicity. Antibiotics should be administered for a minimum of five days,[62] initially intravenously. A paracentesis should be repeated in 48 to 72 hours to assess response to therapy. Patients with evidence of resolution of symptoms, or a decrease in ascites fluid PMN to < 250 cells/mm^3 on a repeat paracentesis after 48 hours of therapy, can be changed to oral antibiotics.[28] The approach to the diagnosis and treatment of SBP is summarized in Figure 13.5.

The increased use of antibiotic prophylaxis to prevent SBP has led to an increased number of gram positive cocci infections in cirrhotics, including quinolone and trimethoprim/sulfamethoxazole-resistant organisms. In addition, there has been an increased rate of methicillin-resistant *Staphylococcus aureus* (MRSA) infections in cirrhotics with prior norfloxacin prophylaxis.[28] Cefotaxime continues to be active against quinolone-resistant *E. coli* infections, and a large retrospective study confirmed that cefotaxime is equally effective in the treatment of SBP developing in patients on previous chronic antibiotic prophylaxis compared to those on no prior antibiotics.[63] Given the increased incidence of MRSA infection in patients on norfloxacin prophylaxis,[64] the addition of vancomycin to the initial antibiotic regimen of highly symptomatic patients should be considered while awaiting final culture results.

Renal dysfunction develops in up to a third of patients with SBP and is the most important predictor of death in patients with SBP. A recent prospective studied demonstrated that the use of albumin infusion in addition to cefotaxime reduced the number of patients exhibiting renal dysfunction and improved in-hospital and three-month mortality rates compared to cefotaxime alone.[65] Beneficial effects of albumin were most notable among patients with serum bilirubin levels over 4 mg/dL and any evidence of renal impairment such as a blood urea nitrogen (BUN) >30 g/dL or creatinine >1.0 mg/dL at the time SBP was diagnosed. Recommended dose of albumin is 1.5 g/kg of body weight at time of diagnosis and a second dose of 1 g/kg 72 hours later.

Recurrence of SBP after the first episode is common, with a recurrence rate of 70% at one year. Thus, antibiotic prophylaxis should be considered in all patients that have recovered from an episode of SBP. Daily norfloxacin at a dose

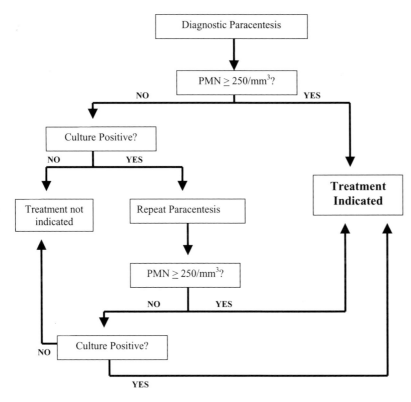

PMN = polymorphonuclear cells

Figure 13.5. Diagnosis and treatment of spontaneous bacterial peritonitis
PMN = Polymorphonuclear Cells.

of 400 mg/day decreases the risk of recurrent SBP from 68% to 20% at one year.[66] Prophylaxis using weekly doses of quinolones is no longer recommended due to a lower efficacy and an increased incidence of quinolone-resistant organisms, compared to daily norfloxacin.[67] Trimethoprim/sulfamethoxazole prophylaxis, one double-strength tablet five days a week appears to also be effective, although it has not been extensively studied.

HEPATORENAL SYNDROME

Hepatorenal syndrome (HRS) describes the development of functional renal failure occurring in patients with advanced liver disease, in the absence of other known causes of renal dysfunction. The diagnosis of HRS is one of exclusion, criteria for the diagnosis of HRS exist[68] and are listed on Table 13.3. Strict adherence to these criteria and careful exclusion of other causes of renal failure in cirrhosis is of paramount importance, as in most cases the diagnosis of HRS is incorrect. Most patients with HRS in the setting of cirrhosis have ascites at the time when HRS is diagnosed. The probability of developing HRS in patients with ascites and cirrhosis is 20% at one year and increases to 40% at five years.[69]

Two types of HRS have been observed[68] Type I, which is less common, is an aggressive form with a very poor prognosis. It is defined by a doubling of

---

Table 13.3. Diagnostic Criteria of Heptorenal Syndrome

Major criteria*
1. Low glomerular filtration rate, as indicated by serum creatinine >1.5 mg/dL.
2. Exclusion of shock, ongoing bacterial infection, volume depletion, and use of nephrotoxic drugs including NSAIDs
3. No improvement in renal function despite stopping diuretics and volume repletion with 1.5 Liters of saline
4. No proteinuria or ultrasonographic evidence of obstructive uropathy or parenchyma renal disease.

Minor criteria*
1. Urine volume <500 ml/day
2. Urine sodium <10 mEq/L
3. Urine osmolality > plasma osmolality
4. Urine red blood cells <50 per high power field
5. Serum sodium concentration <130 meq/L

---

*All major criteria are necessary for the diagnosis of hepatorenal syndrome, minor criteria do not need to be present but provide useful supportive evidence.
Source: From Arroyo V, et al. Reference #68.

---

the initial serum creatinine to a level higher than 2.5 mg/dL or a 50% reduction of the initial 24-hour creatinine clearance in less than two weeks to a level of <20 ml/min. HRS type I is associated with a median survival time of two weeks. Type II hepatorenal syndrome develops much more slowly and is defined as an impairment in renal function (serum creatinine >1.5 mg/dL) that does not meet criteria for type I HRS, the median survival is six months.

The pathophysiologic hallmark of HRS is severe renal vasoconstriction leading to a severe reduction in glomerular filtration rate and functional renal insufficiency.[70] Severe renal vasoconstriction is often triggered by events that worsen splanchnic and peripheral vasodilation such as sepsis, SBP or large-volume paracentesis without albumin infusion. Once renal vasoconstriction develops, intrarenal mechanisms perpetuate HRS leading to progressive renal failure.

The management of HRS is evolving. Until recently, HRS was considered to be a terminal event without effective medical therapy with the exception of liver transplantation. Recently, the use of vasoconstrictor therapy has resulted in reversal of HRS in some instances. The most studied vasoconstrictor is terlipressin, which is not currently available in the United States. The administration of terlipressin and albumin is associated with a significant improvement of GFR and reduction in serum creatinine to below 1.5 mg/dL in approximately 60–75% of patients with type I HRS.[71] An approach that is available in the United States is the combination of midodrine, octreotide and albumin infusion. Although this regimen has only been studied in a small number of patients, there was a marked improvement in renal perfusion and GFR, as well as suppression of rennin, aldosterone, and norepinephrine, indicating reversal of the pathophysiologic mechanisms that led to HRS.[72,73]

Hemodialysis is usually avoided in HRS due to a high incidence of severe side effects including hypotension, coagulopathy, gastrointestinal bleeding and increased mortality. Continuous arterio-venous or veno-venous hemofiltration are better tolerated but their efficacy has yet to be determined. In some instances, renal replacement therapy can be used as a bridge to liver transplantation. Although there are scattered reports of TIPS use for the treatment of HRS, at this time its use remains investigational and should not be considered an option in this situation.

HEPATIC ENCEPHALOPATHY

Hepatic encephalopathy (HE) is a disturbance in central nervous system function caused by hepatic insufficiency. Most theories regarding the pathogenesis of HE revolve around the principle that nitrogenous substances derived from the gut adversely affect brain function. HE is a diagnosis of exclusion; other metabolic disorders, infectious diseases and intracranial events may present with similar symptoms and signs and must be excluded. Although most theories consider ammonia as a key factor in the pathogenesis of HE, it is clear that ammonia is not the only compound responsible for the neuropsychiatric alterations associated with cirrhosis.[74] Although determination of serum ammonia may help in the evaluation of the obtunded patient, there is no role in serial ammonia level determinations or measuring ammonia levels in patients with cirrhosis and no evidence of neuropsychiatric impairment.

Treatment of hepatic encephalopathy is tailored to the clinical situation and shown in Figure 13.6. To asses for improvement or worsening, it is important to stage encephalopathy using a scale such as the one depicted in Table 13.4. Adequate supportive care is crucial at all stages of encephalopathy. For stage 3 and 4 encephalopathy, prophylactic tracheal intubation should be considered. Adequate nutrition should be provided during the period of altered mental status. One of the early goals of management is identification and correction of potential precipitating factors such as gastrointestinal hemorrhage, infections, electrolyte disturbances, use of psychoactive medications, constipation, or excess dietary protein.[75] Laxatives and nonabsorbable disaccharides reduce the nitrogenous load from the gut and help hasten recovery. Lactulose, given orally or via nasogastric tube is initiated at 45 cc hourly until evacuation occurs. The dose is then adjusted to produce two or three soft stools per day; the usual maintenance dose is 15–45 cc two to three times per day. Protracted diarrhea from lactulose therapy may result in hypertonic dehydration with hypernatremia and worsening of HE. Lactulose retention enemas, prepared as 300 ml of lactulose in 1 liter of water, can be used for patients who cannot tolerate oral feedings. The patient is placed in Trendeleburg position and the enema is retained for one hour.[76]

Neomycin, a non-absorbable antibiotic alters the intestinal flora to decrease production of nitrogenous waste and improve encephalopathy. The usual dose is 3–6 grams per day orally, not to exceed a period of two weeks. Although it may prove beneficial in the short term, chronic use of neomycin is discouraged. Despite its poor absorption, chronic neomycin therapy can cause auditory loss and renal impairment. Metronidazole, starting at a dose of 250 mg twice a day, affects a different bacterial population than neomycin and can be used as single agent or in combination with neomycin. Chronic use of metronidazole may lead to neurotoxicity which can be severe in patients with cirrhosis, who may

Table 13.4. Stages of Hepatic Encephalopathy

Stage 0   Lack of detectable changes in personality or behavior.
Stage 1   Trivial lack of awareness, shortened attention span. Hypersomnia, insomnia or inversion of sleep pat Asterixis can be detected.
Stage 2   Lethargy or apathy. Disorientation. Inappropriate behavior. Slurred speech. Obvious asterixis
Stage 3   Gross disorientation. Bizarre behavior. Semistupor to stupor. Asterixis generally absent.
Stage 4   Coma

From Blei AT and Cordoba J, reference #75.

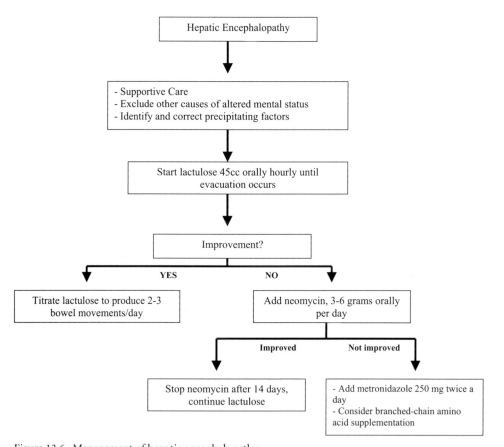

Figure 13.6. Management of hepatic encephalopathy.

have impaired clearance of the drug.[77] Newer nonabsorbable antibiotics such as rifaximin appear promising for the treatment of HE, but their recommendation awaits results of randomized, placebo-controlled trials.

Nutrition support is crucial during treatment of HE. In case of deep encephalopathy, oral intake is withheld for 24–48 hours and intravenous glucose is provided. Enteral nutrition should be started after 48 hours if the patient is unable to eat. Protein should be provided initially at a dose of 0.5 g/kg/day, with progressive increase to 1–1.5g/kg/day. The use of special branched-chain amino acid enteral formulas is rarely required and is reserved for patients with refractory encephalopathy in whom nutritional needs cannot be met.

SUMMARY

Cirrhosis is a chronic, progressive disease with predictable complications resulting from portal hypertension and liver insufficiency. A thorough knowledge of the pathophysiology and natural history of these complications allows for a targeted approach to the patient to institute timely preventive and therapeutic measures that may lead to improvement in quality of life and survival.

REFERENCES

1. Kochanek KD, Murphy SL, Anderson RN. Deaths: Final data for 2002. In National Center for Health Statistics. National Vital Statistics Report. Vol 53, No. 5, Hyatsville, MD. National Center for Health Statistics 2004.
2. Davis GL, Albright JE, Cook SF, Rosenberg DM. Projecting future complications of chronic hepatitis C in the United States. Liver Transpl 2003;9:331–8.
3. United Network for Organ Sharing and Organ Procurement and Transplant Network, Richmond, VA. Current U.S. waiting list for liver transplantation. In: United Network for Organ Sharing; 2006. Available at http://www.unos.org/data. Accessed on November 26, 2006.
4. D'Amico G, Garcia-Tsao G, Pagliaro L. Natural history and prognostic indicators of survival in cirrhosis: A systematic review of 118 studies. J Hepatol 2006;44:217–31.
5. Fattovich G, Giustina G, Degos F, et al. Morbidity and mortality in compensated cirrhosis type C: A retrospective follow-up study of 384 patients. Gastroenterology 1997;112:463–72.
6. Alberti A, Chemelo L, Benvegnu L. Natural history of hepatitis C. J Hepatol 1999;31(Suppl. 1):17–24.
7. Christensen E. Prognostic models including the Child-Pugh, MELD and Mayo risk scores – Where are we and where should we go? J Hepatol 2004;41:344–50.
8. Pugh RN, Murray-Lyon IM, Dawson JL, Peitroni MC, Williams R. Transection of the esophagus for bleeding esophageal varices. Br J Surg 1973;60:646–49.
9. Kamath PS, Wiesner RH, Malinchoc M, et al. A model to predict survival in patients with end-stage liver disease. Hepatology 2001;33:464–70.
10. Gores GJ, Wiesner RH, Dickson ER, Zinsmeister AR, Jorgensen RA, Langworthy A. Prospective evaluation of esophageal varices in primary biliary cirrhosis: development, natural history and influence on survival. Gastroenterology 1989;96:1552–9.
11. Kamath PS. Esophageal variceal bleeding: Primary prophylaxis. Clinical Gastroenterol Hepatology 2005;3:90–3.
12. Thuluvath PJ, Kirshnan A. Primary prophylaxis of variceal bleeding. Gastrointest Endosc 2003;58:558–67.
13. D'Amico G, Pagliaro L, Bosch J. The treatment of portal hypertension: a meta-analytic review. Hepatology 1995;22:332–54.
14. Poynard T, Cales P, Pasta L, Ideo G, Pascal JP, Pagliaro L, Lebrec D. Beta-adrenergic antagonists in the prevention of first gastrointestinal bleeding in patiens with cirrhosis and esophageal varices. Analysis of data and prognostic factors in 589 patients from four randomized clinical trials. N Engl J Med 1991;324:1532–38.
15. Plevris JN, Elliot R, Mills PR, Hislop WS, Davies JM, Bouchier IA, Hayes PC. Effect of propranolol on prevention of first variceal bleed and survival in patients with chronic liver disease. Aliment Pharmacol Ther 1994;8:63–70.

16. Groszmann RJ, Garcia-Tsao G, Bosch J, et al. Beta-blockers to prevent gastroesophageal varices in patients with cirrhosis. N Engl J Med 2005;353:2254–61.

17. Beppu K, Inokuchi K, Koyanagi N, Nakayama S, Sakata H, Kitano S, et al. Prediction of variceal hemorrhage by esophageal endoscopy. Gastrointest Endosc 1981;27: 213–8.

18. Adams PC, Arthur MJ, Boyer TD, DeLeve LD, Di Bisceglie AM, Hall M, et al. Screening in liver disease: Report of an AASLD workshop. Hepatology 2004;39:1204–12.

19. Grace ND. Diagnosis and treatment of gastrointestinal bleeding secondary to portal hypertension. American College of Gastroenterology Practice Parameters Committee. Am J Gastroenterol 1997;92:1081–91.

20. ASGE. ASGE Guideline: the role of endoscopy in the management of variceal hemorrhage, updated July 2005. Gastointest Endosc 2005;62:651–55.

21. D'Amico G, Pasta L, Madonia S, Tarantino G, Mancuso A, Malizia G, Giannuoli GC, Pagliaro L. The incidence of esophageal varices in cirrhosis Gastroenterology 2001;120:A-2 (abstract).

22. Bosch J, Abraldes JG, Groszmann R. Current management of portal hypertension. J Hepatol 2003;38:554–68.

23. Abraczinskas DR, Ookubo R, Grace ND, Groszmann RJ, Bosch J, Garcia-Tsao G, et al. Propranolol for prevention of first esophageal variceal hemorrhage – A lifetime commitment? Hepatology 2001;34:1096–102.

24. Jensen DM. Endoscopic screening for varices in cirrhosis: Findings, implications and outcomes. Gastroenterology 2002;122:1620–30.

25. Carbonell N, Pauwels A, Serfaty L, et al. Improved survival after variceal bleeding in patients with cirrhosis over the past two decades. Hepatology 2004;40:652–9.

26. Ejlersen E, Melsen T, Ingerslev J, et al. Recombinant activated factor VIIa corrects prothrombin time in cirrhotic patients: a preliminary study. Gastroenterology 2001;36:1081–5.

27. Bernard B, Grange JD, Khac EN, Amiot X, Opolon P, Poynard T. Antibiotic prophylaxis for the prevention of bacterial infection in cirrhotic patients with gastrointestinal bleeding: a meta–analysis. Heptology 1999;29:1655–61.

28. Garica-Tsao G. Bacterial infections in cirrhosis: treatment and prophylaxis. J Hepatol 2005;S85–92.

29. Corley DA, Cello JP, Adkisson W, et al. Octreotide for acute esophageal variceal bleeding: a meta-analysis. Gastroenterology 2001;120:946–54.

30. Bosch J, Lebrec D, Jenkis SA. Development of analogues: successes and failures. Scand J Gastroenterol Suppl 1998;226:3–13.

31. Lo GH, Lai KH, Cheng JS, Lin CK, Huang JS, Hsu PL, et al. Emergency banding ligation versus sclerotherapy for the control of active bleeding from esophageal varices. Hepatology 1997;25:1101–4.

32. D'Amico G, Pagliaro L, Bosch J. The treatment of portal hypertension: a meta-analytic review. Hepatology 1995;22:332–54.

33. Garcia-Tsao G. Current management of the complications of cirrhosis and portal hypetension: Variceal hemorrhage, ascites and spontaneous bacterial peritonitis. Gastroenterology 2001;120:726–48.

34. D'Amico G, Plagiaro L, Bosch J. Pharmacological treatment of portal hypertension: an evidence-based approach. Semin Liv Dis 1999;19:475–505.

35. Patch D, Sabin CA, Goulis J, et al. A randomized, controlled trial of medical therapy versus endoscopic ligation for the prevention of variceal rebleeding in patients with cirrhosis. Gastroenterology 2002;123:1013–19.

36. de la Peña J, Brullet E, Sanchez-Hernandez E, et al. Variceal ligation plus nadolol compared with ligation for prophylaxis of variceal rebleeding: a multicenter trial. Hepatology 2005;41:572–8.

37. Abraldes JG, Angermayr B, Bosch J. The management of portal hypertension. N A Clin Liv Dis 2005;9:685–713.

38. Lo GH, Lai KH, Cheng JS, et al. A prospective randomized trial of butyl cyanoacrylate injection versus band ligation in the management of bleeding gastric varices. Hepatology 2001;33:1060–4.
39. Gines P, Quintero E, Arroyo V, Teres J, Bruguera M, Rimola A, Caballeria J, et al. Compensated cirrhosis: natural history and prognostic factors. Hepatology 1987;7:12–18.
40. Schrier RW, Arroyo V, Bernaqrdi M, et al. Peripheral arterial vasodilation hypothesis: a proposal for the initiation of renal sodium and water retention in cirrhosis. Hepatology 1988;8:1151–7.
41. Runyon BA. Care of the patient with ascites. N Engl J Med 1994;330:337–42.
42. Pinzello G, Simonetty RG, Craxi A, di Piazza S, Spano C, Pagliaro L. Spontaneous bacterial peritonitis: a prospective investigation in predominantly nonalcoholic patients. Hepatology 1983;3:545–9.
43. Runyon BA. Paracentesis of ascitic fluid: a safe procedure. Arch Intern Med 1986; 146:2259–61.
44. Lin CH, Shih FY, Ma MH, et al. Should bleeding tendency deter abdominal paracentesis? Dig Liv Dis 2005;37:946–51.
45. Thomsen TW, Shaffer RW, White B, Setnik GS. Paracentesis. N Engl J Med 2006;355:e21.
46. Habeeb KS, Herrera JL. Management of ascites. Paracentesis as a Guide. Postgrad Med 1997;101:191–200.
47. Runyon BA, Montano AA, Akriviadis EA, Antillon MR, Irving MA, McHutchison JG. The serum-ascites albumin gradient is superior to the exudates-transudate concept in the differential diagnosis of ascites. Ann Intern Med 1992;117:215–20.
48. Llach J, Rimola A, Navasa M, et al. Incidence and predictive factors of first episode of spontaneous bacterial peritonitis in cirrhosis with ascites: relevance of ascitic fluid protein concentration. Hepatology 1992;16:724–27.
49. Soriano G, Guarner C, Teixido M, et al. Selective intestinal decontamination prevents spontaneous bacterial peritonitis. Gastroenterology 1991;100:477–81.
50. Runyon BA, Hoefs JC, Morgan TR. Ascitic fluid analysis in malignancy-related ascites. Hepatology 1988;8:1104–9.
51. Stiehm AJ, Mendler MH, Runyon BA. Detection of diuretic resistance or diuretic sensitivity by the spot urine Na/K ratio in 729 specimens from cirrhotics with ascites: approximately 80% accuracy as compared to 24 hour urine Na excretion. Hepatology 2002:36:222A [abstract]
52. Perez-Ayuso RM, Arroyo V, Plans R, Gaya J, Bory F, Rimola A, Rivea F, et al. Randomized comparative study of efficacy of furosemide vs. spironolactone in nonazotemic cirrhosis with ascites. Gastroenterology 1983;84:961–8.
53. Santos J, Planas R, Pardo A, Durandez R, Cabre E, Mrillas RM, et al. Spironolactone alone or in combination with furosemide in the treatment of moderate ascites in nonazotemic cirrhosis. A randomized comparative study of efficacy and safety. J Hepatol 2003;39:187–92.
54. Runyon BA. Management of adult patients with ascites due to cirrhosis. Hepatology 2004;39:841–56.
55. Fitzgerald GA, Patrono C. The coxibs, selective inhibitors of cyclooxygenase-2. N Engl J Med 2001;345:433–42.
56. Claria J, Kent JD, Lopez-Parra M, Escolar G, Ruiz del Arbol L, Gines P, et al. Effects of celecoxib and naproxen on renal function in nonazotemic patients with cirrhosis and ascites. Hepatology 2005;41:579–87.
57. Gines P, Tito L, Arroyo V, Planas R, Viver J, et al. Randomized comparative study of therapeutic paracentesis with and without intravenous albumin in cirrhosis. Gastroenterology 1988;94:1493–501.
58. Sanyal A, Genning C, Reddy KR, Wong F, Kowdley KV, Benner K, et al. The North American study for the treatment of refractory ascites. Gastroenterology 2003;124:634–41.

59. Gines P, Arroyo V, Vargas V, Plans R, Casafont F, Panes J, Hoyos M, et al. Paracentesis with intravenous infusion of albumin as compared with peritoneovenous shunting in cirrhosis with refractory ascites. N Engl J Med 1991;325:829–35.

60. Moore KP, Aithal GP. Guidelines on the management of ascites in cirrhosis. Gut 2006;55:1–12.

61. Felisart J, Rimola A, Arroyo V, Perez-Ayuso RM, Quintero E, Gines P, et al. Cefotaxime is more effective than is ampicillin-tobramycin in cirrhotics with severe infections. Hepatology 1985;5:457–62.

62. Runyon BA, McHutchison JG, Antillon MR, et al. Short-course versus long-course antibiotic treatment of spontaneous bacterial peritonitis: a randomized controlled study of 100 patients. Gastroenterology 1991;100:1737–42.

63. Llovet JM, Rodriguez-Iglesias P, Moitinho E, Planas R, Bataller R, Navasa M, et al. Spontaneous bacterial peritonitis in patients with cirrhosis undergoing selective intestinal decontamination. A retrospective study of 229 spontaneous bacterial peritonitis episodes. J Hepatol 1997;26:88–95.

64. Campillo B, Richardet JP, Kheo T, Dupeyron C. Nosocomial spontaneous bacterial peritonitis and bacteremia in cirrhotic patients: impact of isolate type on prognosis and characteristics of infection. Clin Infect Dis 2002;35:1–10.

65. Sort P, Navasa M, Arroyo V, Aldeguer X, Planas R, Ruiz del Arbol L, et al. Effects of intravenous albumin on renal impairment and mortality in patients with cirrhosis and spontaneous bacterial peritonitis. N Engl J Med 1999;341:403–9.

66. Gines P, Rimola A, Planas R, Vargas V, Marco F, Almela M. Norfloxacin prevents spontaneous bacterial peritonitis recurrence in cirrhosis: results of a double-blind, placebo-controlled trial. Hepatology 1990;12:716–24.

67. Bauer TM. Follo A, Navasa M, Vila J, Plans R, Clemente G, et al. Daily norfloxacin is more effective than weekly rufloxacin in prevention of spontaneous bacterial peritonitis recurrence. Dig Dis Sci 2002;47:1356–61.

68. Arroyo V, Gines P, Berges A, et al. Definition and diagnostic criteria of refractory ascites and hepatorenal syndrome in cirrhosis. Hepatology 1996;23:164–76.

69. Gines A, Escorsell A, Gines P, et al. Incidence, predictive factors and prognosis of hepatorenal syndrome in cirrhosis. Gastroenterology 1993;105:229–36.

70. Cardenas, A. Hepatorenal syndrome: A dreaded complication of end-stage liver disease. Am J Gastroenterol 2005;100:460–7.

71. Ortega R, Gines P, Uriz J, et al. Terlipressin therapy with and without albumin for patients with hepatorenal syndrome. Results of a prospective, non-randomized study. Hepatology 2002;36:941–8.

72. Angeli P, Volpin R, Gerunda G, Craighero R, Roner P, Merenda R, et al. Reversal of type 1 hepatorenal syndrome with the administration of midodrine and octreotide. Hepatology 1999;29:1690–7.

73. Wong F, Pantea L, Sniderman K. Midodrine, octreotide, albumin and TIPS in selected patiens with cirrhosis and type 1 hepatorenal syndrome. Hepatology 2004;40:55–64.

74. Butterworth RF. The neurobiology of hepatic encephalopathy. Semin Liv Dis 1996;16:235–44.

75. Blei AT, Cordoba J. Hepatic Encephalopathy. Am J Gastroenterol 2001;96:1968–76.

76. Uribe M, Campollo A, Vargas F, et al. Acidifying enemas (lactitol and lactose) vs. non-acidifiying enemas (tap water) to treat acute portal-systemic encephalopathy. A double-blind randomized clinical trial. Hepatology 1987;7:639–43.

77. Loft S, Sonne J, Dossing M, Andreasen PB. Metronidazole pharmacokinetics in patients with hepatic encephalopathy. Scand J Gastroenterol 1987;22:117–23.

Liver Transplantation

Robert L. Carithers, Jr., MD

BACKGROUND

Liver transplantation is the most effective treatment for many patients with acute or chronic liver failure. Survival after liver transplantation has improved steadily during the past 20 years. Most transplant centers have one-year survival rates of 85–90% and five-year survival rates of 75–80%.[1] Transplant recipients have the opportunity for extended survival with excellent quality of life despite the many complications that can occur during or after the procedure.[2] Most patients have been able to return to work, and physically active recipients have returned to vigorous endeavors such as snowboarding, basketball, and marathon running. Furthermore, the costs of liver transplantation have steadily declined, making it accessible to more and more patients.[3]

Indications for Liver Transplantation

Liver transplantation should be considered in patients with acute or chronic liver failure from any cause. The most common indications for transplantation include:

1. Cirrhosis secondary to chronic hepatitis B and C infection
2. Alcoholic cirrhosis
3. Cirrhosis due to cholestatic disorders such as primary biliary cirrhosis and sclerosing cholangititis
4. Cirrhosis and liver failure from autoimmune hepatitis
5. Cirrhosis and liver failure resulting from metabolic disorders including:
   a. Non-alcoholic steatohepatitis (NASH),
   b. Wilson disease,
   c. Alpha-1-antitripsin deficiency, and
   d. Hemochromotosis
6. Hepatocellular carcinoma, and
7. Fulminant hepatic failure

Less common reasons for transplantation include the Budd-Chiari syndrome, cystic fibrosis, amyloidosis, and polycystic liver disease.

Evaluation of the Potential Transplant Recipient

When considering a patient for liver transplantation, it is important to systematically address the following questions:

1. Does the patient need transplantation?
2. Are there alternative treatments that may be as effective as transplantation?
3. Does the patient have the potential for a reasonable outcome following transplantation?

1. DETERMINING THE NEED FOR LIVER TRANSPLANTATION

To address this important issue the natural history of the patient's disease must be carefully compared to the anticipated survival following transplantation. The clinical tools most widely used to do this include the prognostic Model for End Stage Liver Disease (MELD), the Child-Turcotte-Pugh classification, plus the impact of specific complications of cirrhosis on patient survival. Because none of these tools is perfect, they should be considered complimentary measures, which, when used in combination, give the most accurate estimate of the prognosis of most patients with chronic liver disease.

The Model of End-stage Liver Disease (MELD) was originally derived from a study of patients undergoing transjugular intrahepatic portosystemic shunt (TIPS) procedures. Serum bilirubin, international normalized ratio of prothrombin time (INR), serum creatinine, and the underlying diagnosis of liver disease were found to be the best predictors of post-TIPS survival.[4] Subsequent studies of this model demonstrated its utility as an effective tool for determining the prognosis in patients with chronic liver disease.[5] The MELD score also has been found useful in predicting short-term survival in patients on the waiting list for liver transplantation as well as estimating the risk of post-operative mortality.[6,7] A simplified MELD model is now used to prioritize patients for donor allocation in the United States. In this model, patients are assigned scores from 6 to 40, which equate to estimated three-month survival rates without transplantation ranging from 90% to 7%, respectively.[4]

The Child-Turcotte-Pugh (CTP) classification, originally designed to determine the risk of portacaval shunt surgery, also has been used to determine the prognosis of patients with chronic liver disease (Table 14.1).[8]

The CTP score can be quite effective in determining short-term prognosis among groups of patients awaiting liver transplantation.[10] More than one-third of those with CTP scores $\geq$ 10 can be expected to die within a year.[10,11] In contrast, patients with CTP scores of 7–9 have an 80% chance of surviving five years, and those with CTP scores of 5–6 have a 90% chance of surviving more than five years without transplantation.[11–13]

Complications of cirrhosis such as ascites, variceal bleeding, hepatic encephalopathy, hepatocellular carcinoma, hepatopulmonary syndrome, spontaneous bacterial peritonitis, and hepatorenal syndrome also can have a significant impact on the prognosis of patients with cirrhosis. The five-year survival

Table 14.1. Child-Turcotte-Pugh (CTP) Scoring System

Points	1	2	3
Encephalopathy (grade)*	None	1 and 2	3 and 4
Ascites	Absent	Slight	Moderated
Bilirubin (mg/dL)	1–2	2–3	>3
Albumin (g/dL)	3.5	2.8–3.5	<2.8
Prothrombin time (seconds prolonged)	1–4	4–6	>6
Or (INR)	<1.7	1.7–2.3	>2.3
For primary biliary cirrhosis: bilirubin (mg/dL)	1–4	4–10	>10

*According to grading of Trey, Burns, and Saunders[9]

Table 14.2. Assessing the Need for Liver Transplantation

MELD Score	CTP Score	Clinical Summary
>16	>10	The need for transplantation is unequivocal.
10–16	7–10	Clinical judgement required. Transplantation indicated only if a patient has complications such as intractable ascites, hepatic hydrothorax, severe encephalopathy, spontaneous bacterial peritonitis, hepatopulmonary syndrome, or hepatocellular carcinoma.
<10	<7	Transplantation usually indicated only if a patient has hepatocellular carcinoma.

rate of individuals who develop any of these complications is only 20–50% of that of patients with compensated cirrhosis.[14-16] The most ominous complications are spontaneous bacterial peritonitis (SBP) and rapid-onset (Type I) hepatorenal syndrome. Less than half of those who develop SBP can be expected to survive a year without transplantation, whereas the median survival among patients with Type I hepatorenal syndrome is less than two weeks.[17,18]

Liver transplantation provides patients with MELD scores ≥ 16 and CTP scores ≥ 10 the greatest chance for improved survival.[10,19] Transplantation in patients with MELD scores of 10–16 and CTP scores of 7–10 should be reserved primarily for those with one of more of the major complications of cirrhosis. Finally, transplantation should rarely if ever be considered in patients with MELD <10 and CTP < 7 unless they have hepatocellular carcinoma.[20] These principles are summarized in Table 14.2.

Decision making regarding transplantation versus continued medical therapy can be even more challenging in patients with fulminant hepatic failure (FHF). If given appropriate critical care support, most patients with fulminant hepatic failure spontaneously recover.[21] Recovery is typically complete, with no evidence of residual liver injury. Factors useful in determining the probability of spontaneous recovery include the patient's age, the underlying etiology of disease, the degree of encephalopathy, prolongation of INR values, and elevated APACHE II scores.[21,22] Most young people with acetaminophen hepatotoxicity or hepatitis A infection recover spontaneously without the need for transplantation.[23] In contrast, older patients with idiosyncratic drug reactions or FHF of unknown etiology are far less likely to recover without transplantation and patients with fulminant Wilson disease invariably require urgent transplantation if they are to survive.[24] Patients with FHF can improve rapidly or develop cerebral edema, multiorgan failure, or cardiovascular collapse within days to weeks after clinical presentation.[25] As a consequence, hour-to-hour assessment by experienced clinicians is required to optimize decisions regarding urgent transplantation versus continued medical management in these critically ill patients.

2. EXPLORING ALTERNATIVE FORMS OF TREATMENT

Because of the need for long-term immunosuppressive therapy, liver transplantation can be associated with higher mortality and long-term morbidity than alternative treatments for some chronic liver diseases. As a result, every therapeutic option should be carefully considered before committing a patient to transplantation. Examples include immunosuppressive therapy for patients with severe autoimmune hepatitis, chelation therapy for patients with chronic Wilson disease, antiviral therapy for patients with decompensated cirrhosis secondary to chronic hepatitis B, portocaval shunt surgery or transjugular intrahepatic shunts (TIPS) for patients with well compensated cirrhosis and intractable variceal bleeding, mesocaval shunts or TIPS procedures for patients with Budd-Chiari syndrome, and hepatic resection or radiofrequency ablation for patients with hepatocellular carcinoma and preserved liver function. However, if the outcome of these treatments remains in doubt, it is reasonable to begin evaluation for transplantation while continually assessing the results of the alternative form of therapy.

3. DETERMINING THE POTENTIAL FOR SUCCESSFUL LIVER TRANSPLANTATION

Once it has been determined that a patient is sick enough for transplantation and that no other alternative treatments are available, a careful evaluation should be performed to address the following fundamental questions:

A. Can the patient survive the operation and the immediate postoperative period?
B. Does the patient have other comorbid conditions that could so limit survival that transplantation would be futile?
C. Does the patient have an adequate support system and the emotional strength and discipline to comply with the required medical regimen after transplantation?

A. Assessment of Operative and Perioperative Survival

A variety of factors can impact a patient's chance of surviving liver transplantation. These most important of these are neuropsychiatric disorders, cardiopulmonary status, body weight, underlying renal function, and patency of the portal vein.

Patients with severe neurologic or cardiopulmonary disease usually cannot withstand the stress of transplant surgery and the early postoperative period. Perioperative mortality is particularly high in patients with coronary

Table 14.3. Contraindications to Liver Transplant Surgery	
Condition	*Comments*
Severe neuropsychiatric disease	These patients can rarely tolerate the stress of major surgery and immunosuppression
Coronary artery disease	Perioperative mortality high
Severe pulmonary hypertension	Reduced perioperative survival unless medical control can be achieved
Severe hypoxia	Excessive perioperative mortaliy
Morbid obesity	Significantly reduced survival
Chronic renal failure	Perioperative mortality high unless combined liver-kidney transplant utilized
Extensive portal vein thrombosis	Graft and patient survival reduced

artery disease.[26] Severe pulmonary hypertension is associated with high perioperative mortality and, if not successfully treated, is a contraindication to transplantation.[27–29] Patients with severe hypoxia from the hepatopulmonary syndrome or emphysema also have increased perioperative mortality.[30,31] The median survival of these patients is less than 12 months.[32] Obesity, an increasingly common problem among patients being considered for liver transplantation, also has an adverse impact on both immediate and long-term survival. Morbid obesity (BMI $> 40\,kg/m^2$) is associated with decreased 30-day, one-year, and two-year postoperative survival.[33]

Elevated serum creatinine is an independent risk factor for both the development of renal failure and decreased survival following liver transplantation.[34] Although acute renal failure from the hepatorenal syndrome usually improves dramatically after liver transplantation, patients with pre-existing chronic renal disease have diminished survival and an increased risk of requiring dialysis after transplantation. Unfortunately, it can be quite difficult to distinguish these two conditions in patients with severe liver disease.[35] Combined liver and renal transplantation is very effective in selected patients with pre-existing renal disease who develop liver failure.[36,37] However, this approach can only be used sparingly, given the large number of patients on renal transplant waiting lists.[38]

The most commonly encountered surgical contraindication to liver transplantation is absence of a viable splanchnic venous inflow system, usually from extensive portal vein thrombosis. If the entire portal venous system is occluded, transplantation is associated with a high risk of graft loss and perioperative mortality.[39,40]

The most common contraindications to liver transplant surgery are summarized in Table 14.3.

B. Conditions Affecting Long-Term Survival (Table 14.4)

Other conditions, which do not influence periopertive mortality, can reduce long-term survival to such an extent that they are considered to be either absolute or relative contraindications to transplantation. Included among these are intrahepatic and extrahepatic malignancies, HIV infection, cigarette smoking, and iron overload.

Table 14.4. Factors Affecting Long-Term Survival After Liver Transplantation

Condition	Comment
Hepatocellular carcinoma > 5 cm, more than 3 tumors, extrahepatic spread	90% of patients with large tumors or portal vein invasion have recurrent disease within 2 years after transplantation
Cholangiocarcinoma	High recurrence rate. Contraindicated except in special research centers
Extrahepatic malignancies	Transplantation should be delayed for 1–5 years after cure of tumor
Uncontrolled drug and alcohol addiction	Compliance poor and survival diminished

Liver transplantation has become one of the most effective treatments for hepatocellular carcinoma (HCC). The best outcomes are seen in patients with a single lesion ≥ 2 cm and < 5 cm in size, or no more than three lesions, the largest of which is < 3 cm in size, with no radiographic evidence of extrahepatic disease.[41] Patients with larger tumors often have nodal involvement or subtle extrahepatic spread.[42] More than 90% of these patients develop recurrent disease within two years of transplantation.[43] As a consequence, larger and more extensive HCC is a contraindication to transplantation. The exception is the fibrolamellar variant, which has a much better prognosis.[44,45] Patients with HCC who are optimal candidates for transplantation are currently assigned increased MELD scores in the United States to facilitate early transplantation.[46]

Liver transplantation for cholangiocarcinoma remains a frustrating enigma. Even small tumors with no evidence of local invasion almost invariably recur within a few years after transplantation.[47] Although highly selected patients may benefit from aggressive preoperative radiotherapy and chemotherapy followed by transplantation, this approach remains experimental.[48] Otherwise, cholangiocarcinoma remains a contraindication to liver transplantation.

Patients with a history of extrahepatic malignancies such as breast cancer or lymphomas risk severe recurrent disease after liver transplantation because of the immunosuppression required. Thus, it is reasonable to defer transplantation for a reasonable period after cure of any such malignancy. This may range from one to five years, based on the tumor type. Decisions to transplant these patients require close consultation between transplant physicians and the patient's oncologist.

A number of other conditions are associated with decreased survival after transplantion. However, these are considered by most transplant programs to be only relative contraindications to transplantation. Examples include HIV infection in patients with HCV-associated cirrhosis and hemochromatosis.

Survival following transplantation in patients with HIV infection well controlled with HAART therapy is comparable to that seen in HIV negative recipients.[49] However, severe recurrent hepatitis C has been observed in a number of these patients and remains an ongoing concern.[50]

Patients with hemochromatosis have diminished survival compared to patients transplanted for other conditions.[51] These suboptimal results appear to result from a high rate of postoperative infections as well as occasional deaths from cardiac failure or recurrent hepatocellular carcinoma.

C. Psychosocial Issues

Psychosocial issues often are the greatest deterrent to successful liver transplantation. Significant psychiatric disorders must be under excellent medical control with assurance that the patient can be compliant after the transplant. In addition, patients must have adequate support from family or friends during the perioperative period. The most frequently encountered contraindication to transplantation is continued destructive behavior due to drug and alcohol addiction.

Liver Transplantation: The Operation

Most liver transplants are performed using a whole liver from a deceased donor (deceased donor transplant). However, the unique anatomical organization of the liver allows surgeons to divide organs and transplant two recipients with one donor organ (split liver transplantation).[52,53] The same surgical techniques are used for living donor transplantation, in which only a portion of the donor organ is removed for transplantation. Living donor transplantation for children, in which a relatively small portion of the left lobe is used, is a well-established procedure.[54] Living donor transplantation in adults, which requires removal of the right lobe, also is performed at many transplant centers, although donor safety remains an ongoing concern.[55-57] Perioperative complications are slightly higher with split-liver or living donor techniques; however, long-term survival appears comparable to deceased donor transplants.[53,58]

The transplant operation consists of: (1) removal of the diseased organ; (2) replacement with the donor organ; (3) vascular reconstruction of the hepatic artery, the portal vein, and the hepatic venous drainage to the inferior vena cava; and (4) biliary reconstruction, which usually is accomplished using an end-to-end or side-to-side anastomosis of the proximal donor bile duct to the distal recipient duct. In recipients with diseased ducts (in patients with biliary atresia or sclerosing cholangitis), the donor duct is anastomosed to the jejunum using a Roux-en-Y loop. This same technique is used in retransplants and in other special circumstances, such as mismatch or donor and recipient duct size or insufficient length of the donor bile duct.

Although simple in concept, liver transplantation is a technically demanding operation.[59] Numerous modifications of the procedure have been employed over the years in efforts to improve hemodynamic stability in the operating room, to reduce the duration of the operation, and to minimize periopertive complications. The classical technique includes *en block* resection and removal of the vena cava with the diseased liver, cross clamping of the vena cava and portal vein (often followed by a venovenous bypass to maintain blood pressure and reduce intestinal swelling), anastamoses of the donor vena cava to the recipient vessel above and below the liver, hepatic artery reconstruction, portal vein anastamosis, and drainage of the bile duct using a T tube. In recent years many surgeons have abandoned the venovenous bypass and T tube drainage, and have replaced the classical vena caval anastamosis with a "piggyback technique," in which the recipient vena cava is preserved.[60–62]

Immediate Post-Operative Complications

The most serious complication seen immediately after liver transplantation is primary nonfunction of the graft, which occurs in 5–10% of cases. This dramatic failure of the liver to function after the transplant is easily recognized by its clinical features, which include persistent encephalopathy, coagulapathy, progressive jaundice, and metabolic acidosis. Advanced donor age, donation after cardiac death, and the use of split grafts each increase the risk of graft failure following transplantation.[63] Emergent retransplantation is the only option for these patients.

The two most common post-transplant surgical complications include hepatic artery thrombosis and biliary tract complications, which are often interrelated. Biliary tract complications such as anastamotic strictures and leaks can be effectively managed by endoscopy.[64] Hepatic artery thrombosis (HAT) can result in more serious biliary tract complications including diffuse intrahepatic strictures resembling sclerosing cholangitis as well as necrosis of the intrahepatic bilary radicals. This latter complication usually results in recurrent bilomas and requires retransplantation. A variety of surgical and nonsurgical factors are associated with increased risk for HAT including transient postoperative hypercoagulability, tobacco use, and cytomegalovius infection.[65]

Other less common surgical complications include hepatic artery stenosis, aneurysms of the hepatic artery, splenic artery rupture, vena caval stenosis, and portal vein thrombosis. Hepatic artery stenosis can result in the same biliary tract complications as HAT. Aneurysms of the hepatic artery, which generally result from bacterial infection at the anastamosis, can be fatal; urgent excision of the aneurysm and revascularization of the graft with an alternative blood supply is the most effective treatment. Splenic artery aneurysms are common in patients with cirrhosis. Rupture following transplantation is usually a rapidly fatal event. Management options include surgical treatment of the aneurysms during the transplant operation and coil embolization in those discovered after transplantation.[66,67] Hepatic vein occlusion and portal vein thrombosis are unusual complications after transplantation.

Infections remain among the most serious medical complications encountered after transplantation. Potential pathogens such as pneumocystis and cytomegalovirus can usually be prevented by aggressive prophylaxis with trimethoprim/sulfa and ganciclovir or valganciclovir during the first six months after the operation.[68] The best methods of preventing other infections include optimizing the timing of the operation, avoiding prolonged intensive care unit stay, and minimizing immunosuppressive therapy. Many of the most serious postoperative infections occur in debilitated, critically ill patients. Invasive candidiasis and aspergillosis, which are the most serious of the infections to occur in the early postoperative period, are often fatal.[69] Infections with antimicrobial-resistant bacteria, such as methicillin-resistant *Staphylococcus aureus* or vancomycin-resistant *Enterococcus faecium*, also are associated with increased postoperative mortality.[70]

Table 14.5. Commonly Used Immunosuppressive
Protocols

Induction Therapy	Double-Drug Regimens	Triple-Drug Regimens
ATG	Cyclosporine or	Cyclosporine or
ALG	tacrolimus* and	tacrolimus*
OKT3, or	Corticosteroids	Corticosteroids, and
Basiliximab or		Azathioprine or
daclvzimab		mycophenolate mofetil

*Sirolimus substituted for calcineurin inhibitors in patients with renal failure.

Immunosuppressive Agents and Their Complications

A number of immunosuppressive agents are available for use after solid-organ transplantation. These agents include cyclosporine, tacrolimus, azathioprine, mycophenolate mofetil, sirolimus, and corticosteroids, as well as various polyclonal or monoclonal antilymphocyte preparations.[71] Most transplant programs use two or three immunosuppressive agents with different mechanisms of action (double-drug or triple-drug protocols). Double-drug protocols usually combine a calineurin inhibitor such as cyclosporine or tacrolimus with corticosteroids. Commonly used triple-drug protocols include a calcineurin inhibitor and corticosteroids plus and antimetabolite (either azathioprine or mycophenolate mofetil). Sirolimus can be used *in lieu* of calcineurin inhibitors in patients with renal failure.[72] In addition, some programs use a short peritransplant induction regime including either antithymocyte globulin (ATG), anti-lymphocyte globulin (ALG), OKT3 (a monoclonal antibody preparation directed against the CD3 component of the T-cell receptor), or an IL-2 antagonists, such as basiliximab or daclvzimab. The more commonly used regimens are summarized in Table 14.5.

Cyclosporine and tacrolimus are both associated with a number of complications including renal dysfunction, neurological toxicity, hypertension, and a variety of metabolic abnormalities including hyperlipidemia, hyperkalemia, and hyperuricemia. Renal failure occurs within 10 years in 10% of patients who take cyclosporine or tacrolimus after transplantation.[73] The highest risk patients are those with preexisting renal disease at the time of transplantation and those with a glomerular filtration rate less than 40 ml per minute a year after the operation. Some patients who receive either cyclosporine or tacrolimus develop severe neuropsychiatric complications, including psychosis, seizures, and apraxia.[74] Many patients complain of headaches, tremors, and severe musculoskeletal pains. Hypertension, which is thought to result from peripheral and renal vasoconstriction, is quite common in patients who take either cyclosporine or tacrolimus.[75] Pancreatic damage with development of type 1 diabetes (insulin-dependent) also is common in patients who take tacrolimus. Patients who take either drug can experience hyperkalemia, hyperuricemia, and elevated cholesterol and/or triglyceride levels.[76] Tacrolimus appears to induce less severe hyerlipidemias than cyclosporine.[77] Cyclosporine is associated with gingival hyperplasia and excessive hair growth, particularly on the arms and face, whereas patients who take tacrolimus are generally spared these complications.

Both azathioprine and mycophenolate mofetil can cause bone marrow suppression with leukopenia, thrombocytopenia, and anemia. Many patients who take mycophenolate mofetil also complain of gastrointestinal side effects including nausea, abdominal pain, and diarrhea. Long-term corticosteroid therapy is associated with obesity, hypertension, glucose intolerance, cataracts, osteoporosis, and hypercholesterolemia. Side effects of sirolimus include gastrointestinal symptoms and marked elevation of serum lipids, particularly when the drug is used in combination with cyclosporine.[78]

These various immunosuppressive agents are associated with a numerous drug-drug interactions.[71] Both cyclosporine and tacrolimus are metabolized intrahepatically, primarily via the cytochrome P-450 IIIA enzyme. Inhibitors or inducers of this enzyme can have profound affects of the blood levels of these two agents. The most striking examples include interactions with ketoconazole and phenytoin. Ketoconazole inhibits P-450 IIIA and can dramatically increase circulating levels of cyclosporine and tacrolimus. In contrast, phenytoin, which induces the enzyme, with resulting enhanced metabolism of cyclosporine and tacrolimus, can profoundly depress circulating levels of either drug. Another important interaction is that between allopurinol and azathioprine. This commonly used agent for the prevention of gout can interfere with azathioprine metabolism, resulting in profound, life-threatening leucopenia. Awareness of these various interactions is important in managing post-transplant patients.

Acute Cellular Rejection: Assessment and Treatment

Cellular rejection, which occurs within the first year in 20–40% of liver transplant recipients, is usually manifested primarily by elevated aminotransferase levels in an asymptomatic patient. If the diagnosis is delayed, patients may experience malaise, anorexia, and right upper quadrant pain and develop fever and jaundice. The diagnosis is confirmed by liver biopsy, which reveals cellular inflammatory invasion of the small bile ducts and vascular endothelium.[79] Most patients with rejection respond rapidly to boluses of corticosteroid therapy administered over three to five days. Only 5–10% of patients fail to respond to such therapy; treatment of these patients generally requires more aggressive treatment with an antilymphocyte agent such as ALG or OKT3. Rejection refractory to these agents is extremely rare.

Differentiating cellular rejection from recurrent hepatitis C is one of the most common and difficult challenges for clinicians and pathologists who care for liver transplant recipients. The clinical features are indistinguishable and there is considerable overlap in the histological features of the two conditions. Hepatitis C is characterized histologically by dense portal inflammation and expansion of the portal tracts plus diffuse intralobular inflammation and necrosis with prominent acidophilic bodies. However, a number of these patients also have bile duct injury and endothelial injury, which can make differentiation from cellular rejection extremely difficult, even for the most experienced pathologist.[80] This a critically important issue because excessive immunosuppression used to treat rejection, especially with anti-lymphocytic agents such as OKT3, can accelerate the progression of recurrent hepatitis C.[81,82] As a consequence, an extremely cautious approach to treating suspected episodes of rejection in patients with hepatitis C (even to the extent of performing multiple biopsies to confirm the diagnosis) is prudent.[83]

Long-Term Complications

Although delayed allograft rejection and surgical complications can occur, most long-term complications seen after liver transplantation are secondary to the continued use of immunosuppressive drugs, the underlying medical condition of the recipient, or recurrence of the original disease.

MEDICAL COMPLICATIONS

The most common long-term complications seen after liver transplantation include: (1) obesity and the associated metabolic issues of diabetes and dyslipidemias; (2) hypertension and renal failure; (3) hyperuricemia and gout; (4) osteoporosis; and, (5) various malignancies.[84] Cardiovascular disease and malignancies are the two leading causes of death in long-term survivors.[85]

OBESITY AND METABOLIC ISSUES

Obesity has emerged as one of the most common complications seen after liver transplantation. Weight gain is common, particularly within the first two years after the operation.[86] Approximately 20% of liver transplant recipients are obese and up to 60% are overweight. Factors associated with rapid weight gain and obesity include the pretransplant body mass index, the cumulative dose of corticosteroids, and the absence of rejection.[86] Obese patients are particularly prone to the development of diabetes, dyslipidemias, and hypertension. As a consequence, aggressive dietary counseling and exercise beginning the early post-operative period is extremely important.[87]

Diabetes is extremely common in liver transplant recipients, particularly in those with pretransplant diagnoses of hepatitis C and non-alcoholic steatohepatitis.[88,89] Obesity, high-dose corticosteroid therapy and tacrolimus are the immunosuppressive agents with the strongest association with post-transplant diabetes.[90,91] Because post-transplant diabetes is associated with increased morbidity and mortality, aggressive management with weight reduction and early reduction and/or elimination of corticosteroids are important goals to pursue.[90,92]

Although common, both hypercholesterolemia and hypertryglyceridemia are seen less frequently after liver transplantation than after other solid organ transplants.[93] Furthermore, it has not been clearly documented that these abnormalities increase the cardiovascular risk of liver transplant recipients. Nevertheless, there is a general consensus that these lipid abnormalities should be aggressively treated. Specific risk factors for dyslipidemias after liver transplantation include corticosteroid therapy, calcineurin inhibitors, and sirolimus, particularly when used in combination with cyclosporine.[78,91,93] Therefore a prudent approach to immunosuppressive therapy is to minimize the use of corticosteroids and if used, to combine sirolimus with an immunosuppressive agent other than cyclosporine.[78,90] Among the available lipid lowering agents, pravastatin and cerivastatin have been shown to be safe in transplant recipients and have few drug-drug interactions with immunosuppressive agents.[94–96]

HYPERTENSION AND RENAL FAILURE

Risk factors for hypertension, which is common in transplant recipients, include obesity, corticosteroids, and the use of calcineurin inhibitors. Treatment in posttransplant patients must be considered in context with the various interactions between antihypertensives and immunosuppressive agents. Thiazides can exacerbate elevated uric acid levels and ACE inhibitors and diuretics can increase potassium levels in patients taking calcineurin inhibitors. A number of calcium channel blockers have significant drug-drug interactions with tacrolimus, cyclosporine, and sirolimus. Nicardipine, verapamil, and mebefradil should be used with caution for this reason.[97] The safest and most effective management of hypertension in the patients includes minimizing corticosteroid and calcineurin inhibitor therapy in combination with judicious use of calcium channel blockers such as amlodipine or nifedipin.[98,99] Even when these agents are used, however, it is prudent to monitor blood levels of cyclosporine tacrolimus and sirolimus for two to three months after initiation of therapy to insure that appropriate immunosuppression is maintained.

The most important long-term adverse effect of cyclosporine and tacrolimus is nephrotoxicity, which can lead to chronic renal failure and the need for dialysis. In the subset of patients who develop progressive renal insufficiency, it may be useful to replace calcineurin inhibitors with either mycophenolate mofetil or sirolimus, although there is an increased risk of rejection with either of these approaches.[72,100]

HYPERURICEMIA AND GOUT

Hyperuricemia, although a common complication seen after liver transplantation, is not as profound as in other solid organ recipients.[101] The mechanism appears to be calcineurin inhibitor-induced reduction in glomerular filtration rate and tubular secretion of uric acid. Despite the high prevalence of hyperuricemia, clinical manifestations of gout occur in less than 5% of patients. Nevertheless, management of patients with hyperuricemia and gout can be quite challenging as most commonly used treatments have significant interactions with immunosuppressive agents. Nonsteroidal anti-inflammatory drugs can increase the nephrotoxicity of calcineurin inhibitor and allopurinol can interfere with the metabolism of azathioprine, resulting in severe bone marrow suppression. The safest agent for acute gout attacks is colchicin. Allopurinol, the best long-term treatment of hyperuricemia, has been shown to improve renal function in patients with increased serum creatinine.[102]

OSTEOPOROSIS

Osteoporosis is a common complication of cirrhosis. Although most common in post-menopausal women, it can be seen in patients with cholestatic disorders such as PBC and PSC, and patients who have received prolonged corticosteroid therapy. Osteoporosis is also common in patients with chronic hepatitis C and alcoholic cirrhosis.[103] Preexisting osteoporosis frequently is accelerated within the first three to six months after transplantation with progressive bone resorption and increased risk for pathological fractures; however, bone mass generally returns to pretransplant levels within the ensuing six months.[104,105] Risk factors for accelerated post-operative bone loss include preexisting osteoporosis, postoperative immobilization, and the use of corticosteroids and calcineurin inhibitors. Management includes minimal doses and duration of corticosteroid therapy, physical activity, cessation of smoking, calcium and vitamin D therapy and, in appropriate patients, hormone replacement therapy.[106] Biphosphonates should be considered in patients with severe osteoporosis or pathological fractures.

MALIGNANCIES

Malignancies are the second leading cause of death in long-term survivors after liver transplantation.[85] Skin cancers are the most common malignancies encountered.[107,108] These tumors tend to be more aggressive with higher rates of invasion and metastases than in the general population. Furthermore, metastatic disease in these patients is associated with considerable morbidity and mortality.[109] Risk factors include pretransplant cutaneous malignancies, fair skin, increased age, exposure to ultraviolet radiation, and the intensity of immunosuppression.[110] Patient education regarding the importance of protective clothing and sunscreen plus aggressive surveillance and management of any new lesions are extremely important.[111]

Less common but even more ominous is the development of post-transplant lymphoproliferative disorder (PTLD), a non-Hodgkin's lymphoma, usually associated with Epstein-Barr infection induced by immunosuppressive therapy.[112] PTLD commonly presents with involvement of the GI tract and central nodes, with sparing of peripheral nodes. The prognosis varies considerably from patient to patient. Older patients who have a delayed presentation and monoclonal proliferation have the worst prognosis.[113] Treatment generally includes reduction of immunosuppressive therapy, antiviral therapy, and/or chemotherapy.[114]

Other less common tumors include oropharygeal and gastrointestinal tumors (which are particularly common in patients with alcoholic liver disease), lung tumors in chronic smokers, and colon cancer, particularly in patients with PSC and inflammatory bowel disease.[115,116] The latter patients need intensive annual screening to facilitate early diagnosis and management of this potentially rapidly fatal malignancy.[116]

DISEASE REOCCURRENCE

Disease reoccurrence can also result in significant morbidity and mortality after liver transplantation. By far, the most common and serious condition is recurrence of hepatitis C. Most patients with chronic hepatitis C virus infection have persistent viremia after transplantation. Although many patients experience little if any histological damage associated with chronic HCV infection, approximately 15% develop cirrhosis within five to seven years after transplantation. Long-term survival of these patients is significantly worse than for patients who receive transplantation for other conditions.[117] Risk factors for severe recurrent hepatitis C include the use of older donor organs, delayed graft function, and aggressive treatment of rejection, particularly with anti-lymphocyte preparations.[118] Although some patients have responded to interferon and ribavirin therapy, many cannot tolerate these agents. As a result, the optimal management of these patients remains unclear.[119]

Recurrent hepatitis B is uncommon in patients who are compliant with hepatitis B immune globulin and antiviral therapy with lamivudine, or adefovir. However, patients with a high viral load at the time of transplantation and those who receive inadequate prophylaxis can have recurrent infection, which can be quite severe, particularly if the diagnosis is delayed.[120] Continuous monitoring of anti-HBs and HBV DNA levels with early and aggressive treatment of recurrent disease is critical to the long-term management of these patients.[121,122]

Recurrent autoimmune hepatitis, primary biliary cirrhosis, and primary sclerosing cholangitis can also occur. However, recurrence of these disorders infrequently impacts post-transplant survival. More concerning is recurrence of nonalcoholic steatohepatitis, which is being reported with increasing frequency.[123,124] The overall impact of recurrent disease on long-term survival and the optimal management of these patients are unknown.

Given the stringent selection criteria currently used, recurrent hepatocellular carcinoma is uncommon after liver transplantation. Poorly differentiated tumors with vascular invasion observed in the diseased liver removed at the time of transplantation are those most likely to recur.[125] The optimal management of these high-risk patients is unclear.

SUMMARY

Liver transplantation has dramatically improved the outcome for patients with acute or chronic liver failure and for patients with hepatocellular carcinoma. Judicious selection of potential recipients and improved perioperative and long-term care have resulted in continuous improvements in long-term survival. As a result, liver transplantation is now considered the ultimate treatment for many liver disorders.

REFERENCES

1. Murray KF, Carithers RL, Jr. AASLD practice guidelines: Evaluation of the patient for liver transplantation. Hepatology 2005;41:1407–32.
2. Belle SH, Porayko MK, Hoofnagle JH, Lake JR, Zetterman RK. Changes in quality of life after liver transplantation among adults. National Institute of Diabetes and Digestive and Kidney Diseases (NIDDK) Liver Transplantation Database (LTD). Liver Transpl Surg 1997;3:93–104.

3. Best JH, Veenstra DL, Geppert J. Trends in expenditures for Medicare liver transplant recipients. Liver Transpl 2001;7:858–62.

4. Malinchoc M, Kamath PS, Gordon FD, Peine CJ, Rank J, ter Borg PC. A model to predict poor survival in patients undergoing transjugular intrahepatic portosystemic shunts. Hepatology 2000;31:864–71.

5. Kamath PS, Wiesner RH, Malinchoc M, Kremers W, Therneau TM, Kosberg CL, D'Amico G, Dickson ER, Kim WR. A model to predict survival in patients with end-stage liver disease. Hepatology 2001;33:464–470.

6. Wiesner R, Edwards E, Freeman R, Harper A, Kim R, Kamath P, Kremers W, Lake J, Howard T, Merion RM, Wolfe RA, Krom R. Model for end-stage liver disease (MELD) and allocation of donor livers. Gastroenterology 2003;124:91–6.

7. Freeman RB, Wiesner RH, Edwards E, Harper A, Merion R, Wolfe R. Results of the first year of the new liver allocation plan. Liver Transpl 2004;10:7–15.

8. Pugh RNH, Murray-Lyon IM, Dawson JL, Pietroni MC, Williams R. Transection of the oesophagus for bleeding oesophageal varices. Brit J Surg 1973;60:646–8.

9. Trey C, Burns DG, Saunders SJ. Treatment of hepatic coma by exchange blood transfusion. N Engl J Med 1966;274:473–81.

10. Oellerich M, Burdelski M, Lautz H-U, Binder L, Pichlmayr R. Predictors of one-year pretransplant survival in patients with cirrhosis. Hepatology 1991;14: 1029–34.

11. Shetty K, Rybicki L, Carey WD. The Child-Pugh classification as a prognostic indicator for survival in primary sclerosing cholangitis. Hepatology 1997;25:1049–53.

12. Propst A, Propst T, Sangeri G, Ofner D, Judmaier G, Vogel W. Prognosis and life expectancy in chronic liver disease. Dig Dis Sci 1995;40:1805–15.

13. Lucey MR, Brown KA, Everson GT, Fung JJ, Gish R, Keeffe EB, Kneteman NM, Lake JR, Martin P, McDiarmid SV, Rakela J, Shiffman ML, So SK, Wiesner RH. Minimal criteria for placement of adults on the liver transplant waiting list: a report of a national conference organized by the American Society of Transplant Physicians and the American Association for the Study of Liver Diseases. Liver Transpl Surg 1997;3: 628–37.

14. Fattovich G, Giustina G, Degos F, Tremolada F, Diodati G, Almasio P, Nevens F, Solinas A, Mura D, Brouwer JT, Thomas H, Njapoum C, Casarin C, Bonetti P, Fuschi P, Basho J, Tocco A, Bhalla A, Galassini R, Noventa F, Schalm SW, Realdi G. Morbidity and mortality in compensated cirrhosis type C: a retrospective follow-up study of 384 patients. Gastroenterology 1997;112:463–72.

15. Gines P, Quintero E, Arroyo V, Teres J, Bruguera M, Rimola A, Caballeria J, Rodes J, Rozman C. Compensated cirrhosis: natural history and prognosis factors. Hepatology 1987;7:122–8.

16. Llovet JM, Fuster J, Bruix J. Prognosis of hepatocellular carcinoma. Hepatogastroenterology 2002;49:7–11.

17. Andreu M, Sola R, Sitges SA, Alia C, Gallen M, Vila MC, Coll S, Oliver MI. Risk factors for spontaneous bacterial peritonitis in cirrhotic patients with ascites. Gastroenterology 1993;104:1133–8.

18. Gines A, Escorsell A, Gines P, Sal'o J, Jim'enez W, Inglada L, Navasa M, Claria J, Rimola A, Arroyo V, et a. Incidence, predictive factors, and prognosis of the hepatorenal syndrome in cirrhosis with ascites. Gastroenterology 1993;105:229–36.

19. Merion RM, Schaubel DE, Dykstra DM, Freeman RB, Port FK, Wolfe RA. The survival benefit of liver transplantation. Am J Transplant 2005;5:307–13.

20. Lucey MR, Brown KA, Everson GT, Fung JJ, Gish R, Keeffe EB, Kneteman NM, Lake JR, Martin P, Rakela J, Shiffman ML, So S, Wiesner RH. Minimal criteria for placement of adults on the liver transplant waiting list: a report of a national conference organized by the American Society of Transplant Physicians and the American Association for the Study of Liver Diseases. Transplantation 1998;66:956–62.

21. Lee WM. Acute liver failure in the United States. Semin Liver Dis 2003;23:217–26.

22. Bailey B, Amre DK, Gaudreault P. Fulminant hepatic failure secondary to acetaminophen poisoning: a systematic review and meta-analysis of prognostic criteria determining the need for liver transplantation. Crit Care Med 2003;31:299–305.

23. Larson AM, Polson J, Fontana RJ, Davern TJ, Lalani E, Hynan LS, Reisch JS, Schiodt FV, Ostapowicz G, Shakil AO, Lee WM. Acetaminophen-induced acute liver failure: results of a United States multicenter, prospective study. Hepatology 2005;42:1364–72.

24. Roberts EA, Schilsky ML. A practice guideline on Wilson disease. Hepatology 2003;37:1475–92.

25. McCormick PA, Treanor D, McCormack G, Farrell M. Early death from paracetamol (acetaminophen) induced fulminant hepatic failure without cerebral oedema. J Hepatol 2003;39:547–51.

26. Plotkin JS, Scott VL, Pinna A, Dobsch BP, De Wolf AM, Kang Y. Morbidity and mortality in patients with coronary artery disease undergoing orthotopic liver transplantation. Liver Transpl Surg 1996;2:426–30.

27. Ramsay MA, Simpson BR, Nguyen AT, Ramsay KJ, East C, Klintmalm GB. Severe pulmonary hypertension in liver transplant candidates. Liver Transpl Surg 1997;3:494–500.

28. Krowka MJ, Plevak DJ, Findlay JY, Rosen CB, Wiesner RH, Krom RA. Pulmonary hemodynamics and perioperative cardiopulmonary-related mortality in patients with portopulmonary hypertension undergoing liver transplantation [In Process Citation]. Liver Transpl 2000;6:443–50.

29. Starkel P, Vera A, Gunson B, Mutimer D. Outcome of liver transplantation for patients with pulmonary hypertension. Liver Transpl 2002;8:382–8.

30. Collisson EA, Nourmand H, Fraiman MH, Cooper CB, Bellamy PE, Farmer DG, Vierling JM, Ghobrial RM, Busuttil RW. Retrospective analysis of the results of liver transplantation for adults with severe hepatopulmonary syndrome. Liver Transpl 2002;8:925–31.

31. Arguedas MR, Abrams GA, Krowka MJ, Fallon MB. Prospective evaluation of outcomes and predictors of mortality in patients with hepatopulmonary syndrome undergoing liver transplantation. Hepatology 2003;37:192–7.

32. Schenk P, Schoniger-Hekele M, Fuhrmann V, Madl C, Silberhumer G, Muller C. Prognostic significance of the hepatopulmonary syndrome in patients with cirrhosis. Gastroenterology 2003;125:1042–52.

33. Nair S, Verma S, Thuluvath PJ. Obesity and its effect on survival in patients undergoing orthotopic liver transplantation in the United States. Hepatology 2002;35:105–9.

34. Nair S, Verma S, Thuluvath PJ. Pretransplant renal function predicts survival in patients undergoing orthotopic liver transplantation. Hepatology 2002;35:1179–85.

35. Davis CL, Gonwa TA, Wilkinson AH. Pathophysiology of renal disease associated with liver disorders: implications for liver transplantation. Part I. Liver Transpl 2002;8:91–109.

36. Grewal HP, Brady L, Cronin DC, Loss GE, Siegel CT, Oswald K, Fisher JS, Bruce DS, Aronson AJ, Woodle ES, Millis JM, Thistlethwaite JR, Newell KA. Combined liver and kidney transplantation in children. Transplantation 2000;70:100–5.

37. Rogers J, Bueno J, Shapiro R, Scantlebury V, Mazariegos G, Fung J, Reyes J. Results of simultaneous and sequential pediatric liver and kidney transplantation. Transplantation 2001;72:1666–70.

38. Davis CL, Gonwa TA, Wilkinson AH. Identification of patients best suited for combined liver-kidney transplantation: part II. Liver Transpl 2002;8:193–211.

39. Sobhonslidsuk A, Reddy KR. Portal vein thrombosis: a concise review. Am J Gastroenterol 2002;97:535–41.

40. Mitchell A, John PR, Mayer DA, Mirza DF, Buckels JA, de Ville dG. Improved technique of portal vein reconstruction in pediatric liver transplant recipients with portal vein hypoplasia. Transplantation 2002;73:1244–47.

41. Mazzaferro V, Regalia E, Doci R, Andreola S, Pulvirenti A, Bozzetti F, Montalto F, Ammatuna m, Morabito A, Gennari L. Liver transplantation for the treatment of small hepatocellular carcinomas in patients with cirrhosis. N Engl J Med 1996;334:693–9.

42. Pawlik TM, Delman KA, Vauthey JN, Nagorney DM, Ng IO, Ikai I, Yamaoka Y, Belghiti J, Lauwers GY, Poon RT, Abdalla EK. Tumor size predicts vascular invasion and histologic grade: Implications for selection of surgical treatment for hepatocellular carcinoma. Liver Transpl 2005;11:1086–92.

43. Bismuth H, Majno PE, Adam R. Liver transplantation for hepatocellular carcinoma. Semin Liver Dis 1999;19:311–22.

44. El Serag HB, Davila JA. Is fibrolamellar carcinoma different from hepatocellular carcinoma? A US population-based study. Hepatology 2004;39:798–803.

45. Makhlouf HR, Ishak KG, Goodman ZD. Epithelioid hemangioendothelioma of the liver: a clinicopathologic study of 137 cases. Cancer 1999;85:562–82.

46. Sharma P, Balan V, Hernandez JL, Harper AM, Edwards EB, Rodriguez-Luna H, Byrne T, Vargas HE, Mulligan D, Rakela J, Wiesner RH. Liver transplantation for hepatocellular carcinoma: The MELD impact. Liver Transpl 2004;10:36–41.

47. Goldstein RM, Stone M, Tillery GW, Senzer N, Levy M, Husberg BS, Gonwa T, Klintmalm G. Is liver transplantation indicated for cholangiocarcinoma? Am J Surg 1993;166:768–71.

48. Heimbach JK, Gores GJ, Nagorney DM, Rosen CB. Liver transplantation for perihilar cholangiocarcinoma after aggressive neoadjuvant therapy: a new paradigm for liver and biliary malignancies? Surgery 2006;140:331–4.

49. Roland ME, Stock PG. Liver transplantation in HIV-infected recipients. Semin Liver Dis 2006;26:273–84.

50. Stock PG, Roland ME, Carlson L, Freise CE, Roberts JP, Hirose R, Terrault NA, Frassetto LA, Palefsky JM, Tomlanovich SJ, Ascher NL. Kidney and liver transplantation in human immunodeficiency virus-infected patients: a pilot safety and efficacy study. Transplantation 2003;76:370–5.

51. Kowdley KV, Brandhagen DJ, Gish RG, Bass NM, Weinstein J, Schilsky ML, Fontana RJ, McCashland T, Cotler SJ, Bacon BR, Keeffe EB, Gordon F, Polissar N. Survival after liver transplantation in patients with hepatic iron overload: the national hemochromatosis transplant registry. Gastroenterology 2005;129:494–503.

52. Keeffe EB. Liver transplantation: current status and novel approaches to liver replacement. Gastroenterology 2001;120:749–62.

53. Renz JF, Emond JC, Yersiz H, Ascher NL, Busuttil RW. Split-liver transplantation in the United States: outcomes of a national survey. Ann Surg 2004;239:172–81.

54. Malago M, Hertl M, Testa G, Rogiers X, Broelsch CE. Split-liver transplantation: future use of scarce donor organs. World J Surg 2002;26:275–82.

55. Trotter JF, Wachs M, Everson GT, Kam I. Adult-to-adult transplantation of the right hepatic lobe from a living donor. N Engl J Med 2002;346:1074–82.

56. Surman OS. The ethics of partial-liver donation. N Engl J Med 2002;346:1038.

57. Trotter JF, Adam R, Lo CM, Kenison J. Documented deaths of hepatic lobe donors for living donor liver transplantation. Liver Transpl 2006;12:1485–88.

58. Settmacher U, Theruvath T, Pascher A, Neuhaus P. Living-donor liver transplantation – European experiences. Nephrol Dial Transplant 2004;19 Suppl 4:iv16–21.

59. Eghtesad B, Kadry Z, Fung J. Technical considerations in liver transplantation: what a hepatologist needs to know (and every surgeon should practice). Liver Transpl 2005;11:861–71.

60. Chari RS, Gan TJ, Robertson KM, Bass K, Camargo CA, Jr., Greig PD, Clavien PA. Venovenous bypass in adult orthotopic liver transplantation: routine or selective use? J Am Coll Surg 1998;186:683–90.

61. Scatton O, Meunier B, Cherqui D, Boillot O, Sauvanet A, Boudjema K, Launois B, Fagniez PL, Belghiti J, Wolff P, Houssin D, Soubrane O. Randomized trial of choledochocholedochostomy with or without a T tube in orthotopic liver transplantation. Ann Surg 2001;233:432–7.

62. Belghiti J, Ettorre GM, Durand F, Sommacale D, Sauvanet A, Jerius JT, Farges O. Feasibility and limits of caval-flow preservation during liver transplantation. Liver Transpl 2001;7:983–7.

63. Feng S, Goodrich NP, Bragg-Gresham JL, Dykstra DM, Punch JD, DebRoy MA, Greenstein SM, Merion RM. Characteristics associated with liver graft failure: the concept of a donor risk index. Am J Transplant 2006;6:783–90.

64. Moser MA, Wall WJ. Management of biliary problems after liver transplantation. Liver Transpl 2001;7:S46–52.

65. Pastacaldi S, Teixeira R, Montalto P, Rolles K, Burroughs AK. Hepatic artery thrombosis after orthotopic liver transplantation: a review of nonsurgical causes. Liver Transpl 2001;7:75–81.

66. Heestand G, Sher L, Lightfoote J, Palmer S, Mateo R, Singh G, Moser J, Selby R, Genyk Y, Jabbour N. Characteristics and management of splenic artery aneurysm in liver transplant candidates and recipients. Am Surg 2003;69:933–40.

67. Lupatelli T, Garaci FG, Sandhu C, Tisone G, Simonetti G. Endovascular treatment of giant splenic aneurysm that developed after liver transplantation. Transpl Int 2003;16:756–60.

68. Kalil AC, Levitsky J, Lyden E, Stoner J, Freifeld AG. Meta-analysis: the efficacy of strategies to prevent organ disease by cytomegalovirus in solid organ transplant recipients. Ann Intern Med 2005;143:870–80.

69. Rabkin JM, Oroloff SL, Corless CL, Benner KG, Flora KD, Rosen HR, Olyaei AJ. Association of fungal infection and increased mortality in liver transplant recipients. Am J Surg 2000;179:426–30.

70. Singh N, Gayowski T, Rihs JD, Wagener MM, Marino IR. Evolving trends in multiple-antibiotic-resistant bacteria in liver transplant recipients: a longitudinal study of antimicrobial susceptibility patterns. Liver Transpl 2001;7:22–6.

71. Levy GA. Long-term immunosuppression and drug interactions. Liver Transpl 2001;7:S53–9.

72. Fairbanks KD, Eustace JA, Fine D, Thuluvath PJ. Renal function improves in liver transplant recipients when switched from a calcineurin inhibitor to sirolimus. Liver Transpl 2003;9:1079–85.

73. Cohen AJ, Stegall MD, Rosen CB, Wiesner RH, Leung N, Kremers WK, Zein NN. Chronic renal dysfunction late after liver transplantation. Liver Transpl 2002;8:916–21.

74. Beresford TP. Neuropsychiatric complications of liver and other solid organ transplantation. Liver Transpl 2001;7:S36–45.

75. Textor SC, Taler SJ, Canzanello VJ, Schwartz L, Augustine JE. Posttransplantation hypertension related to calcineurin inhibitors. Liver Transpl 2000;6:521–30.

76. Charco R, Cantarell C, Vargas V, Capdevila L, Lazaro JL, Hidalgo E, Murio E, Margarit C. Serum cholesterol changes in long-term survivors of liver transplantation: a comparison between cyclosporine and tacrolimus therapy. Liver Transpl Surg 1999;5:204–8.

77. Neal DA, Gimson AE, Gibbs P, Alexander GJ. Beneficial effects of converting liver transplant recipients from cyclosporine to tacrolimus on blood pressure, serum lipids, and weight. Liver Transpl 2001;7:533–9.

78. Trotter JF, Wachs ME, Trouillot TE, Bak T, Kugelmas M, Kam I, Everson G. Dyslipidemia during sirolimus therapy in liver transplant recipients occurs with concomitant cyclosporine but not tacrolimus. Liver Transpl 2001;7:401–8.

79. Demetris AJ, Batts KP, Dhillon AP, Ferrell L, Fung J, Geller SA, Hart J, Hayry P, Hofmann WJ, Hubscher S, Kemnitz J, Koukoulis G, Lee RG, Lewin KJ, Ludwig J, Markin RS, Petrovic LM, Phillips MJ, Portmann B, Rakela J, Randhawa P, Reinhold FP, Reynes M, Robert M, Schlitt H, Solez K, Snover D, Taskinen E, Thung SN, Tillery GW, Wiesner RH, Wight DGD, Williams JW, Yamabe H. Banff schema for grading liver allograft rejection: an international consensus document. Hepatology 1997;25:658–63.

80. Demetris AJ, Eghtesad B, Marcos A, Ruppert K, Nalesnik MA, Randhawa P, Wu T, Krasinskas A, Fontes P, Cacciarelli T, Shakil AO, Murase N, Fung JJ, Starzl TE.

Recurrent hepatitis C in liver allografts: prospective assessment of diagnostic accuracy, identification of pitfalls, and observations about pathogenesis. Am J Surg Pathol 2004;28:658–69.

81. Rosen HR, Shackleton CR, Higa L, Gralnek IM, Farmer DA, McDiarmid SV, Holt C, Lewin KJ, Busuttil RW, Martin P. Use of OKT3 is associated with early and severe recurrence of hepatitis C after liver transplantation. Am J Gastroenterol 1997;92:1453–57.

82. Neumann UP, Berg T, Bahra M, Puhl G, Guckelberger O, Langrehr JM, Neuhaus P. Long-term outcome of liver transplants for chronic hepatitis C: a 10-year follow-up. Transplantation 2004;77:226–31.

83. Burton JR, Jr., Rosen HR. Acute rejection in HCV-infected liver transplant recipients: The great conundrum. Liver Transpl 2006;12:S38–47.

84. Sheiner PA, Magliocca JF, Bodian CA, Kim-Schluger L, Altaca G, Guarrera JV, Emre S, Fishbein TM, Guy SR, Schwartz ME, Miller CM. Long-term medical complications in patients surviving > or = 5 years after liver transplant. Transplantation 2000;69:781–9.

85. Fung JJ, Jain A, Kwak EJ, Kusne S, Dvorchik I, Eghtesad B. De novo malignancies after liver transplantation: a major cause of late death. Liver Transpl 2001;7:S109–18.

86. Everhart JE, Lombardero M, Lake JR, Wiesner RH, Zetterman RK, Hoofnagle JH. Weight change and obesity after liver transplantation: incidence and risk factors. Liver Transpl Surg 1998;4:285–96.

87. Reuben A. Long-term management of the liver transplant patient: diabetes, hyperlipidemia, and obesity. Liver Transpl 2001;7:S13–21.

88. Baid S, Cosimi AB, Farrell ML, Schoenfeld DA, Feng S, Chung RT, Tolkoff-Rubin N, Pascual M. Posttransplant diabetes mellitus in liver transplant recipients: risk factors, temporal relationship with hepatitis C virus allograft hepatitis, and impact on mortality. Transplantation 2001;72:1066–72.

89. Khalili M, Lim JW, Bass N, Ascher NL, Roberts JP, Terrault NA. New onset diabetes mellitus after liver transplantation: the critical role of hepatitis C infection. Liver Transpl 2004;10:349–55.

90. Stegall MD, Everson GT, Schroter G, Karrer F, Bilir B, Sternberg T, Shrestha R, Wachs M, Kam I. Prednisone withdrawal late after adult liver transplantation reduces diabetes, hypertension, and hypercholesterolemia without causing graft loss. Hepatology 1997;25:173–77.

91. Levy G, Villamil F, Samuel D, Sanjuan F, Grazi GL, Wu Y, Marotta P, Boillot O, Muehlbacher F, Klintmalm G. Results of lis2t, a multicenter, randomized study comparing cyclosporine microemulsion with C2 monitoring and tacrolimus with C0 monitoring in de novo liver transplantation. Transplantation 2004;77:1632–8.

92. John PR, Thuluvath PJ. Outcome of patients with new-onset diabetes mellitus after liver transplantation compared with those without diabetes mellitus. Liver Transpl 2002;8:708–13.

93. Fernandez-Miranda C, de la CA, Morales JM, Guijarro C, Aranda JL, Gomez-Sanz R, Gomez-Izquierdo T, Larumbe S, Moreno E, Rodicio JL, del PA. Lipoprotein abnormalities in long-term stable liver and renal transplanted patients. A comparative study. Clin Transplant 1998;12:136–41.

94. Dresser GK, Spence JD, Bailey DG. Pharmacokinetic-pharmacodynamic consequences and clinical relevance of cytochrome P450 3A4 inhibition. Clin Pharmacokinet 2000;38:41–57.

95. Imagawa DK, Dawson S, III, Holt CD, Kirk PS, Kaldas FM, Shackleton CR, Seu P, Rudich SM, Kinkhabwala MM, Martin P, Goldstein LI, Murray NG, Terasaki PI, Busuttil RW. Hyperlipidemia after liver transplantation: natural history and treatment with the hydroxy-methylglutaryl-coenzyme A reductase inhibitor pravastatin. Transplantation 1996;62:934–42.

96. Zachoval R, Gerbes AL, Schwandt P, Parhofer KG. Short-term effects of statin therapy in patients with hyperlipoproteinemia after liver transplantation: results of a randomized cross-over trial. J Hepatol 2001;35:86–91.

97. Duvoux C, Cherqui D, Di M, V, Metreau JM, Salvat A, Lauzet JY, Fagniez PL, Dhumeaux D. Nicardipine as antihypertensive therapy in liver transplant recipients: results of long-term use. Hepatology 1997;25:430–3.

98. Gomez R, Moreno E, Colina F, Loinaz C, Gonzalez-Pinto I, Lumbreras C, Perez-Cerda F, Castellon C, Garcia I. Steroid withdrawal is safe and beneficial in stable cyclosporine-treated liver transplant patients. J Hepatol 1998;28:150–56.

99. Kuypers DR, Neumayer HH, Fritsche L, Budde K, Rodicio JL, Vanrenterghem Y. Calcium channel blockade and preservation of renal graft function in cyclosporine-treated recipients: a prospective randomized placebo-controlled 2-year study. Transplantation 2004;78:1204–11.

100. Schlitt HJ, Barkmann A, Boker KH, Schmidt HH, Emmanouilidis N, Rosenau J, Bahr MJ, Tusch G, Manns MP, Nashan B, Klempnauer J. Replacement of calcineurin inhibitors with mycophenolate mofetil in liver-transplant patients with renal dysfunction: a randomised controlled study. Lancet 2001;357:587–91.

101. Shibolet O, Elinav E, Ilan Y, Safadi R, Ashur Y, Eid A, Zamir G, Fridlander M, Bdolah-Abram T, Shouval D, Admon D. Reduced incidence of hyperuricemia, gout, and renal failure following liver transplantation in comparison to heart transplantation: a long-term follow-up study 106. Transplantation 2004;77:1576–80.

102. Neal DA, Tom BD, Gimson AE, Gibbs P, Alexander GJ. Hyperuricemia, gout, and renal function after liver transplantation. Transplantation 2001;72:1689–91.

103. Carey EJ, Balan V, Kremers WK, Hay JE. Osteopenia and osteoporosis in patients with end-stage liver disease caused by hepatitis C and alcoholic liver disease: not just a cholestatic problem. Liver Transpl 2003;9:1166–73.

104. Trautwein C, Possienke M, Schlitt HJ, Boker KH, Horn R, Raab R, Manns MP, Brabant G. Bone density and metabolism in patients with viral hepatitis and cholestatic liver diseases before and after liver transplantation. Am J Gastroenterol 2000;95:2343–51.

105. Leslie WD, Bernstein CN, LeBoff MS. AGA technical review on osteoporosis in hepatic disorders. Gastroenterology 2003;125:941–66.

106. Josephson MA, Schumm LP, Chiu MY, Marshall C, Thistlethwaite JR, Sprague SM. Calcium and calcitriol prophylaxis attenuates posttransplant bone loss. Transplantation 2004;78:1233–6.

107. Saigal S, Norris S, Muiesan P, Rela M, Heaton N, O'Grady J. Evidence of differential risk for posttransplantation malignancy based on pretransplantation cause in patients undergoing liver transplantation. Liver Transpl 2002;8:482–7.

108. Sanchez EQ, Marubashi S, Jung G, Levy MF, Goldstein RM, Molmenti EP, Fasola CG, Gonwa TA, Jennings LW, Brooks BK, Klintmalm GB. De novo tumors after liver transplantation: a single-institution experience. Liver Transpl 2002;8:285–91.

109. Martinez JC, Otley CC, Stasko T, Euvrard S, Brown C, Schanbacher CF, Weaver AL. Defining the clinical course of metastatic skin cancer in organ transplant recipients: a multicenter collaborative study. Arch Dermatol 2003;139:301–6.

110. Haagsma EB, Hagens VE, Schaapveld M, van den Berg AP, de Vries EG, Klompmaker IJ, Slooff MJ, Jansen PL. Increased cancer risk after liver transplantation: a population-based study. J Hepatol 2001;34:84–91.

111. Stasko T, Brown MD, Carucci JA, Euvrard S, Johnson TM, Sengelmann RD, Stockfleth E, Tope WD. Guidelines for the management of squamous cell carcinoma in organ transplant recipients. Dermatol Surg 2004;30:642–50.

112. Paya CV, Fung JJ, Nalesnik MA, Kieff E, Green M, Gores G, Habermann TM, Wiesner RH, Swinnen JL, Woodle ES, Bromberg JS. Epstein-Barr virus-induced post-transplant lymphoproliferative disorders. ASTS/ASTP EBV-PTLD Task Force and The Mayo Clinic Organized International Consensus Development Meeting. Transplantation 1999;68:1517–25.

113. Manez R, Breinig MC, Linden P, Wilson J, Torre-Cisneros J, Kusne S, Dummer S, Ho M. Posttransplant lymphoproliferative disease in primary Epstein-Barr virus infection after liver transplantation: the role of cytomegalovirus disease. J Infect Dis 1997;176:1462–7.

114. Preiksaitis JK. New developments in the diagnosis and management of posttransplantation lymphoproliferative disorders in solid organ transplant recipients. Clin Infect Dis 2004;39:1016–23.

115. Herrero JI, Lucena JF, Quiroga J, Sangro B, Pardo F, Rotellar F, Alvarez-Cienfuegos J, Prieto J. Liver transplant recipients older than 60 years have lower survival and higher incidence of malignancy. Am J Transplant 2003;3:1407–12.

116. Fabia R, Levy MF, Testa G, Obiekwe S, Goldstein RM, Husberg BS, Gonwa TA, Klintmalm GB. Colon carcinoma in patients undergoing liver transplantation. Am J Surg 1998;176:265–9.

117. Forman LM, Lewis JD, Berlin JA, Feldman HI, Lucey MR. The association between hepatitis C infection and survival after orthotopic liver transplantation. Gastroenterology 2002;122:889–96.

118. Lake JR, Shorr JS, Steffen BJ, Chu AH, Gordon RD, Wiesner RH. Differential effects of donor age in liver transplant recipients infected with hepatitis B, hepatitis C and without viral hepatitis. Am J Transplant 2005;5:549–57.

119. Davis GL. The challenge of progressive hepatitis C following liver transplantation. Liver Transpl 2006;12:19–21.

120. Marzano A, Gaia S, Ghisetti V, Carenzi S, Premoli A, bernardi-Venon W, Alessandria C, Franchello A, Salizzoni M, Rizzetto M. Viral load at the time of liver transplantation and risk of hepatitis B virus recurrence. Liver Transpl 2005;11:402–9.

121. Roche B, Feray C, Gigou M, Roque-Afonso AM, Arulnaden JL, Delvart V, Dussaix E, Guettier C, Bismuth H, Samuel D. HBV DNA persistence 10 years after liver transplantation despite successful anti-HBS passive immunoprophylaxis. Hepatology 2003;38:86–95.

122. Terrault N, Roche B, Samuel D. Management of the hepatitis B virus in the liver transplantation setting: a European and an American perspective. Liver Transpl 2005;11:716–32.

123. Contos MJ, Cales W, Sterling RK, Luketic VA, Shiffman ML, Mills AS, Fisher RA, Ham J, Sanyal AJ. Development of nonalcoholic fatty liver disease after orthotopic liver transplantation for cryptogenic cirrhosis. Liver Transpl 2001;7:363–73.

124. Sanjeevi A, Lyden E, Sunderman B, Weseman R, Ashwathnarayan R, Mukherjee S. Outcomes of liver transplantation for cryptogenic cirrhosis: a single-center study of 71 patients. Transplant Proc 2003;35:2977–980.

125. Zavaglia C, De CL, Alberti AB, Minola E, Belli LS, Slim AO, Airoldi A, Giacomoni A, Rondinara G, Tinelli C, Forti D, Pinzello G. Predictors of long-term survival after liver transplantation for hepatocellular carcinoma. Am J Gastroenterol 2005;100:2708–716.

Novel Technologies in Studying Chronic Liver Diseases

Ancha Baranova, PhD,[1,2] Emanuel Petricoin III, PhD,[1,3] Lance Liotta, MD, PhD,[1,3] and Zobair M. Younossi, MD, MPH, FACG, FACP[1,4]

BACKGROUND

A "high-throughput revolution," unfolding in modern clinical science, has led to a significant increase in knowledge describing genome, transcriptome, and proteome in complex human diseases, including chronic liver diseases.

Genome-based methods of the assessment of the cellular functioning highlight the differences between individuals known as Single Nucleotide Polymorphisms (SNPs). SNPs are a DNA sequence variations of a single nucleotide – A, T, C, or G – that are commonly present in a healthy human population. For example, two sequenced DNA fragments from different individuals, AATCC-CTA and AATGCCTA, contain a difference in a single nucleotide. In this case, we usually say that there are two SNP alleles: C and G. SNPs may fall within coding sequences of genes or their noncoding, regulatory regions. SNPs that are not in protein coding regions may still have consequences for the alternative splicing of the mRNA, for the transcription factor binding to the promoter, or to the annealing of the gene-regulating noncoding RNA. Often, noncoding SNPs lead to the alterations in the cellular levels of the mRNA encoded for the particular protein, and, consequently, to the changes in the protein concentrations. As the concentrations of the proteins differ between individuals, humans differ in their degree of predisposition to various chronic diseases, including chronic liver diseases (CLD).

Transcriptomics and proteomics methods of cellular function assessment aim at the collection of the molecular "snapshots" reflecting relative levels of the mRNAs (transcriptome) or proteins (proteome) in the particular human tissues. Normal tissue profiles are most often compared to ones corresponding to that of the tissues affected by pathological changes. The statistically significant differences in the concentrations of certain proteins or mRNAs may accompany the progression of the disease ("bystander changes") or even point to its origin ("causal changes"). In both cases, identification of significant molecular changes is helping to advance clinical management of the disease: "causal changes" highlight the novel therapeutic targets suitable for correction, while "bystander changes" may be used as surrogate markers allowing prediction of the disease outcomes.

An important milestone in any project approaching complex liver pathology by high-throughput techniques is the development of a database integrating transcriptome and/or proteome profiles with clinical parameters and outcomes. Proper integration of the clinical, genomic, and proteomic platforms produces terabyte levels of data, making fast query response times a challenge.[1,2] Hopefully, recent advances in biomedical informatics will improve the ability of researchers to examine possible links between cellular circuits (gene expression and proteomics data) and phenotypes (clinical and outcomes data).

Despite obvious difficulties with data analysis, high-throughput functional assessment of the hepatic function in the patients with various CLDs already prompted significant advancements in understanding of the CLD etiology and the improvements of the patients' care. Ultimately, the decrease in the cost of the application of such methods and their introduction into the clinic's routine will bring the era of the individualized medicine, when the patient's treatment will be tailored to the particular characteristic changes in the cellular genome, transcriptome, proteome, and metabolome observed in the every diseased liver.

POLYMORPHISMS OF THE HUMAN GENOME INFLUENCE LIVER FUNCTION AND OUTCOMES OF CHRONIC LIVER DISEASE

One clear outcome of the international efforts on human genome sequencing and genotyping is the clear understanding that the common polymorphisms present in the human DNA indeed influence the incidence, the phenotypes, and the outcomes of the complex human diseases. An illustrative example of this kind is the viral hepatitis caused by HBV or HCV viruses. Genetic predisposition studies have examined five aspects of the viral hepatitis: (1) susceptibility to viral infection; (2) viral persistence and clearance; (3) response to the therapy; (4) evolution to cirrhosis and fibrosis; (5) rate of the conversion to the liver malignancy.

Most of the hepatitis C-related human polymorphisms described to date are located in the coding or regulatory areas of the genes involved in the host cytokine system and immune response. Patients with hepatitis C have elevated serum levels of Tumor Necrosis Factor (TNF)-α and TNF-β, encoded by genes TNF and LTA, respectively.[3] Both cytokines are potent multifunctional immune modulators that play a critical role in the control of viral infection by recruiting and activating macrophages, NK cells, and T-cells and by regulating the processing of the antigens, their transport, and the expression of the Major Histocompatibility Complex (MHC) molecules. The functional efficacy of TNF-mediated cell death may influence the course and the outcomes of the chronic HCV infection. A number of studies demonstrated the linkage between TNFβ intron 1 AA genotype, the susceptibility to hepatitis C and the severity of the disease[4] as well as between TNF-α GG genotypes at positions −308 and −238, lower pretreatment viral RNA levels and higher mean fibrosis scores.[5] Additional, ethnically stratified studies revealed that in the black subjects the common wild-type haplotype −863C/−308G is associated with viral persistence (odds ratios (OR) 1.91, 95% confidence interval (CI) 1.24–2.95), while the presence of the allele − 863A, characterized by reduced promoter activity, is linked to the viral clearance (OR 0.52, 95% CI 0.29–0.93).[6] Among other genetic polymorphisms associated with persistent hepatitis C viremia are these located in IL4, IL8RB, IL10RA, PRL, ADA, NFKB1, GRAP2, CABIN1, IFNAR2, IFI27, IFI41, TNFRSF1A, ALDOB, AP1B1, SULT2B1, EGF, EGFR, TGFB1, LTBP2, and CD4 genes.[7]

Often, a particular polymorphism or a combination of the polymorphisms used to predict treatment response or the disease outcome. For example, combined genotyping of 26 SNPs in the set of seven human genes (ADAR, CASP5, FGF1, ICSBP1, IFI44, TAP2, and TGFBRAP1) predicts responsiveness to a combination of interferon (IFN)-α and ribavirin with sensitivity of 62.8% and specificity of 67.2%.[8] When the viral genotype information was added to the model, the performance of the test improved to 80.7% sensitivity and 67.2% specificity.[8] The proposed model might be advanced further by taking into consideration additional SNP markers characterized in other studies. Among potential candidates are polymorphisms located at the positions −443 and −1748 in the osteopontin (OPN) gene[9], at the −88 position in the myxovirus resistance protein 1 encoding gene (MxA)[10], in the 3' UTR of the low-density lipoprotein receptor (LDLR) gene[11], and in the promoter of the Interleukin-10 encoding (IL10) gene.[12] In order to create highly specific and sensitive multiplexed assay, these and other polymorphisms need to be assessed in large, demographically stratified populations of the patients infected with hepatitis C. In the future, genotype based assays might become a part of the pretreatment evaluation in order to maximize the efficacy.

Other polymorphisms may influence fibrosis progression in chronic hepatitis C. For example, carriers of the homozygous genotype 2/2 defined as a certain number of the GT repeat units in the promoter of the solute carrier family 11 member 1 (SLC11A1) exerts a protective effect against cirrhosis development, while the combination of TNF − 238A/G and the presence of allele 3 is conducive to progression to pre-cirrhotic or cirrhotic stages of the disease.[13] Another study demonstrated that hepatitis C patients carrying missense SNP in the DEAD box polypeptide 5 (DDX5) gene are at an increased risk of developing advanced fibrosis, whereas those with a missense SNP in the carnitine palmitoyltransferase 1A (CPT1A) gene are at a decreased risk.[14] Other studies pointed toward an importance of the minor variants of the LDLR[11], interleukin 12B (IL12B)[15], tumor growth factor TGF-β1[16], and cytochrome CYP2D6.[17] The presence of the -670G allele in the promoter region of the FAS gene is shown to be associated with necrosis in periportal areas[18], while the presence of the UDP-glucuronosyltransferase (UGT) low-activity genotypes[19], −308A TNF-α promoter allele[20], and CYP2D6 fast metabolizer genotypes[21] were more common in the patients with hepatitis C-related hepatocellular carcinoma (HCC). One may envision the compilation of all these genotyping efforts in a single multiplexed assay allowing the prediction of the long-term outcomes of the hepatitis C infection. Studies with similar design were performed in the cohorts of patients infected with hepatitis B.[22]

The studies describing the inherited predispositions to noninfectious liver diseases are less common. A number of the polymorphic alleles were found to be associated with various manifestations of the alcoholic liver disease, including the presence of the ADH1B∗2 allele[23], the −159T allele in the promoter region of the CD14 gene[24] and the −238A allele in the TNF-α encoding gene.[25] In case of the nonalcoholic steatohepatitis (NASH) positive associations were revealed for the −493G allele in the microsomal triglyceride transfer protein (MTP) promoter that leads to decreased MTP transcription, less export of triglyceride from hepatocytes, and greater intracellular triglyceride accumulation and the 1183T allele in MnSOD mitochondrial targeting sequence responsible for the diminished transport of MnSOD to the mitochondria.[26] Another important finding describes the association of the amino-terminal polymorphisms in codon 27 of the beta2-adrenergic receptor gene with hypertryglyceridemia and the development of NASH.[27] In addition to that, a functional polymorphism in cytrochrome CYP17 encoding gene that is associated with circulating estrogen is a risk factor for the tamoxifen-induced hepatic steatosis in breast cancer patients.[28]

A number of studies reviewed an influence of various SNPs on the pharmacokinetics of the common therapeutics modulating liver physiology, for example, lipid-lowering agents. The main target organ of statins, the liver, is also the major site of cholesterol synthesis. Pravastatin, a hydrophilic HMG-CoA reductase inhibitor, is taken up efficiently from the circulation into the liver by organic anion-transporting polypeptide 1B1 (OATP1B1) that is expressed on the baso-lateral membrane in the hepatocytes. Recently, the SLCO1B1∗17 allele containing −11187 G>A, 388 A>G and 521T>C nucleotide changes was associated with the decreased acute effect of pravastatin on cholesterol synthesis.[29] Later, heterozygous carriers of the SLCO1B1∗15 allele (a combination of 388 A>G and 521 T>C substitutions) have been demonstrated to have lower response than non-carriers (percent of the low-density lipoprotein cholesterol (LDL-C) reduction: −14.1 vs. −28.9%); however, the genotype-dependent difference in the cholesterol-lowering effect disappeared after 1 year of treatment.[30] In addition, combined genotyping of CYP7A1 -204 A>C and APOE e4 variants were shown to be instrumental for predicting the long-term clinical outcomes of pravastatin.[30]

Another important direction of the SNP association studies is the prediction and the minimization of the adverse side effects. Genotype-based prescribing may lead to improvement of the overall efficacy rates and a decrease in the secondary complications of the therapy, heralding a new era of the individualized medicine. Major hepatic events are the most common reason for the withdrawal of the drug from the market accounting for 26–37% of recent safety related drug withdrawals.[31] During the three years to 2005, at least seven other drugs attracted hepatotoxicity warnings reflected at the labels (leflunomide, nevirapine, nefadozone, rituximab, interferon-β1b, duloxetine, atomoxetine).[31] High prevalence of the hepatotoxic effects is not surprising as hepatocytes serving as primary points of the drug absorption and activation are constantly exposed to the drug and to its metabolite (s). The rate of the metabolite formation is mostly defined by hepatic cytochromes, glutathione–S transferases, N-acetyltransferases, and other activating/deactivating enzymes. In human genome, the genes encoding drug-metabolizing enzymes are highly polymorphic and produce phenotypes characterized by extensive metabolism (EM) or poor metabolism (PM) of certain drug. In the circulation and the tissues of the EM and PM patients half-lives of the drug may differ up to 5–7 times, leading to necessity of the dose adjustments. Lack of pre-treatment genotyping produces overtreatment of the predisposed group of the patients increasing their chances to develop adverse effects. When genotyping techniques will become a routine of the lab diagnostics, precise adjustments of the therapy to the individual' metabolizing capacity will dramatically decrease a number of major hepatotoxic events and remove some "external xenobiotic pressure" clearly contributing to CLD development and progression. All together, these effects will lead to the decrease of the non-infectious CLD cases and longer event-free periods in already monitored patients. The recent clinical introduction of AmpliChip allowing simultaneous pre-treatment testing for 29 CYP2D6 and 2 CYP32D19 mutations was welcomed as a start in the described direction.[31,32]

Another interesting approach to the problem of the hepatotoxicity of common drugs is "pharmaco-metabonomic approach" based on a combination of pre-treatment metabolite profiling and chemometrics taking into account both genotypic and environmental components rather than on straightforward genome assessment. The "proof-of principle" study of this kind has been recently completed on the model of liver damage resulted from paracetamol (acetaminophen) administration to rats.[33]

TRANSCRIPTOME PROFILING IN PATIENTS WITH CHRONIC LIVER DISEASE

Most of the quantitative molecular data collected so far are related to the states of the cellular transcriptomes representing a variety of the mRNAs produced on the templates of the human genes expressed in the particular tissue. Transcriptomics aims at the simultaneous detection of the relative expression levels of large numbers of genes and gene fragments in given tissue. Among the common methods of study of the cellular transcriptomes are expression microarrays[33-35] and SAGE.[37-41] Microarray platforms colud be based on short (25–30mer) oligonucleotides (e.g., Affymetrix GeneChip and NimbleGen) or long (60–70mer) oligonucleotides and cDNAs. Individual arrays can be commercially pre-printed en masse, or custom-designed to answer particular scientific or clinical questions. SAGE techniques involve quantification of the gene-specific sequences 9–13 nt in length known as SAGE tags. SAGE method allows physical ligation of these tags for simultaneous automated sequencing, facilitating quantification of the SAGE results. This technique does not allow pre-fabrication, and, therefore, limited to the specialized labs. Each variety of the transcriptome profiling technique has its own advantages and disadvantages, and the diversity of protocols interferes with cross-platform reproducibility. Analysis of the data obtained in the high-throughput expression profiling experiments is always a challenge due to necessity of unification of the sample processing, the strict quality control procedures, and careful choice of the statistical tests. One current challenge of microarray studies in human tissue is to develop databases that integrate clinical and molecular data, allowing researchers to examine potential links between patient genotypes (gene expression data) and phenotypes (clinical parameters and outcomes). A second challenge is the development of the universal approach to the sample processing and data analysis allowing independent validation of the obtained results.

Typically, transcriptomics based methods identify mRNA molecules differentially expressed in the diseased tissue samples in comparison to the normal (control) samples. Before profiling, mRNAs are extracted from surgical excision specimens, characterized by heterogeneous cellular composition. For example, typical liver biopsy specimen, in addition to hepatocytes, includes sinusoidal endothelial cells, stellate cells, red blood cells, microvasculature, cholangiocytes, and intrahepatic lymphocytes. Due to its complexity, liver is second only to brain in transcriptome size, with 25–40% of human genes expressed in the hepatic milieu[42,43] The exact percentage of the desired cellular component may change depending on physiological factors such as inflammation. Invention of laser capture microdissection (LCM)[44,45] greatly improved scientific and clinical value of the expression profiling in complex diseases.

To distinguish disease-specific changes in transcriptome or from changes related to the disturbance in tissue composition, standard expression signatures of specific cell types must be identified. Such signatures can be obtained by profiling cultured cell lines. However, the process of cell culturing itself can lead to perturbation of expression signatures. For example, when the gene expression profile of HepG2 cells was compared to that of primary hepatocytes, it has been found that 31% of the HepG2 transcriptome was unique to the cell line.[46] A number of genes were found to be expressed in primary liver cells only, and apparently silenced during culture.[46]

One approach to resolve this problem is assessment of gene expression patterns in "healthy tissue." However, given the logistic and ethical issues involved in obtaining "healthy tissue," these studies are quite limited. Authors aware of a handful of high-throughput attempts to assess individual variability of gene expression in non-diseased human livers. A profiling of four surgically excised liver specimens revealed that 1212 of 2418 (50%) of the profiled genes were similarly expressed.[36] Another study used the novel AFLP-based (Amplified Fragment Length Polymorphism) method of transcript imaging called GeneTag. In four adult human liver samples studied, between 2.6% and 4.6% of the analyzed transcripts showed more than 2.5-fold changes in expression level for at least one sample compared to all others. Some transcripts could be found in one specimen while entirely absent in another.[47] Study of Harris et al. revealed similar picture when individual specimens taken from three male donors were compared.[46] Recent studies suggest gender-specific gene expression differences in nonreproductive organs.[48] A study of Delongchamp et al. demonstrated gender-specific differences for 8% of the genes expressed in 18 human livers.[49] On the other hand, registered differences were relatively small, less than two-fold.[49] As some of the samples were taken from individuals known to have died in a hospital where they were administered drugs in a failed attempt to stabilize their condition, relevance of these findings to the normal physiology of the liver remains unknown.

Unresolved problems with interindividual variability difficulties are further exacerbated by "location-specific variations" in patterns of gene expressions. For example, whole genome expression profiling in left and right liver lobes of the mid-gestational baboon fetuses revealed 875 differentially expressed genes that belong to multiple molecular pathways.[50] Authors explained these observations by differences in the vascular supply of two lobes in developing embryo.[50] It has been suggested earlier that these differences may result in long-term programming of hepatic function following *in utero* challenges.[51,52] According to these findings, human liver could not be considered as homogeneous organ; therefore the choice of the site for the liver biopsy could influence the study results.

A majority of the high-throughput attempts of the transcriptome profiling in CLD were aimed at characterization of the hepatic responses to the infection with HCV or HBV. For example, recent study of Walters et al. concentrated at the comparisons of the hepatic gene expression in HCV-infected individuals with and without HIV co-infection.[53] The intrahepatic global gene expression profiles of these patients were similar to each other. Interestingly, authors identified a subset of patients who shared specific pattern of gene expression comprised of increased levels of the lymphocytic adhesion molecules, impaired FAS apoptosis pathway, and lack of IFN-γ induction. This pattern was similar to that of the patients who developed fibrosis within one year of receiving a liver transplant.[53] Described data further strengthened a hypothesis implying diagnostic utility of the potentially predictive fibrosis signature previously found in patients infected with HCV only.[54–56] Another study of HCV infected patients revealed three distinct hierarchical gene expression clusters associated with early, mid-stage, and advanced fibrosis, respectively. At the fibrosis stage 0 deregulated genes mostly found among these involved in glycolipid metabolism, 1 and 2 stages of the fibrotic process were associated with changes in the levels of genes related to oxidative stress, apoptosis, inflammation, proliferation and matrix degradation, whereas transcripts increased in stages 3 and 4 were associated mostly with brogenesis per se and cellular proliferation, consistent with a predisposition to cancer.[57]

A number of observations point that specific gene-expression signatures in non-cancerous or liver tissue may help accurately predict the risk for developing hepatocellular carcinoma (HCC). One of the diagnostic systems relies on the quantification of mRNAs for 36 genes commonly associated with both primary multicentric HCC and multicentric recurrence.[58] Another study showed that a gene expression profile comprising 14 genes discriminative for vascular invasion can predict the recurrence of HCC after liver resection.[59] Transcriptome assessments are also instrumental for preoperative staging of HCC allowing optimization of the use of the scarce liver transplant resources.[60] One of the newest approaches to the transcriptome profiling of the HCC concentrates on the quantitative evaluation of the miRNAs – a non-coding family of genes involved in post-transcriptional gene regulation and associated with cell proliferation, differentiation, and death.[61] Similarly to hepatic cancers developed because of HCV infection, HBV derived HCCs were also profiled in a number of studies.[62] Interestingly, high-throughput methods of the transcription profiling fail to distinguish HCC samples derived from HCV and HBV infected cells, while easy discriminating samples representing various nonmalignant CLDs.[61]

Studies of liver transcriptome performed at the tissue samples of CLD patients support widely accepted assumption that that various types of liver diseases often serve as confounding factor for each other. Indeed, most CLDs, including NASH, viral hepatitis, and even hepatocellular carcinomas (HCCs) share common features including inflammation, lymphocytic infiltration, hepatocytes necrosis, fibrosis, and cirrhosis. In accordance with this statement, one of the high-throughput studies of CLDs uncovered that end-stage liver cirrhosis of various etiologies possesses HCC-like changes in gene expression.[63] It has been suggested that CLDs may be able to "precondition" hepatic tissue for malignization.

On the other hand, transcriptome analysis allows classification of similar CLDs with different etiologies. For example, profiling of liver biopsies from patients with cirrhosis caused by either chronic alcohol consumption or HCV revealed that latter type of cirrhosis is characterized by uniform expression independent of Child-Turcotte-Pugh (CTP) stage and induction of the innate antiviral immune response.[64] In case of the alcohol-related cirrhosis differential expression signature was revealed for less severe CTP class A cirrhosis.[64] A majority of the classifying genes were involved in the modification of lipids and the response to oxidative stress. Sreekumar et al. examined gene expression levels in three distinct groups of cirrhotic patients: NASH with cirrhosis (n = 6), HCV-related cirrhosis (n = 6), cirrhosis-related to primary biliary cirrhosis (n = 6)[56]), and a group of healthy controls (n = 6).[65] Sixteen genes were differentially expressed in patients with cirrhotic-stage NASH when compared to all other groups. Authors observed the suppression of the genes important for maintaining mitochondrial function, including copper/zinc superoxide dismutase SOD1, aldehyde oxidase, and catalase. Genes involved in fatty acid and glucose metabolisms were also repressed in the NASH patients.[65]

Younossi et al. performed a high-throughput study of gene expression in NASH using a cDNA array of 5220 genes. A total of 29 NASH patients, 7 obese non-NAFLD patients, and 6 non-obese control samples[66] were analyzed. To exclude genes specifically related to obesity rather than NASH, an additional comparison was made between the obese patients without NAFLD and the lean control subjects. Nineteen out of 34 genes differentially expressed in NASH remained significantly deregulated after excluding confounding factors, including genes related to lipid metabolism and extracellular matrix remodeling. This analysis also highlighted deregulation of the triglyceride formation in the liver and the ketogenesis pathway in NASH patients. Downregulation of IGFBP1 was found to be a hallmark of steatosis, but not typical for a fully developed NASH. Among NASH specific findings a decrease in expression of FGL1, involved in liver regeneration, and adrenomedullin, which protects the liver against organ damage via oxidative stress, were registered. Activities of oxidative stress related genes CAT and glutathione S-transferase A4 (GSTA4) genes were prominent in both NASH and non-NAFLD livers of obese controls, but not in the livers of the nonobese controls. This finding suggests that the altered expression of stress related genes in NASH may be a reflection of increase in ROS production that usually accompanies obesity. Similarly, a group of anti-inflammatory genes found to be under-expressed in the obese subjects.[66]

Most recent high-throughput study of the steatohepatitis concentrated on steatosis.[67] Nine normal and nine steatotic livers without microscopic signs of inflammation or fibrosis were profiled by Affymetrix HG-U133A arrays containing 22 283 sequences. A total of 34 additional human samples including normal, HCV-related steatosis or steatohepatitis associated with alcohol consumption or obesity were used as controls. Among 110 genes differentially expressed in non-alcoholic steatosis a large group encoded proteins involved in the mitochondrial respiratory chain or capable to interfere with mitochondrial metabolism.[67] In steatohepatitis, an increase of the gene and protein expression of mitochondrial antigens, interleukin 1 receptor (IL-1R1), insulin growth factor (IGF2), and tumor growth factor-β (TGFB1) was also observed, with IL-1R1 being always strongly expressed in steatohepatitis linked to alcohol or obesity.[67] Authors concluded that activation of inflammatory pathways is present at a very early stage of steatosis, even if no morphological sign of inflammation is observed.[67]

PROTEOME PROFILING IN PATIENTS WITH CHRONIC LIVER DISEASE

The ability to translate information about differentially expressed mRNAs as molecular markers for CLDs to quantitative PCR is certainly an attraction to the use of that technology for biomarker discovery. Despite the low cost of PCR diagnostics, the reliability of this method in clinical settings awaits major improvement. One major impediment to routine use of this approach is the necessity of clean-room procedures adding significant cost to the test. Conversely, protein-based tests, such as widely used immunochemical methods, are the preferred measurement method in the clinic as immunoassay measurements underpin most routinely ordered clinical tests. Moreover, differential mRNA expression registered in the liver biopsy sample does not guarantee that the corresponding protein product could be useful as serum marker. Therefore, the further development of protein-based diagnostics is warranted. Unfortunately, expression patterns of mRNAs detected by both expression microarrays and SAGE method does not necessarily reflect corresponding changes in their cognate proteins. Simultaneous gene expression and proteomics studies performed in both cell lines[68] and primary tissue samples[69] revealed that the differential expression of mRNA (up or down) can capture no more than 40% of the variation of protein expression, with most of the concordance being found in highly abundant structural proteins.

Taking into account issues discussed above, some recent studies of chronic liver pathologies concentrate on the direct high-throughput profiling of tissue proteomes. The least technologically demanding method of this kind is two-dimensional polyacrylamide gel electrophoresis (2D-PAGE). 2D-PAGE gels separated proteins based on the charge of the protein (pI) and its molecular weights.[70] As these two protein characteristics are not related to each other, protein molecules migrate across the gel and form a recognizable "spotty" pattern that could be detected by a staining with Coomassie blue, silver staining, or with fluorescent dyes.[71] Differentially expressed proteins spots could be excised, subjected to proteolytic or chemical digestion, and analyzed by mass-spectrometry (MS). 2D-PAGE proteomics profiling is convincingly simple, but laborious and requires a large amount of sample material. Moreover, it loses resolution when proteins with low and high molecular weight, hydrophobicity, and isoelectric points are compared.[72]

Some proteins do not resolve well in 2D-PAGE due to their physico-chemical properties. The only way to identify them is a proteolytic digestion into comprising peptides. The resulting fragments peptides are resolved by two-dimensional capillary liquid chromatography (LC-LC) following by subsequent database searching with algorithms such as SEQUEST.[73] Both 2D-PAGE and LC-LC are used in conjunction with a variety of MS methods.

In the past decade, mass spectrometry (MS) has become one of the most important tools for biomarker discovery in complex diseases. MS-based methods of peptide fragment separations include matrix-assisted laser desorption ionization (MALDI), surface-enhanced laser desorption/ionization (SELDI), quadruple ion-trap-MS (e.g., LCQ-MS), and Fourier transform ion cyclotron resonance (FTICR)-MS.[74] Although MALDI mass spectrometer is a powerful tool for the accurate mass determination of peptide mixtures, the quality of MALDI data depends on the choice of suitable solvents and the method of sample preparation.[74]SELDI spectrometers analyze protein mixtures subsets that selectively bind to a chemically modified surface such that retantate chromatography is achieved (e.g., cation exchange) prior to MS.[75] A major advantage of SELDI is the small sample requirements (typically 1–2 microliter per analysis), which is ideal for core needle liver biopsy that could be studied in a high-throughput settings.[76] SELDI does not allow direct identification of resolved proteins, but generates peak profiles that could be either used as diagnostic inputs themselves or subjected to protein extraction with subsequent identification. "Classical" SELDI-TOF is unable to separate ions that are close in mass/charge, resulting in the peak coalescence. An enhancement of SELDI technology is achieved by its interfacing it with quadruple QqTOF mass spectrometer, instead of simple TOF.[77] Recently developed Fourier transform ion cyclotron resonance (FTICR) MS allows very high-accuracy measurements suitable for direct protein identification.[78]

Focused proteomics studies involve protein arrays of immobilized proteins, which are typically antibodies. These arrays are incubated with the test samples that may contain various analytes.[79] A major limiting factor in a focused proteomic approach of this type is the unavailability of specific and high-affinity antibodies for a range of interesting targets.[79–80] The affinity behavior of immobilized antibodies is much less predictable than DNA hybridization, so multiple probes needs to be pre-tested in order to find the most reliable preparation allowing high-fidelity quantification. PCR-like amplification methods are unavailable for proteins, so low abundance molecules may not be detected. Pre-fractionation of the proteins[80], use of nanoparticles[81] and an extraction of the potential biomarkers from the circulating high molecular mass carrier proteins[82] have been suggested to solve this problem. Another interesting high-throughput method of the complex sample evaluation is reverse phase protein arrays (RPPA). RPPAs represent nanogram to attogram amounts of lysates derived from patients' tissue queried with a single antibody. This technique allows one to achieve a multiplex measurement of hundreds of proteins simultaneously and to profile the state of multiple signaling pathway targets.[83]

Recently, international efforts aimed at the characterization of the human liver proteome were taken into coordination by HLPP (The Human Liver Proteome Project) that was launched in October 2002. The scientific objectives of this initiative are the identification, characterization, and integration of the human liver proteome: expression profiles, modification profiles, protein-protein interaction maps, proteome localization maps, and definition of an ORFeome, physiome, and pathome of the liver.[84] Current outputs of HLPP include the identification of 2053 proteins and 15426 mRNA transcripts produced in the healthy liver. HLPP liver diseases subproject initiated in June 2005 concentrates on hepatocellular carcinoma and associated chronic conditions such as chronic hepatitis, fibrosis, and cirrhosis.[84] One of the HLPP coordinated attempt of the comparative landscaping of the liver proteome involved multidimensional protein identification technology (MudPIT)[85] that relies on gel-free fractionation procedures performed prior to MS.[86] In the cited study, normal human liver samples were compared to samples from the brain, heart, lung, muscle, pancreas, spleen, and testes tissues resulting in 1,713 high confidence protein identifications.[85] One of the major finding of the study is that protein profile of human liver most closely resembles that of pancreas ($P < 0.01$) and testes ($P < 0.001$).[85] The largest numbers of tissue-specific mRNAs and proteins appears to be expressed exclusively in liver. Interestingly, a number of proteins and their corresponding mRNAs found to be discordant in their relative levels exclusively in the liver.[85] This finding points to existence of liver-specific post-translational control processes.

Similarly to liver mRNAs, the expression levels of liver proteins fluctuate inter-individually. The range of fluctuations is less pronounced than in case of mRNAs: the mean CV values (SD/mean $\times$ 100) of standardized abundance for the protein spots revealed by 2D electrophoresis in healthy state is 19%.[87] A number of proteins is fluctuating among normal individuals at larger scale, with CVs over 50%, namely, translationally controlled tumor protein (TCPC), haptoglobin precursor (HAP), superoxide dismutase (SOD), peroxiredoxin 6 (PRDX6), 10-for-myltetrahydrofolate dehydrogenase, apolipoprotein C1, tetrahydrofolatesynthase, and 4-aminobutyrate aminotransferase.[87] Use of these proteins as CLD markers might lead to unreliable conclusions. The remedy for the problem of interindividual variability is the pooling of studied samples, with no less than eight samples in each pool.[87]

All modifications of the described technology are expensive and labor intensive. That is why the attempts of its application to CLDs are still limited. Gallagher and co-authors used classical proteomics methods to perform "focused" study of three human hepatic mitochondrial alpha class GST isoforms.[88] High-resolution HPLC with subsequent electrospray ionization-mass spectrometry (ESI/MS) and octagonal matrix-assisted laser description/ionization time of flight mass spectrometry (oMALDI-TOF MS) was employed for identification of particular GST subunits in the mitochondrial fraction of the liver cells.[88] Three distinct HPLC peaks revealed by chromatograms were identified as the products of GSTP1, GSTA1, and GSTA2 genes.[88] The mitochondrial targeting of these GSTs is suggestive of a role in the metabolism of lipid peroxidation products serving as a major source of oxidative damage involved in the pathogenesis of NAFLD.

Another focused study concentrated on human liver cytochromes P450 and their redox partners (NADPH-cytochrome P450 reductase and cytochrome b5) by using the biochemical analysis of microsomes in a combination with scanning of images obtained after protein separation in gels followed by mass spectrometric protein identification.[89] This study compared preparations of normal human liver with seemingly normal liver tissue surrounding colon carcinoma metastasis. Eleven distinct enzymes including nine cytochromes P450 were identified from the liver samples in control and 13 enzymes including 10 cytochromes P450 from the liver samples in pathology. Eight cytochromes P450 – CYPs 2A6, 2C8,

2C9, 2C10, 2D6, 2E1, 3A4, and 4F2 – were found in all cases. The microsomal CYP enzymes 1B1 and 4A11 were not seen in controls as opposed to pathology; however, the control experiments revealed the presence of cytochrome 1A2.[89]

To date, focused proteomics-based assays provided a number of valuable diagnostic markers related to HCC, including members of the aldoketoreductase (AKR) family, tissue ferritin light chain, and aldehyde dehydrogenase.[90–92] All of these markers were identified by 2D-PAGE, the oldest and most widely used technology for global proteome analysis. Other CLDs that underwent detailed characterization by 2D-PAGE with subsequent MS identifications of the excised spots include HCV and HBV-induced chronic hepatites[93], HCC[93–95], and primary hepatolithiasis.[96] Newer technologies representing "true" high-throughput methods, e.g., SELDI-TOF, easily demonstrate "proof-of-principle" but produce results that are challenging for interpretation. For example, a recent study attempting profiling of the polyclonal regenerative and monoclonal neoplastic cirrhotic nodules with SELDI-TOF technology on Q10 Cypergen Protein Chips revealed three protein peaks overexpressed in monoclonal versus polyclonal nodules.[97] M/z ratios of these peaks were measured as 10,092, 54,025, and 62,133 Da, but identities of the corresponding proteins remain to be determined.[97]

Most SELDI-based experiments aimed at the discovery of the molecular markers of CLDs are performed on serum samples rather than on microdissected liver cells. Serum profiling is more attractive for researchers as its successful implementation may yield the molecular markers suitable for noninvasive diagnostics. It is important that the collected proteome profiles of the serum possess independent diagnostic value, even when corresponding proteins remain unidentified. For example, in the one of the latest studies SELDI-TOF profiling of serum proteome of the patients with HCV infection was able to distinguish HCC from pre-cirrhotic liver disease and advanced cirrhosis.[98] Another study of the HCC proteome allowed the development of the six-peaks algorithm correctly classifying patients' samples according to the presence or absence of HCC with 92% of accuracy.[99] The highest discriminating peak (8,900 Da) was purified further and was characterized as the C-terminal part of the V10 fragment of vitronectin resulted from the cleavage with metalloproteinase MMP-2.[99] Interestingly, tumor-specific changes in SELDI-based protein profiles do not revert to normal after cytoreduction therapy. This conclusion has been made in the study of the serial serum samples from 37 hepatitis C patients before development of HCC, with HCC and following radiotherapy.[100] It is possible, that the characteristic SELDI profile is not linearly related to tumor burden but reflect the progression of underlying liver disease or the emergence of precancerous lesions. Cited study identified b2-microglobulin as the most significant proteomic feature associated with HCC.[100]

An interesting application of proteome analysis to HCC is the detection of autoantibodies that also could serve as diagnostic markers for HCC. In this case 2D-PAGE assays are paired with SEREX (serologic analysis of recombinant cDNA expression libraries) technique. After analysis of the corresponding immunoreactive proteins by LC-MS/MS, heat shock 70kDa protein 1 (HSP70), peroxiredoxin, and manganese superoxide dismutase (Mn-SOD) were identified and corresponding autoantibodies were confirmed as novel HCC biomarkers.[101]

Despite obvious necessity of the developments of noninvasive methods for the detection of nonmalignant CLDs, serum proteome studies of these conditions are less common. One of such studies concentrated on nonalcoholic fatty liver disease (NAFLD). SELDI-TOF proteome profilings have been performed in liver biopsy specimens from 98 bariatric surgery patients.[102] Among these samples, seven were classified as having normal histology, 12 were characterized by steatosis alone, 52 had steatosis with the presence of nonspecific inflammation and 27 had fully developed NASH. Each group of NAFLD patients was compared with the obese controls. A total of 12 protein peaks showed significant changes in expression when sera from three NAFLD groups were compared with the obese controls separately. One of the peaks, with a mass-to-charge ratio between 64,907 Da and 65,042 Da was increased in the steatosis with nonspecific inflammation group, and in the NASH cohort, but not in patients with steatosis alone. Another peak corresponding to protein with 10,048–10,073 Da in mass-to-charge ratio was most prominent in steatosis patients, with a relatively moderate increase in NASH patients and no significant changes in patients with steatosis and nonspecific inflammation.[102] When serum protein masses were matched with the masses of 1,440 previously identified serum proteins[103] one of the collected steatosis-specific peaks with a mass between 48,460 and 48,601 Da was provisionally identified as fibrinogen-gamma.

Another study of the NAFLD spectrum diseases has been performed on the omental adipose tissue, a biologically active organ secreting adipokines and cytokines that may play a role in the development of liver steatosis. In this case researchers primarily sought to test the hypothesis that insights into liver pathogenesis could be obtained from adipose tissue from the affected patient, and that the adipose tissue may be an active participant in the liver disease process. In this study, the investigators employed reverse phase protein microarrays (RPA) for multiplexed cell signaling analysis of 54 different kinase substrates and cell signaling endpoints.[104] Surprisingly, the components of insulin receptor-mediated signaling pathway were able to differentiate most of the conditions on the NAFLD spectrum. For example, PKA and AKT/mTOR pathway derangement accurately discriminates patients with NASH from the non-progressive forms of NAFLD, while PKCδ, AKT, and SHC phosphorylation changes occurred only in patients with simple steatosis. Amounts of the FKHR phosphorylated at S256 residue were significantly correlated with AST/ALT ratio in all morbidly obese patients.[104] Furthermore, amounts of cleaved caspase 9 and pp90RSK S380 were positively correlated in patients with NASH. These findings provided direct evidences for the role of omental fat in the pathogenesis, and potentially, the progression of NAFLD.[104]

Another knowledge-oriented facet of the CLD proteomics is the study of the serum subproteomes associated with various protein carriers, especially carriers implicated in the CLD development themselves. For example, 2D-PAGE analysis of the proteins associated with adiponectin, potent anti-inflammatory and anti-diabetic molecule produced in adipose, revealed co-transport and co-distribution of thrombospondin-1, histidine-rich glycoprotein HGRP, kininogen 1, fibronectin, and α2-macroglobulin also involved in CLD-related processes.[105] Further studies are needed to validate the specificities of these interactions and CLD related changes in the composition of theadiponectin-containing protein complexes.

SUMMARY

The recent completion of the human genome and the development of proteomic tools that reach beyond the genome have revolutionized our approach to translational research and scientific discovery. Multiplexing of the genomics, transcriptomics, and proteomics assays is approaching near global scale and provides for detailed dissections of the molecular cascades involved in the development of the chronic liver diseases on a systems level. As a consequence, a growing number of novel molecular markers have been discovered, including these present in the serum, and allowing noninvasive diagnostics of the chronic conditions. Development of the genotyping techniques and proteomic analysis of the drug targets themselves is generating enormous opportunity for individualized medicine, whose promise is the effective stratification of therapy to those most likely to respond and the minimization of the adverse side effects. However, despite the seeming accessibility of these promising techniques, a cautionary approach is necessary in the interpretation of the data. There are universal caveats that preclude meta-analysis of the data collected. Major obstacles still exist in the areas of tissue collection, processing and handling, in the heterogeneity of the samples (and the pathology itself) and the lack of correlation between mRNA and protein levels. Nevertheless, significant progress is being made in the understanding of CLDs much of it due to data accumulated in these high-throughput genomic and preoteomic projects.

REFERENCES

1. Hu H, Brzeski H, Hutchins J, Ramaraj M, Qu L, Xiong R, et al. Biomedical informatics: development of a comprehensive data warehouse for clinical and genomic breast cancer research. Pharmacogenomics 2004; 5(7): 933–41.

2. Berman JJ. Nomenclature-based data retrieval without prior annotation: facilitating biomedical data integration with fast doublet matching. In Silico Biol 2005; 5(3): 313–22.

3. Shapiro S, Gershtein V, Elias N, Zuckerman E, Salman N, Lahat N. mRNA cytokine profile in peripheral blood cells from chronic hepatitis C virus (HCV)-infected patients: effects of interferon-alpha (IFN-alpha) treatment. Clin Exp Immunol 1998 Oct;114(1): 55–60.

4. Goyal A, Kazim SN, Sakhuja P, Malhotra V, Arora N, Sarin SK. Association of TNF-beta polymorphism with disease severity among patients infected with hepatitis C virus. J Med Virol 2004 Jan;72(1):60–5.

5. Dai CY, Chuang WL, Lee LP, Chen SC, Hou NJ, Lin ZY, Hsieh MY, Hsieh MY, Wang LY, Chang WY, Yu ML. Associations of tumour necrosis factor alpha promoter polymorphisms at position -308 and -238 with clinical characteristics of chronic hepatitis C. J Viral Hepat 2006 Nov;13(11):770–4.

6. Thio CL, Goedert JJ, Mosbruger T, Vlahov D, Strathdee SA, O'Brien SJ, Astemborski J, Thomas DL. An analysis of tumor necrosis factor alpha gene polymorphisms and haplotypes with natural clearance of hepatitis C virus infection. Genes Immun 2004 Jun;5(4):294–300.

7. Saito T, Ji G, Shinzawa H, Okumoto K, Hattori E, Adachi T, Takeda T, Sugahara K, Ito JI, Watanabe H, Saito K, Togashi H, Ishii K, Matsuura T, Inageda K, Muramatsu M, Kawata S. Genetic variations in humans associated with differences in the course of hepatitis C. Biochem Biophys Res Commun 2004 Apr 30;317(2):335–41.

8. Hwang Y, Chen EY, Gu ZJ, Chuang WL, Yu ML, Lai MY, Chao YC, Lee CM, Wang JH, Dai CY, Shian-Jy Bey M, Liao YT, Chen PJ, Chen DS. Genetic predisposition of responsiveness to therapy for chronic hepatitis C. Pharmacogenomics 2006 Jul;7(5):697–709.

9. Naito M, Matsui A, Inao M, Nagoshi S, Nagano M, Ito N, Egashira T, Hashimoto M, Mishiro S, Mochida S, Fujiwara K. SNPs in the promoter region of the osteopontin gene as a marker predicting the efficacy of interferon-based therapies in patients with chronic hepatitis C. J Gastroenterol 2005 Apr;40(4):381–8.

10. Suzuki F, Arase Y, Suzuki Y, Tsubota A, Akuta N, Hosaka T, Someya T, Kobayashi M, Saitoh S, Ikeda K, Kobayashi M, Matsuda M, Takagi K, Satoh J, Kumada H. Single nucleotide polymorphism of the MxA gene promoter influences the response to interferon monotherapy in patients with hepatitis C viral infection. J Viral Hepat 2004 May;11(3):271–6.

11. Hennig BJ, Hellier S, Frodsham AJ, Zhang L, Klenerman P, Knapp S, Wright M, Thomas HC, Thursz M, Hill AV. Association of low-density lipoprotein receptor polymorphisms and outcome of hepatitis C infection. Genes Immun 2002 Sep;3(6):359–67.

12. Yee LJ, Tang J, Gibson AW, Kimberly R, Van Leeuwen DJ, Kaslow RA. Interleukin 10 polymorphisms as predictors of sustained response in antiviral therapy for chronic hepatitis C infection. Hepatology 2001 Mar;33(3):708–12.

13. Romero-Gomez M, Montes-Cano MA, Otero-Fernandez MA, Torres B, Sanchez-Munoz D, Aguilar F, Barroso N, Gomez-Izquierdo L, Castellano-Megias VM, Nunez-Roldan A, Aguilar-Reina J, Gonzalez-Escribano MF. SLC11A1 promoter gene polymorphisms and fibrosis progression in chronic hepatitis C. Gut 2004 Mar;53(3):446–50.

14. Huang H, Shiffman ML, Cheung RC, Layden TJ, Friedman S, Abar OT, Yee L, Chokkalingam AP, Schrodi SJ, Chan J, Catanese JJ, Leong DU, Ross D, Hu X, Monto A, McAllister LB, Broder S, White T, Sninsky JJ, Wright TL. Identification of two gene variants associated with risk of advanced fibrosis in patients with chronic hepatitis C. Gastroenterology 2006 May;130(6):1679–87.

15. Suneetha PV, Goyal A, Hissar SS, Sarin SK. Studies on TAQ1 polymorphism in the 3'untranslated region of IL-12P40 gene in HCV patients infected predominantly with genotype 3. J Med Virol 2006 Aug;78(8):1055–60

16. Fishman S, Lurie Y, Peretz H, Morad T, Grynberg E, Blendis LM, Leshno M, Brazowski E, Rosner G, Halpern Z, Oren R. Role of CYP2D6 polymorphism in predicting liver fibrosis progression rate in Caucasian patients with chronic hepatitis C. Liver Int 2006 Apr;26(3):279–84.

17. Wang H, Mengsteab S, Tag CG, Gao CF, Hellerbrand C, Lammert F, Gressner AM, Weiskirchen R. Transforming growth factor-beta1 gene polymorphisms are associated with progression of liver fibrosis in Caucasians with chronic hepatitis C infection. World J Gastroenterol 2005 Apr 7;11(13):1929–36.

18. Aguilar-Reina J, Ruiz-Ferrer M, Pizarro MA, Antinolo G. The -670A > G polymorphism in the promoter region of the FAS gene is associated with necrosis in periportal areas in patients with chronic hepatitis C. J Viral Hepat 2005 Nov;12(6):568–73.

19. Tseng CS, Tang KS, Lo HW, Ker CG, Teng HC, Huang CS. UDP-glucuronosyltransferase 1A7 genetic polymorphisms are associated with hepatocellular carcinoma risk and onset age. Am J Gastroenterol 2005 Aug;100(8):1758–63.

20. Ho SY, Wang YJ, Chen HL, Chen CH, Chang CJ, Wang PJ, Chen HH, Guo HR. Increased risk of developing hepatocellular carcinoma associated with carriage of the TNF2 allele of the -308 tumor necrosis factor-alpha promoter gene. Cancer Causes Control 2004 Sep;15(7):657–63.

21. Silvestri L, Sonzogni L, De Silvestri A, Gritti C, Foti L, Zavaglia C, Leveri M, Cividini A, Mondelli MU, Civardi E, Silini EM. CYP enzyme polymorphisms and susceptibility to HCV-related chronic liver disease and liver cancer. Int J Cancer 2003 Apr 10;104(3):310–7.

22. Wang FS. Current status and prospects of studies on human genetic alleles associated with hepatitis B virus infection. World J Gastroenterol 2003 Apr;9(4):641–4.

23. Lorenzo A, Auguet T, Vidal F, Broch M, Olona M, Gutierrez C, Lopez-Dupla M, Sirvent JJ, Quer JC, Santos M, Richart C. Polymorphisms of alcohol-metabolizing enzymes and the risk for alcoholism and alcoholic liver disease in Caucasian Spanish women. Drug Alcohol Depend 2006 Sep 15;84(2):195–200.

24. Campos J, Gonzalez-Quintela A, Quinteiro C, Gude F, Perez LF, Torre JA, Vidal C. The -159C/T polymorphism in the promoter region of the CD14 gene is associated with advanced liver disease and higher serum levels of acute-phase proteins in heavy drinkers. Alcohol Clin Exp Res 2005 Jul; 29(7):1206–13.

25. Pastor IJ, Laso FJ, Romero A, Gonzalez-Sarmiento R. -238 G>A polymorphism of tumor necrosis factor alpha gene (TNFA) is associated with alcoholic liver cirrhosis in alcoholic Spanish men. Alcohol Clin Exp Res 2005 Nov; 29(11):1928–31.

26. Namikawa C, Shu-Ping Z, Vyselaar JR, Nozaki Y, Nemoto Y, Ono M, Akisawa N, Saibara T, Hiroi M, Enzan H, Onishi S. Polymorphisms of microsomal triglyceride transfer protein gene and manganese superoxide dismutase gene in non-alcoholic steatohepatitis. J Hepatol 2004 May;40(5):781–6.

27. Iwamoto N, Ogawa Y, Kajihara S, Hisatomi A, Yasutake T, Yoshimura T, Mizuta T, Hara T, Ozaki I, Yamamoto K. Gln27Glu beta2-adrenergic receptor variant is associated with hypertriglyceridemia and the development of fatty liver. Clin Chim Acta 2001 Dec; 314(1–2):85–91.

28. Ohnishi T, Ogawa Y, Saibara T, Nishioka A, Kariya S, Fukumoto M, Onishi S, Yoshida S. CYP17 polymorphism and tamoxifen-induced hepatic steatosis. Hepatol Res 2005 Oct; 33(2):178–80.

29. Niemi M, Neuvonen PJ, Hofmann U, Backman JT, SchwabM, LutjohannD, von-BergmannK, EichelbaumM, KivistoKT. Acute effects of pravastatin on cholesterol synthesis are associated with SLCO1B1 (encoding OATP1B1) haplotype *17. Pharmacogenet Genomics 2005;15: 303–9.

30. Takane H, Miyata M, Burioka N, Shigemasa C, Shimizu E, Otsubo K, Ieiri I. Pharmacogenetic determinants of variability in lipid-lowering response to pravastatin therapy. J Hum Genet 2006;51(9):822-6.

31. Shah RR. Can pharmacogenetics help rescue drugs withdrawn from the market? Pharmacogenomics 2006 Sep;7(6):889–908. Review.

32. Jain KK. Applications of AmpliChip CYP450. Mol Diagn. 2005;9(3):119–27.

33. Clayton TA, Lindon JC, Cloarec O, Antti H, Charuel C, Hanton G, Provost JP, LeNet JL, Baker D, Walley RJ, Everett JR, Nicholson JK. Pharmaco-metabonomic phenotyping and personalized drug treatment. Nature 2006;440:1073-7.

34. Zhang LH, Ji JF. Molecular profiling of hepatocellular carcinomas by cDNA microarray. World J Gastroenterol 2005 January 28; 11(4):463–8.

35. Baranova A, Schlauch K, Gowder S, Collantes R, Chandhoke V, Younossi ZM. Microarray technology in the study of obesity and non-alcoholic fatty liver disease. Liver Int 2005 Dec;25(6):1091–6. Review.

36. Yano N, Habib NA, Fadden KJ, Yamashita H, Mitry R, Jauregui H, Kane A, Endoh M, Rifai A. Profiling the adult human liver transcriptome: analysis by cDNA array hybridization. J Hepatol 2001 Aug;35(2):178–86.

37. Kaneko S, Kobayashi K. Clinical application of a DNA chip in the field of liver diseases. J Gastroenterol 2003 Mar; 38 Suppl 15:85–8.

38. Yamashita T, Kaneko S, Hashimoto S, Sato T, Nagai S, Toyoda N, Suzuki T, Kobayashi K, Matsushima K. Serial analysis of gene expression in chronic hepatitis C and hepatocellular carcinoma. Biochem Biophys Res Commun 2001 Mar 30;282(2):647–54.

39. Yamashita T, Hashimoto S, Kaneko S, Nagai S, Toyoda N, Suzuki T, Kobayashi K, Matsushima K. Comprehensive gene expression profile of a normal human liver. Biochem Biophys Res Commun 2000 Mar 5;269(1):110–6.

40. Ruijter JM, Van Kampen AH, Baas F. Statistical evaluation of SAGE libraries: consequences for experimental design. Physiol Genomics 2002 Oct 29; 11(2):37–44. Review.

41. Yamamoto M, Wakatsuki T, Hada A, Ryo A. Use of serial analysis of gene expression (SAGE) technology. J Immunol Methods 2001 Apr; 250(1–2): 45–66. Review.

42. Shackel NA, Seth D, Haber PS, Gorrell MD, McCaughan GW. The hepatic transcriptome in human liver disease. Comp Hepatol. 2006 Nov 7; 5:6.

43. Shackel NA, Gorrell MD, McCaughan GW. Gene array analysis and the liver. Hepatology 2002 Dec;36(6):1313–25.

44. Emmert-Buck MR, Bonner RF, Smith PD, Chuaqui RF, Zhuang Z, Goldstein SR, Weiss RA, Liotta LA. Laser capture microdissection. Science 1996 Nov 8; 274(5289):998–1001.

45. Banks, R. E., M. J. Dunn, et al. The potential use of laser capture microdissection to selectively obtain distinct populations of cells for proteomic analysis–preliminary findings. Electrophoresis 1999;20(4–5): 689–700.

46. Harris AJ, Dial SL, Casciano DA. Comparison of basal gene expression profiles and effects of hepatocarcinogens on gene expression in cultured primary human hepatocytes and HepG2 cells. Mutat Res 2004 May 18;549(1–2):79–99.

47. Wong LY, Hafeman A, Boyd VL, Bodeau J, Lazaruk KD, Liew SN, Casey P, Belonogoff V, Bit S, Sumner C, Bredo A, Ho N, Chu E, Olson S, Rabkin S, Maltchenko S, Spier G, Gilbert D, Baumhueter S. Assessing gene expression variation in normal human tissues using GeneTag, a novel, global, sensitive profiling method. J Biotechnol 2003 Mar 20;101(3):199–217.

48. Rinn J L, Rozowsky J S, Laurenzi I J et al. Major molecular differences between mammalian sexes are involved in drug metabolism and renal function. Dev Cell 2004; 6: 791–800.

49. Delongchamp RR, Velasco C, Dial S, Harris AJ. Genome-wide estimation of gender differences in the gene expression of human livers: statistical design and analysis. BMC Bioinformatics 2005 Jul 15;6 Suppl 2:S13.

50. Cox LA, Schlabritz-Loutsevitch N, Hubbard GB, Nijland MJ, McDonald TJ, Nathanielsz PW. Gene expression profile differences in left and right liver lobes from mid-gestation fetal baboons: a cautionary tale. J Physiol 2006 Apr 1;572(Pt 1):59–66.

51. Haugen G, Hanson M, Kiserud T, Crozier S, Inskip H, Godfrey KM. Fetal liver-sparing cardiovascular adaptations linked to mother's slimness and diet. Circ Res 2005;96:12–14.

52. Haugen G, Kiserud T, Godfrey K, Crozier S & Hanson M. Portal and umbilical venous blood supply to the liver in the human fetus near term. Ultrasound Obstet Gynecol 2004;24:599–605.

53. Walters KA, Smith MW, Pal S, Thompson JC, Thomas MJ, Yeh MM, Thomas DL, Fitzgibbon M, Proll S, Fausto N, Gretch DR, Carithers RL Jr, Shuhart MC, Katze MG. Identification of a specific gene expression pattern associated with HCV-induced pathogenesis in HCV- and HCV/HIV-infected individuals. Virology 2006 Jul 5;350(2):453–64.

54. Smith MW, Walters, K.-A, Korth, M.J., Fitzgibbon, M., Proll, S.C., Thompson, J.C., Yeh, M.M., Shuhart, M.C., Furlong, J.C., Cox, P.P., Thomas, D.L., Phillips, J.D., Kushner, J.P., Fausto, N., Carithers, R.L., Katze, M.G. Gene expression patterns that correlate with hepatitis C and early progression to fibrosis in liver transplant patients. Gastroenterol 2006;130, 179–87.

55. Einav, S., Koziel, M.J. Immunopathogenesis of hepatitis C virus in the immunosuppressed host. Transplant Infect Dis 2002;4, 85–92.

56. Bieche I, Asselah T, Laurendeau I, Vidaud D, Degot C, Paradis V, Bedossa P, Valla DC, Marcellin P, Vidaud M. Molecular profiling of early stage liver fibrosis in patients with chronic hepatitis C virus infection. Virol 2005 Feb 5; 332(1):130–44.

57. Lau DT, Luxon BA, Xiao SY, Beard MR, Lemon SM. Intrahepatic gene expression profiles and alpha-smooth muscle actin patterns in hepatitis C virus induced fibrosis. Hepatology 2005 Aug; 42(2):273–81.

58. Okamoto M, Utsunomiya T, Wakiyama S, Hashimoto M, Fukuzawa K, Ezaki T, Hanai T, Inoue H, Mori M. Specific gene-expression profiles of noncancerous liver tissue predict the risk for multicentric occurrence of hepatocellular carcinoma in hepatitis C virus-positive patients. Ann Surg Oncol 2006 Jul;13(7):947–54.

59. Ho MC, Lin JJ, Chen CN, Chen CC, Lee H, Yang CY, Ni YH, Chang KJ, Hsu HC, Hsieh FJ, Lee PH. A gene expression profile for vascular invasion can predict the recurrence after resection of hepatocellular carcinoma: a microarray approach. Ann Surg Oncol 2006 Nov;13(11):1474–84.

60. Mas VR, Maluf DG, Archer KJ, Yanek K, Williams B, Fisher RA. Differentially expressed genes between early and advanced hepatocellular carcinoma (HCC) as a potential tool for selecting liver transplant recipients. Mol Med 2006 Apr-Jun;12(4–6):97–104.

61. Murakami Y, Yasuda T, Saigo K, Urashima T, Toyoda H, Okanoue T, Shimotohno K. Comprehensive analysis of microRNA expression patterns in hepatocellular carcinoma and non-tumorous tissues. Oncogene 2006 Apr 20;25(17):2537–45.

62. Tamori A, Yamanishi Y, Kawashima S, Kanehisa M, Enomoto M, Tanaka H, Kubo S, Shiomi S, Nishiguchi S. Alteration of gene expression in human hepatocellular carcinoma with integrated hepatitis B virus DNA. Clin Cancer Res 2005 Aug 15;11(16):5821–6.

63. Kim J W, Ye Q, Forgues M, Chen Y, Budhu A, Sime J, Hofseth LJ, Kaul R, Wang XW. Cancer-associated molecular signature in the tissue samples of patients with cirrhosis. Hepatology 2004: 39: 518–27.

64. Lederer SL, Walters KA, Proll S, Paeper B, Robinzon S, Boix L, Fausto N, Bruix J, Katze MG. Distinct cellular responses differentiating alcohol- and hepatitis C virus-induced liver cirrhosis. Virol J 2006 Nov 22;3:98.

65. Sreekumar R, Rosado B, Rasmussen D, Charlton M. Hepatic gene expression in histologically progressive nonalcoholic steatohepatitis. Hepatology 2003 Jul; 38(1):244–51.

66. Younossi ZM, Gorreta F, Ong JP, Schlauch K, Giacco LD, Elariny H, Van Meter A, Younoszai A, Goodman Z, Baranova A, Christensen A, Grant G, Chandhoke V. Hepatic gene expression in patients with obesity-related non-alcoholic steatohepatitis. Liver Int 2005 Aug;25(4):760–71.

67. Chiappini F, Barrier A, Saffroy R, Domart MC, Dagues N, Azoulay D, Sebagh M, Franc B, Chevalier S, Debuire B, Dudoit S, Lemoine A. Exploration of global gene expression in human liver steatosis by high-density oligonucleotide microarray. Lab Invest 2006 Feb;86(2):154–65.

68. Tian Q, Stepaniants SB, Mao M, Weng L, Feetham MC, Doyle MJ, Yi EC, Dai H,Thorsson V, Eng J, Goodlett D, Berger JP, Gunter B, Linseley PS, Stoughton RB, Aebersold R, Collins SJ, Hanlon WA, Hood LE. Integrated genomic and proteomic analyses of gene expression in Mammalian cells. Mol Cell Proteomics 2004 Oct;3(10):960–9.

69. Chen G, Gharib TG, Huang CC, Taylor JM, Misek DE, Kardia SL, Giordano TJ, Iannettoni MD, Orringer MB, Hanash SM, Beer DG. Discordant protein and mRNA expression in lung adenocarcinomas. Mol Cell Proteomics 2002 Apr;1(4):304–13.

70. Craven R. A., Selby P. J., et al. (2004). Proteomics-Based Approaches: New Opportunities in Cancer Research, Humana Press.

71. Berggren K., Chernokalskaya E., et al. (2000). "Background-free, high sensitivity staining of proteins in one- and two-dimensional sodium dodecyl sulfate-polyacrylamide gels using a luminescent ruthenium complex." Electrophoresis 21: 2509–21.

72. Wulfkuhle J.D., Liotta L.A., et al. "Proteomic applications for the early detection of cancer." Nat Rev Cancer 2003;3(4,): 267–75

73. Sadygov RG, Cociorva D, Yates JR 3rd. Large-scale database searching using tandem mass spectra: looking up the answer in the back of the book. Nat Methods 2004 Dec; 1(3):195–202.

74. Lewis JK, Wei J, et al. Matrix-assisted Laser Desorption/Ionization Mass spectrometry in Peptide and Protein Analysis. Encyclopedia of Analytical Chemistry. R. A. Meyers. Chichester, John Wiley & Sons Ltd. 2000;5880–94.

75. Hutchens, T. W. and T. T. Yip. Rapid Commun. Mass Spectrom 1993;7: 576–80.

76. Grus FH, Joachim SC, et al. "Analysis of complex autoantibody repertoires by surface-enhanced laser desorption/ionization-time of flight mass spectrometry." Proteomics 2003;3(6): 957–61.

77. Guo J, Yang EC, et al. "A strategy for high-resolution protein identification in surface-enhanced laser desorption/ionization mass spectrometry: Calgranulin A and chaperonin 10 as protein markers for endometrial carcinoma." Proteomics 2005;3(6): 957–61.

78. Bogdanov B, Smith RD. "Proteomics by FTICR mass spectrometry: top down and bottom up." Mass Spectrom Reviews 2005;24(2): 168–200.

79. Espina V, Mehta AI, Winters ME, Calvert V, Wulfkuhle J, Petricoin EF 3rd, Liotta LA. Protein microarrays: molecular profiling technologies for clinical specimens. Proteomics 2003 Nov;3(11):2091–100. Review.

80. Poetz O., Schwenk J. M., et al. "Protein microarrays: catching the proteome." Mechanisms of Ageing and Development 2005;126: 161–70.

81. Geho DH, Liotta LA, Petricoin EF, Zhao W, Araujo RP. The amplified peptidome: the new treasure chest of candidate biomarkers. Curr Opin Chem Biol 2006 10(1):50-5.

82. Geho DH, Jones CD, Petricoin EF, Liotta LA. Nanoparticles: potential biomarker harvesters. Curr Opin Chem Biol 2006 10(1):56-61.

83. Tibes R, Qiu Y, Lu Y, Hennessy B, Andreeff M, Mills GB, Kornblau SM. Reverse phase protein array: validation of a novel proteomic technology and utility for analysis of primary leukemia specimens and hematopoietic stem cells. Mol Cancer Ther 2006 Oct;5(10):2512–21.

84. Zheng J, Gao X, Beretta L, He F. The Human Liver Proteome Project (HLPP) workshop during the 4th HUPO World Congress. Proteomics. 2006 Mar;6(6):1716–8.

85. Cagney G, Park S, Chung C, Tong B, O'Dushlaine C, Shields DC, Emili A. Human tissue profiling with multidimensional protein identification technology. J Proteome Res 2005 Sep-Oct;4(5):1757–67.

86. Washburn, M. P.; Wolters, D.; Yates, J. R. III Large-scale analysis of the yeast proteome by multidimensional protein identification technology. Nat. Biotechnol 2001;19:242–247.

87. Zhang X, Guo Y, Song Y, Sun W, Yu C, Zhao X, Wang H, Jiang H, Li Y, Qian X, Jiang Y, He F. Proteomic analysis of individual variation in normal livers of human beings using difference gel electrophoresis. Proteomics 2006 Oct;6(19):5260–8.

88. Gallagher EP, Gardner JL, Barber DS. Several glutathione S-transferase isozymes that protect against oxidative injury are expressed in human liver mitochondria. Biochem Pharmacol 2006 71(11):1619-28

89. Petushkova NA, Kanaeva IP, Lisitsa AV, Sheremetyeva GF, Zgoda VG, Samenkova NF, Karuzina II, Archakov AI. Characterization of human liver cytochromes P450 by combining the biochemical and proteomic approaches. Toxicol In Vitro 2006 20(6):966-74.

90. Zeindl-Eberhart E, Haraida S, Liebmann S, Jungblut PR, Lamer S, Mayer D, Jager G, Chung S, Rabes HM. Detection and identification of tumor-associated protein variants in human hepatocellular carcinomas. Hepatology 2004 Feb;39(2):540–9.

91. Park KS, Kim H, Kim NG, Cho SY, Choi KH, Seong JK, Paik YK. Proteomic analysis and molecular characterization of tissue ferritin light chain in hepatocellular carcinoma. Hepatology 2002 Jun;35(6):1459–66.

92. Park KS, Cho SY, Kim H, Paik YK. Proteomic alterations of the variants of human aldehyde dehydrogenase isozymes correlate with hepatocellular carcinoma. Int J Cancer 2002 Jan 10;97(2):261–5.

93. Kim W, Oe Lim S, Kim JS, Ryu YH, Byeon JY, Kim HJ, Kim YI, Heo JS, Park YM, Jung G. Comparison of proteome between hepatitis B virus- and hepatitis C virus-associated hepatocellular carcinoma. Clin Cancer Res. 2003 Nov 15;9(15):5493–500.

94. Ai J, Tan Y, Ying W, Hong Y, Liu S, Wu M, Qian X, Wang H. Proteome analysis of hepatocellular carcinoma by laser capture microdissection. Proteomics 2006 Jan;6(2):538–46.

95. Kim KA, Lee EY, Kang JH, Lee HG, Kim JW, Kwon DH, Jang YJ, Yeom YI, Chung TW, Kim YD, Yoon do Y, Song EY. Diagnostic accuracy of serum asialo-alpha1-acid glycoprotein concentration for the differential diagnosis of liver cirrhosis and hepatocellular carcinoma. Clin Chim Acta 2006 Jul 15;369(1):46–51.

96. Nabetani T, Tabuse Y, Tsugita A, Shoda J. Proteomic analysis of livers of patients with primary hepatolithiasis. Proteomics 2005 Mar;5(4):1043–61.

97. Guedj N, Dargere D, Degos F, Janneau JL, Vidaud D, Belghiti J, Bedossa P, Paradis V. Global proteomic analysis of microdissected cirrhotic nodules reveals significant biomarkers associated with clonal expansion. Lab Invest 2006 Sep;86(9):951–8.

98. Schwegler EE, Cazares L, Steel LF, Adam BL, Johnson DA, Semmes OJ, Block TM, Marrero JA, Drake RR. SELDI-TOF MS profiling of serum for detection of the progression of chronic hepatitis C to hepatocellular carcinoma. Hepatology 2005 Mar;41(3):634–42.

99. Paradis V, Degos F, Dargere D, Pham N, Belghiti J, Degott C, Janeau JL, Bezeaud A, Delforge D, Cubizolles M, Laurendeau I, Bedossa P. Identification of a new marker of hepatocellular carcinoma by serum protein profiling of patients with chronic liver diseases. Hepatology 2005 Jan;41(1):40–7.

100. Ward DG, Cheng Y, N'Kontchou G, Thar TT, Barget N, Wei W, Martin A, Beaugrand M, Johnson PJ. Preclinical and post-treatment changes in the HCC-associated serum proteome. Br J Cancer 2006 Nov 20;95(10):1379–83.

101. Takashima M, Kuramitsu Y, Yokoyama Y, Iizuka N, Harada T, Fujimoto M, Sakaida I, Okita K, Oka M, Nakamura K. Proteomic analysis of autoantibodies in patients with hepatocellular carcinoma. Proteomics 2006 Jul;6(13):3894–900.

102. Younossi ZM, Baranova A, Ziegler K, Del Giacco L, Schlauch K, Born TL, Elariny H, Gorreta F, VanMeter A, Younoszai A, Ong JP, Goodman Z, Chandhoke V. A genomic and proteomic study of the spectrum of nonalcoholic fatty liver disease. Hepatology 2005 Sep;42(3):665–74.

103. Chan K, Lucas D, Hise D, Schaefer C, Xiao Z, Janini G, et al. Analysis of the human serum proteome. Clinical Proteomics 2004;101–226.

104. Calvert V, Collantes R., Elariny H, Afendy A, Baranova A., Mendoza M., Goodman Z., Liotta L., Petricoin EF, Younossi ZM. A Systems Biology Approach to the Pathogenesis of Obesity-related Non Alcoholic Fatty Liver Disease Using Reverse Phase Protein Microarrays for Multiplexed Cell Signaling Analysis. Hepatology, in press.

105. Wang Y, Xu LY, Lam KS, Lu G, Cooper GJ, Xu A. Proteomic characterization of human serum proteins associated with the fat-derived hormone adiponectin. Proteomics 2006 Jul;6(13):3862–70.

Index

Note: An *f* following a page number denotes a figure on that page; a *t* following a page number indicates a table on that page.

acetaminophen hepatotoxicity, 175, 176, 184*f*, 260
acute liver failure
  drug induced, 175, 175*t*, 176, 178–180, 186*t*, 187, 189
  HAV-related, 5
  HBV-related, 9
  HCV-related, 13, 43
  Wilson's disease and, 134
acute viral hepatitis
  conditions causing, 1, 2*t*
  general considerations, 1
  hepatotropic viruses causing, 1, 2*t*
  serologic diagnosis, 4*t*. *See also*
    Hepatitis A virus; Hepatitis B virus; Hepatitis C virus; Hepatitis D virus; Hepatitis E virus
adefovir (ADV)
  for chronic HBV, 30, 31, 32, 69*t*
  for chronic HBV-HIV co-infection, 68, 69*t*
  for compensated cirrhosis, 33
  for decompensated cirrhosis, 33–34
  patients with ADV resistance, 34
Advisory Committee on Immunization Practices (ACIP), 6, 10
alanine aminotransferase (ALT) levels, 26–27, 31, 46, 47, 52–53, 161, 180
alcohol use
  drug-induced liver disease and, 182
  NAFLD and, 80
alcoholic hepatitis treatment, 101–103
  pathophysiology based treatment, 103

prognosis, 101
prognostic scoring system, 101–103
alcoholic liver disease (ALD), 98–111
  HCV and, 54
  HFE and, 124, 127
  histological characteristics, 99*t*
  inherited predispositions to, 258–259
  mortality, 103*t*
  nutritional guidelines, 109*t*
  pentoxifylline decreased morality in AH, 105*f*
  potential new therapies, 107–108
  prognosis scores, 102*t*
  relative risk, and alcohol intake level, 100*t*
  risk factors, 98–101
    gender, 99–100
    malnutrition and diet, 101
    quantity of alcohol consumed, 98–99
    virus, 100–101
  steroids *vs.* placebo, 104*f*
  survival, 99*t*, 104*f*
  therapeutic algorithm for long-term management, 111*f*
  therapeutic algorithm for management, 107*f*
  treatment, long-term, 108–111
    antiviral therapy, 108
    liver transplantation, 108–111
    nutritional therapy, 108
    other therapies, 108. *See also*
      Alcoholic liver disease (ALD), treatment

alcoholic liver disease (ALD), treatment, 101–108
  alcoholic hepatitis, 101–103
    pathophysiology based treatment, 103
    prognosis, 101
    prognostic scoring system, 101–103
  anti-cytokine therapy, 105–106
    anti-TNF treatment, 106
    entanercept, 106
    pentoxifyllline, 105–106
  antioxidents, 106–107
    S-adenosyl-L-methionine, 106–107
  corticosteroids, 103–105
alcoholic steatohepatitis (ASH), 80
alcoholism, 98, 181t, 184f
allopurinol, 244
alpha-1 antitrypsin deficiency (AAD), 140–152
  cigarette smoking and, 146, 149, 151t
  clinical presentation, 144–147
    liver disease, 144–146
    other conditions, 147
    panniculitis, 144, 146, 147
    pulmonary disease, 146
    vasculitis, 146–147
  diagnosis, 147–148
  general considerations, 140
  genetics of, 141–143
  liver biopsy results
  lung disease and, 143t, 144
  M-type, 141
  management, 148–150
  pathogenesis, 143–144
  PI**MM phenotype, 142
  PI*SS phenotype, 143
  PI*SZ allele, 143
  PI*ZZ allele, 141–142, 145, 146, 151
  prognosis, 151
  schematic of PI types, 142f
  selected PI variants, 141t
alphafetoprotein (AFP) screening, 200, 202
American Indians, decline of HAV among, 3
aminoglycosides, 226
AmpliChip, 260
Amplified Fragment Length Polymorphism (AFLP), 261
aneurysm, of hepatic artery, 242
angiotensin converting enzyme inhibitor (ACEI), 89
angiotensin receptor blocker (ARB), 89
animal studies
  acetaminophen proof-of-principle study, 260

alcoholic liver disease, 105
  location-specific variations in gene expression patterns, 261–262
  NASH, 83
anti-cytokine therapy, 105–106
anti-TNF treatment, 106
antibiotic prophylaxis, 226–227
antioxidants, 87, 88, 89, 106, 108, 138
antiviral therapy
  for acute hepatitis B, 10–11
  for acute hepatitis C, 14–16
  for acute hepatitis D, 17
  for alcoholic liver disease, 108
  for chronic hepatitis B, 29, 30–35
  for chronic hepatitis C, 48–49, 51, 53, 54. See also HIV, and viral hepatitis
ascites, 221–227
  ascitic fluid analysis, 222–223
  ascitic fluid analysis, recommended tests, 223t
  based on total protein and SAAG, 224f
  refractory ascites, 224
  spontaneous bacterial peritonitis
    diagnosis and treatment, 227f
    prevalence, 225–227
  treatment, 224
aspartate aminotransferase (AST), 46, 161
autoimmune hepatitis, 164–170
  classification, 168t
  clinical presentation, 165–166
  diagnosis, 166–167
  management, 167–170
  prednisone treatment, 165f
  therapy, 169t
autoimmune liver disease (AIH), 155–171
  autoimmune hepatitis, 164–170
  ERCP vs MRCP, 157f
  extrahepatic autoimmune diseases, 161t
  general considerations, 155
  overlap syndromes, 170–171
    diagnostic criteria, 170t
  prevalence of ANA in liver disease, 166f
  primary biliary cirrhosis, 159, 159t, 160f, 161t, 162t, 164
  primary sclerosing cholangitis, 155, 156t, 157t, 158f, 158t, 159, 159t
  survival with UDCA therapy, 163f
azathioprine, 244

bariatric surgery, 80, 86–87
Beclere model, 101–102
betaine, 88

biliary cirrhosis, 189
  primary, 158*f*, 159, 159*t*, 161*t*, 162*t*, 164
bilirubin levels, 1, 4, 5
biopsy, liver
  for AAT deficiency, 147–148
  for alpha-1 antitrypsin deficiency
  for chronic hepatitis B diagnosis, 29
  for chronic hepatitis C diagnosis, 45–46,
    52–53
  for cirrhosis, 216
  for drug-induced liver disease, 189
  for hepatocellular carcinoma, 47–48
  for HIV/HBV coinfection, 66
  for NAFLD/NASH diagnosis, 82–83
  for primary biliary cirrhosis, 161–162
  for Wilson's disease, 132, 135
bone marrow suppression, 244, 246
bone marrow transplantation, 187
breast cancer, 240, 259
Budd-Chiari syndrome, 238
burned-out NASH, 77
bystander changes, 256–257

capillary liquid chromatography (LC-LC),
    264–265
causal changes, 256–257
cefotaxime, 226
central nervous system, and hepatic
    encephalopathy, 229–231
Child-Turcotte-Pugh (CTP) score,
    101–102, 216, 236, 237*t*, 263
children
  AAT deficiency in, 144–145
  acute hepatitis A in, 5
  acute hepatitis B in, 10
  chronic HDV and, 35
  decline of HAV in, 3
  hemangioma in, 196
  hepatitis C transmission to, 40
  NAFLD in, 79
  NASH in, 79
cholangiocarcinoma, 157, 158*f*, 240
cholestasis, 187
cholesterol synthesis, 259
chronic hepatitis B (CHB)
  clinical presentation, 27–28, 28*f*
  diagnosis, 28–29
  general considerations, 26
  hepatocellular carcinoma and, 199
  immune tolerant phase, 26–27
  management, 30–35
    chronic hepatitis B, 31–33
    cirrhosis, 33–34
    cirrhosis, compensated, 33
    cirrhosis, decompensated, 33–34, 238

combination antiviral therapies,
    34–35
  HBeAg negative, 31–33
  HBeAg positive, 31
  inactive carrier state, 31
  patients with ADV resistance, 34
  patients with ETV resistance, 34
  patients with LAM resistance, 34
  patients with LdT resistance, 34
  pathogenesis, 26–27
  prevalence and incidence of, 26
  transmission, 26
  treatment algorithm, 30*f*
chronic hepatitis C (CHC), 39–55
  clinical manifestations, 43
  combination therapy contraindications,
    50*t*
  combination therapy predictors, 49*t*
  diagnostic tests, 44–45
  epidemic, 215
  epidemiology and transmission, 39–41
  extrahepatic manifestations, 44*t*
  fibrosis progression in, 258
  general considerations, 39
  histologic features of, 46*t*
  laboratory tests and clinical evaluation,
    43–47
  liver biopsy, 45–46
  natural history of, 42*f*
  pathogenesis of chronic infection,
    41–42
  progression, 42–43
  recommended pretreatment
    investigations, 50*t*
  screening recommendations, 41*t*
  side effects of pegylated interferon plus
    ribavirin, 52*t*
  survival rates, 216
  treatment, 47–55
    alcohol and injecting drug use
      patient, 54
    assessing early treatment response,
      49–51
    children, 53–54
    decisions, 47–48
    future options, 55
    normal serum ALT levels and/or
      minimal liver disease, 52–53
    options, 48–49
    patients with comorbid disease due
      to other causes, 53
    pretreatment assessment and
      evaluation, 49
    relapsers and nonresponders to
      previous treatment, 54–55

chronic hepatitis C (CHC) (*cont.*)
  side effects of antiviral therapy and
    dose reduction, 51
  specific patient populations, 51–55
chronic hepatitis D (CHD), 35–36
  clinical presentation, 35
  diagnosis, 36
  HBV co-/super-infection and, 35
  management, 36
  pathogenesis, 35
  prevalence, 35
  treatment algorithm, 30*f*
cigarette smoking, 146, 149, 151*t*
cirrhosis
  alcoholic, 216
  alcoholic liver disease and, 99*t*
  compensated, 33, 53, 215
  cryptogenic, 77
  decompensated, 33–34, 53, 137, 215,
    238
  HIV/HBV coinfection and, 66
  NASH and, 79
  primary biliary, 157
  survival of different types of cirrhosis,
    99*t*
  Wilson's disease and, 133. *See also*
    Cirrhosis, complications of
cirrhosis, complications of, 215–231
  ascites, 221–227
    ascitic fluid analysis, 222–223
    ascitic fluid analysis, recommended
      tests, 223*t*
    diagnosis based on total protein and
      SAAG, 224*f*
    refractory, 224
    spontaneous bacterial peritonitis,
      225–227, 227*f*
    treatment, 224
  general considerations, 215
  hepatic encephalopathy, 229–231
  hepatorenal syndrome, 227, 228*t*,
    229
  modified Child-Turcotte criteria, 216*t*
  portal hypertension and, 216
  prognosis, 215–216
  variceal hemorrhage, 217–221
    bacterial infections and, 218–219
    balloon tamponade for, 219
    endoscopic therapy for, 219
    gastric varices, 220–221
    management of acute, 220*f*
    non-selective beta blockers for
      treatment, 217–218
    pharmacologic agents for treatment,
      219

prevention of recurrent bleeding,
  219–220
primary prophylaxis, 217–218
prophylaxis of, 218*f*
prophylaxis of recurrent, 221*f*
transjugular intrahepatic
  protosystemic shunts, 219
treatment of acute, 218–219
colchicin, 246
colon cancer, 159
confromational disease, 144
contrast-enhanced ultrasonography
  (CEUS), 82, 197, 198
COPD, 146, 148–149
copper accumulation. *See* Wilson's disease
corticosteroids, 103–105
COX-2 inhibitors, 225
cryptogenic cirrhosis, 77
CT scanning, 81–82, 159, 196, 198,
  200–202
cyclosporine, 243–244, 246
cytochrome P450 (CYP) system, 182–183,
  184
cytotoxic T cells, 5–6
cytotoxic T lymphocytes (CTLs), 27

diabetes
  prevalence of diabetes and NAFLD,
    78*f*
  transplantation and, 245
didanosine, 64
differentially expressed mRNA, 264
drug induced liver disease (DILI), 174–191
  acetaminophen hepatoxicity, 179, 183,
    185
  clinical presentation, 184–188
    cholestasis, 186–187
    clinical and histological patterns, 186*t*
    fibrosis, 187
    granulomas, 187
    hepatitis, 186
    hepatocellular necrosis, 186
    neoplasms, 188
    steatosis and steatohepatitis, 187
    vascular lesions, 187–188
  commonly implicated agents, 176–179
    common groups of agents to cause
      DILI, 178*t*
    FDA regulatory actions due to
      hepatoxicity, 177*t*
    herbal medications associated with
      liver toxicity, 178*t*
  diagnosis, 188–189
    key elements in, 188*t*
  drug development and, 179–180

epidemiology, 174–176
hepatotoxicity background, 174–176
historically reported frequency of
idiosyncratic DILI, 175*t*
management, 189–191
key guidelines, 190*t*
pathogenesis, 182–184
mechanism of acetaminophen
hepatotoxicity, 184*f*
risk factors, 181, 181*t*, 182
troglitazone and, 179, 180
Drug Induced Liver Injury Network
(DILIN), 177
dual energy X-ray absorptiometry
(DEXA), 82

early virological response (EVR), 49–51
emtricitabine, 71
endoscopic ultrasound, to detect
intrahepatic cholangiocarcinoma,
207
entanercept, 106
entecavir (ETV)
for chronic HBV, 30, 31, 32, 69*t*
for chronic HBV-HIV co-infection, 68,
70
for compensated cirrhosis, 33
for decompensated cirrhosis, 33–34
patients with ETV resistance, 34
enzyme immunoassay (EIA), 44
extensive metabolism (EM), of drugs,
259
extrahepatic autoimmune diseases, 161*t*

Fibroscan, 82
fibrosis
drug induced liver disease and, 187
hepatitis C and, 258, 262
NASH and, 79, 84–85
focal nodular hyperplasia (FNH), 196–197
clinical presentation, 197
diagnosis, 197
treatment, 197
folic acid, 89
food contamination, and hepatitis A, 3
Fourier transform ion cyclotron resonance
(FTICR), 265
fulminant hepatic failure (FHF)
acute HBV and, 9
acute HDV and, 18
hepatitis C and, 13
hepatitis E and, 19
lamivudine treatment, 10
transplantation and, 237–238
Wilson's disease and, 133, 137

gender differences
alcoholic liver disease and, 99–100
chronic liver disease and, 261
drug-induced liver disease and,
181–182
gene expression in nonreproductive
organs, 261
hemangioma and, 195
Gene Tag, 261
genetic counseling, and AAT deficiency,
150
genetic disease. *See* Alpha-1 antitrypsin
deficiency
genetic testing, for liver disease with
secondary iron overload, 124
genotype testing, for HCV infection, 45
gout, and liver transplantations, 244,
246

HCV-RNA, 19–20
health care workers, and chronic hepatitis
C, 40
hemangioma, 195–196
clinical presentation, 196
diagnosis, 196
hemophilia, 62
hepatic adenoma, 188, 197–199
clinical presentation, 198
diagnosis, 198
treatment, 199
hepatic artery stenosis, 242
hepatic artery thrombosis (HAT), 242
hepatic encephalopathy (HE), 229–231
management, 230*f*
stages, 230*t*
hepatic fibrogenesis, 43
hepatitis
autoimmune, 164–170
icteric, 9, 19
hepatitis A virus (HAV)
acute, 1–7
clinical presentation, 4–5
decrease in incidence, 1
diagnosis, 4
epidemiology, 3–4
estimated new infections, 1, 2*t*
high prevalence areas, 3
incidence, U.S., 1980-2002 3, 3*f*
management, 6–7
pathogenesis, 5–6
vaccination, 6–7, 7*t*
hepatitis B virus (HBV)
acute, 7–11
antiviral therapy, 10–11
clinical presentation, 9

hepatitis B virus (HBV) (*cont.*)
  decrease in incidence, 1
  diagnosis, 9
  distribution, 7
  epidemiology, 7–9
  estimated new infections, 1, 2*t*
  incidence, 8
  management, 10–11
  outcome according to age at infection,
    8*f*
  pathogenesis, 9–10
  transmission, 8
  vaccination, 10. *See also* Chronic
    hepatitis B; Hepatitis B, in
    HIV-infected patient
hepatitis B, in HIV-infected patient, 65–73
  adefovir, 70–71
  approved FDA medications for chronic
    HBV infections, 68, 69*t*
  combination therapy *vs.* monotherapy,
    72
  diagnosis, 67–68
  emtricitabine, 71
  entecavir, 70
  epidemiology, 65
  lamivudine, 70
  liver-related mortality by HIV and
    HBsAg status, 67*f*
  natural history, 65–67
  prevention, 73
  recurrent, 248
  telbivudine, 71–72
  tenofovir, 71
  tenofovir *vs.* adefovir, 69*t*
  treatment approach, 72–73
hepatitis C virus (HCV)
  acute, 11–16
  alcoholic liver disease and, 100–101
  antiviral therapy, 14–16
  clinical presentation, 13
  decrease in incidence, 1
  diagnosis, 12–13
  distribution/prevalence, 12
  epidemiology, 12
  estimated new infections, 1, 2*t*
  fibrosis progression in chronic, 258
  hepatocellular carcinoma and, 199
  management, 14–16
  occupational exposure management,
    14*t*
  pathogenesis, 13
  polymorphisms, 257–258
  primary biliary cirrhosis and, 162
  recommended routine testing
  recurrent, 247–248

transmission, 12. *See also* Chronic
    hepatitis C; Hepatitis C, in
    HIV-infected patient
hepatitis C, in HIV-infected patient, 61–65
  decompensated liver disease risk, 67*f*
  epidemiology, 61
  management recommendations, 63*t*
  natural history, 62
  treatment, 62, 64*t*, 65
hepatitis D virus (HDV)
  acute, 16–18
  clinical presentation, 17
  diagnosis, 16–17
  distribution, 16
  epidemiology, 16
  management, 18
  pathogenesis, 17. *See also* Chronic
    hepatitis D
hepatitis E virus (HEV)
  acute, 18–20
  clinical presentation, 19
  diagnosis, 19
  distribution, 18
  epidemiology, 18–19
  management, 20
  pathogenesis, 19–20
  transmission, 18–19
  vaccines for, 20
hepatocellular carcinoma (HCC), 199–206
  chronic HBV and, 28
  clinical presentation, 203
  diagnosis, 200
  diagnosis, of small HCC, 200–202
  hepatic tumors and, 188
  HIV/HBV coinfection and, 66
  NAFLD and, 79
  primary biliary cirrhosis and, 162
  proteome assessments and, 267
  screening, 200
  staging of, 204*f*
  transcriptome assessments and, 262
  treatment, 203–206
    chemoembolization, 205
    liver transplantation, 203, 239–240
    local ablation, 205
    other therapy, 205–206
    surgical resection, 203–205
hepatocellular jaundice, 180, 184–185
hepatoma. *See* Hepatocellular carcinoma
hepatorenal syndrome (HRS), 227–229
  diagnostic criteria, 228*t*
hereditary hemochromatosis (HH) and
    iron overload, 117–128
  classification of iron overload
    syndromes, 118*t*

clinical features of HH, 122*t*
clinical presentation, 121–123
diagnosis, 123–125
general considerations, 117
genetics of HFE-linked
    hemochromatosis, 119–120
HFE as common cause of, 118–119
HFE genotype in patients with typical,
    120*t*
iron overload syndromes, 117–119
laboratory findings, 125*t*
management, 125–126
pathophysiologic mechanisms in
    HFE-related, 120–121
    crypt hypothesis, 120–121
    hepcidin, 121
phlebotomy treatment, 126*t*
physical findings, 123*t*
screening, 120*t*, 126–128
    family and population, 126–127
    iron and other liver diseases, 126–127
symptoms, 122*t*
HIV
    educational programs, 40. *See also* HIV,
        and viral hepatitis
HIV, and viral hepatitis, 61–73
    general considerations, 61
    hepatitis B in HIV-infected patient,
        65–73
        adefovir, 70–71
        approved FDA medications, 68, 69*t*
        combination therapy *vs.*
            monotherapy, 72
        diagnosis, 67–68
        emtricitabine, 71
        entecavir, 70
        epidemiology, 65
        lamivudine, 70
        liver-related mortality, 67*f*
        natural history, 65–67
        prevention, 73
        telbivudine, 71–72
        tenofovir, 71
        tenofovir *vs.* adefovir, 69*t*
        treatment approach, 72–73
    hepatitis C in HIV-infected patient,
        61–65
        antiretroviral therapies, 62
        epidemiology, 61
        management recommendations, 63*t*
        natural history, 62
        peginterferon plus ribavirin, 64*t*
        relative risk of decompensated liver
            disease, 67*f*
        treatment, 62–65

Human Liver Proteome Project (HLPP),
    265–266
Hy's Rule, 180
hypertension, and liver transplantations,
    246
hypertriglyceridemia, 77
hyperuricemia, and liver transplantations,
    246
hypothyroidism, 44*t*, 123*t*, 134*t*, 159*t*, 161,
    164

icteric hepatitis, 9, 19
immunization
    hepatitis A, 6–7, 7*t*
    hepatitis B, 10, 73
immunosuppressive agents, and liver
    transplantations, 243–244
inflammatory bowel disease, 155
injection drug use
    as acute hepatitis A risk factor, 3–4
    as chronic hepatitis C risk factor, 40, 54
insulin resistance drugs, 87
interferon therapy
    antiviral therapy, 108
    combined with ribavirin for CHC, 48,
        49*t*
    for acute hepatitis B, 7, 11
    for acute hepatitis C, 15–16
    for chronic hepatitis C, 127
    for chronic hepatitis D, 18
    for HIV/HBV co-infected patients,
        68–69
    for HIV/HCV co-infected patients,
        62–63, 63*t*, 64, 64*t*, 65
    nonresponse to treatment, 127
    PEG-IFN, 48
    predictors of response to, 45, 49*t*, 258
    relapse after, 54–55
    side effects, 52*t*, 54, 55, 248
    treatment trials, 15
interferon-α, 48, 69*t*
interferon-γ, 6, 10
International Autoimmune Hepatitis
    Group Scoring System, 167
international travel, and acute hepatitis A,
    3–4
intrahepatic cholangiocarcinoma (ICC),
    206–207
    clinical presentation, 206
    diagnosis, 206–207
    treatment, 207
iron overload
    chronic HCV and, 53. *See also*
        Hereditary hemochromatosis
        (HH) and iron overload

jaundice
    and acute hepatitis A, 5
    and acute hepatitis B, 9
    and acute hepatitis C, 13
    hepatocellular, 180, 184–185
    primary biliary cirrhosis and, 163

Kaiser Fleischer ring, 132–133
Kasabach-Merritt Syndrome, 196
Kayser-Fleischer rings, 132–133, 135
ketoconazole, 244

lactulose, 229
lamivudine (LAM)
    for chronic HBV, 30, 31, 32, 69t, 70
    for chronic HBV-HIV co-infection, 68,
        69t, 70, 71, 72, 73
    for compensated cirrhosis, 33
    for decompensated cirrhosis, 33–34
    for fulminant hepatitis, 10
    for hepatitis D, 18
    patients with LAM resistance, 34–35
large volume paracentesis (LVP), 225
laser capture microdissection (LCM), 261
life style changes, and NAFLD, 85t, 86
lipid-lowering agents, 88, 246, 259
lipodystrophy, 79, 80
lung disease, and alpha-1 antitrypsin
        deficiency, 141t, 144

Maddrey Discriminate Function (MDF),
        101–102
magnetic resonance spectroscopy, 82
Major Histocompatibility Complex
        (MHC), 257
malnutrition
    alcoholic liver disease and, 101
    drug-induced liver disease and, 182
mass spectrometry (MS), 265
matrix-assisted laser desorption ionization
        (MALDI), 265
metabolic syndrome, 77, 79, 80, 85, 87
metallic bone disease, 157, 162
metformin, 87
metronidazole, 229–230
Milan Criteria, 203
Model for End-Stage Liver Disease
        (MELD) scores, 101–102, 216, 236,
        237
mortality
    and hepatitis B, 9
    and hepatitis C, 19
MRI
    primary sclerosing cholangitis, 159
    to detect hemangioma, 196

to detect hepatocellular carcinoma, 198,
        200–202
to detect intrahepatic
        cholangiocarcinoma, 207
to detect steatosis, 81–82
to measure hepatic triglyceride
        content, 82
Multicenter AIDS Cohort Study (MACS),
        67f
multidimensional protein identification
        technology (MudPIT), 266
mycophenolate mofetil, 244

N-acetyl-p-benzoquinoneamine
        (NAPQI), 183
National Health and Nutrition
        Examination Survey (NHANES), 12
neomycin, 229
non-steroidal anti-inflammatory drugs
        (NSAIDs), 225
nonalcoholic fatty liver disease (NALFD),
        77–90
    algorithm for evaluation, 81f
    antioxidants, 88–89
    clinical presentation, 80–82
    diabetes and, 78f
    drugs targeting insulin resistance, 87
    epidemiology, 77–78
    folic acid and, 89
    HFE mutations and, 128
    histologic diagnosis, 82–83
    life style changes and, 86
    lipid-lowering medications, 88
    natural history, 79–80
    obesity and metabolic issues, 78f
    other novel agents, 89–90
    pathogenesis, 83, 84f
    potential medical and surgical
        strategies, 85t
    proteome assessments, 267–268
    receptor blockers, 89
    treatment, 85
    ursodeoxycholic acid and, 89
    weight loss medications, 86. See also
        Nonalcoholic steatohepatitis
nonalcoholic steatohepatitis (NASH)
    burned-out, 77
    cirrhosis and, 79
    coining of, 77
    HFE mutations and, 128
    in children, 79
    inherited predispositions to, 259
    obesity and metabolic issues, 79
    predictors of NASH, advanced fibrosis,
        mortality, 84–85

type II diabetes and, 79. *See also* Nonalcoholic fatty liver disease
novel technologies, for studying CLDs, 256–269
database development, 257
general considerations, 256–257
polymorphisms, influence on CLD, 257–260
  acetaminophen proof-of-principle animal study, 260
  adverse side effects, 259–260
  hepatitis C, 257–258
  hepatitis C, fibrosis progression in chronic, 258
  hepatotoxicity of common drugs, 259–260
  lipid lowering agents, 259
  pharmaco-metabonomic approach, 260
  predispositions to non-infectious liver disease, 258–259
  treatment response or outcome prediction, 258
  viral hepatitis, 257
proteome profiling, 264–268
  capillary liquid chromatography (LC-LC), 264–265
  cellular function assessment, 256–257
  differentially expressed mRNA, 264
  Human Liver Proteome Project (HLPP), 265–266
  mass spectrometry (MS), 265
  reverse phase protein arrays (RPPA), 265, 268
  two-dimensional polyacrylamide gel electrophoresis (2D-PAGE), 264, 267, 268
Single Nucleotide Polymorphisms, 256
transcriptome profiling, 260–264
  Amplified Fragment Length Polymorphism, 261
  cell culturing, 261
  cellular function, 256–257
  classification schemes, 263
  confounding factors, 262–263
  expression microarrays, 260, 264
  fibrosis and HCV infected patients, 262
  focused studies, 266–267
  gender differences in nonreproductive organs, 261
  gene expression in healthy tissue, 261
  gene expression in NASH, 263
  Gene Tag, 261

hepatocelluar carcinoma and gene expression, 262
  inter-individual fluctuations, 266
  laser capture microdissection (LCM), 261
  location-specific variations, 261–262
  mRNA identification, 260–261, 265–266
  multidimensional protein identification technology, 266
  SAGE techniques, 260, 264
  steatosis, 263–264
nucleoside analogues, 18
  combination therapies and, 34–35
  for chronic HBV, 30, 31, 32–33
  for chronic HBV-HIV co-infection, 68
  for chronic HCV, 48
  for compensated cirrhosis, 33
  for decompensated cirrhosis, 33–34
nutritional therapy, for alcoholic liver disease, 108

obesity and metabolic issues
  drug-induced liver disease and, 182
  in alcoholic liver disease, 101
  in liver transplantations, 245–246
  in NAFLD, 77, 78f, 80, 83, 86
  in NASH, 79
octreotide, 219
omental fat
Orlistat
osteoporosis, 157, 162, 247
oxidative stress, 83

panniculitis, 144, 146, 147
pegylation of intreferon (PEG-IFN), 48
peliosis hepatis, 187–188
penicillamine, and Wilson's disease, 136–138
pentoxifylline, 88–89, 105, 105f, 106, 110
peritoneovenous shunts (PVS), 225
PET scanning, to detect intrahepatic cholangiocarcinoma, 207
pharmaco-metabonomic approach, 260
phenytoin, 244
phlebotomy, therapeutic, 125–126, 127
phospholipidosis, 187
polycystic ovarian syndrome, 79, 80
polymorphisms, and CLD, 257–260
  acetaminophen proof-of-principle animal study, 260
  adverse side effects, 259–260
  hepatitis C, 257–258
  hepatitis C, fibrosis progression in chronic, 258

polymorphisms, and CLD (*cont.*)
  hepatotoxicity of common drugs,
    259–260
  lipid lowering agents, 259
  pharmaco-metabonomic approach, 260
  predispositions to non-infectious liver
    disease, 258–259
  treatment response or outcome
    prediction, 258
  viral hepatitis, 257
poor metabolism (PM), of drugs, 259
porphyria cutanea tarda (PCT), 128
portal hypertension, 162
post-transplant lymphoproliferative
  disorder (PTLD), 247
Prader Willi syndrome, 79
pravastatin, 259
prednisolone treatment, 165*f*
prednisone treatment, 6
pregnancy
  drug-induced liver disease and, 182
  hepatitis E and, 19
  Wilson's disease and, 138
primary biliary cirrhosis (PBC), 157,
  159–160, 164
  AMA negative *vs.* positive PBC, 159*t*
  clinical presentation, 160–161
  complications, 162
  diagnosis, 161–162
  extrahepatic autoimmune diseases, 161*t*
  histologic stages, 162*t*
  management, 163–164
  survival, 160*f*
primary sclerosing cholangitis (PSC),
  155–159
  autoantibodies, 156*t*
  clinical presentation, 155, 156*t*
  complications, 156–157
  diagnosis, 156
  fat soluble deficiencies, 158*t*
  histological findings, 157*t*
  incidence of cholangiocarcinoma, 158*f*
  management, 158–159
  therapies, 159*t*
progressive airway disease, 151
proof-of-principle study, 260
proteome profiling, 264–268
  capillary liquid chromatography,
    264–265
  cellular function assessment, 256–257
  differentially expressed mRNA, 264
  Human Liver Proteome Project,
    265–266
  mass spectrometry, 265
  reverse phase protein arrays, 265, 268

two-dimensional polyacrylamide gel
    electrophoresis, 264, 267, 268
pruritus, 160–161
pulmonary disease. *See* Lung disease, and
    alpha-1 antitrypsin deficiency

quinolones, 226–227

recombinant immunoblot assay (RIBA),
    44–45
refractory ascites, 224
renal dysfunction
  hepatorenal syndrome, 227–229
  spontaneous bacterial peritonitis and,
    226
renal failure
  after liver transplantation, 243
  Wilson's disease and, 133
reverse phase protein arrays (RPPA), 265,
    268
  proteome profiling, 265, 268
reverse transcriptase polymerase chain
    reaction (RTPCR), 45
ribavirin, 48, 51, 54–55
rifaximin, 230
Roussel Uclaf Causality Assessemnt
    Method (RUCAM), 189

S-adenosyl-L-methionine (SAMe),
    106–107
SELDI-TOF, 265, 267–268
serum-ascites albumin gradient (SAAG),
    222–223
sexual activity, as acute hepatitis A risk
    factor, 3
sicca syndrome, 160, 161
Single Nucleotide Polymorphisms (SNPs),
    256, 258
skin cancer, 247
smoking, cigarette, 146, 149, 151*t*
spontaneous bacterial peritonitis (SBP)
  diagnosis and treatment, 227*f*
  prevalence, 225–227
  transplantation and, 237
steatosis
  breast cancer and, 259
  chronic hepatitis C and, 46*t*
  cirrhosis and, 53, 55
  hepatitis C and, 43
  NAFLD and, 77, 79–80, 267–268
  NASH and, 83, 85
  transcriptome profiling and,
    263–264
steroids
  corticosteroids, 103–105

drug-induced liver disease and, 191
hepatic adenomas and, 198
Stevens-Johnson Syndrome, 191
sunflower cataracts, 132–133
surface-enhanced laser
desorption/ionization (SELDI),
265, 267

tacrolimus, 243–244, 245, 246
tamoxifen, 259
telbivudine (LdT), 71–72
for chronic HBV, 30, 31, 32–33, 69t
for chronic HBV-HIV co-infection, 68
resistance to, 34
tenofovir, 69t
terlipressin, 219
tests, diagnostic
AAT deficiency, 147–148
acute hepatitis A, 4
acute hepatitis B, 9
acute hepatitis C, 12–13
acute hepatitis D, 16–17
acute hepatitis E, 19
acute viral hepatitis, 4t
alpha-1 antitrypsin deficiency, 147–148
autoimmune hepatitis, 166–167
chronic hepatitis B, 28–29
chronic hepatitis C, 43–47, 55
chronic hepatitis D, 36
drug induced liver disease, 188–189
drug-induced liver disease, 188–189
focal nodular hyperplasia, 197
hemangioma, 196
hepatic adenoma, 198
hepatitis A virus, 4
hepatitis B, 9
hepatitis B in HIV-infected patient,
67–68
hepatitis C, 12–13
hepatitis D, 16–17
hepatitis E, 19
hepatocellular carcinoma, 200–202
hepatorenal syndrome, 228t
hereditary hemochromatosis, 123–125
intrahepatic cholangiocarcinoma,
206–207
liver disease with secondary iron
overload, 124
nonalcoholic fatty liver disease, 82–83
primary biliary cirrhosis, 161–162
primary sclerosing cholangitis, 156
spontaneous bacterial peritonitis, 227f
Wilson's disease, 134–135, 135t. See also
individual test
therapeutic phlebotomy, 125–126, 127

thiazolidinediones, 87
transcriptome profiling, 260–264
Amplified Fragment Length
Polymorphism, 261
cell culturing, 261
cellular function, 256–257
classification schemes, 263
confounding factors, 262–263
expression microarrays, 260, 264
fibrosis and HCV infected patients, 262
focused studies, 266–267
gender differences in nonreproductive
organs, 261
gene expression in healthy tissue, 261
gene expression in NASH, 263
Gene Tag, 261
hepatocelluar carcinoma and gene
expression, 262
inter-individual fluctuations in gene
expression, 266
laser capture microdissection, 261
location-specific variations, 261–262
mRNA identification, 260–261,
265–266
multidimensional protein
identification, 266
SAGE techniques, 260, 264
steatosis, 263–264
transfusion-associated hepatitis C, 12, 40
transient elastography (Fibroscan), 82
transjugular intrahepatic protosystemic
shunts (TIPS), 219, 225, 236, 238
transplantation, liver, 235–248
AAT deficiency, 144, 150
acute cellular rejection, 244–245
acute hepatitis A, 5
acute hepatitis B, 9, 10
acute hepatitis C, 11
acute hepatitis D, 18
alcoholic liver disease, 108–111
Child-Turcotte-Pugh (CTP) score, 237t
cholangiocarcinoma, 240
chronic hepatitis C, 39, 40, 53
cirrhosis, 225
contraindications to, 239t
diabetes and, 245
disease recurrence, 247–248
for AIH, 170
fulminant hepatic failure, 237–238
general considerations, 235
gout and, 244, 246
hepatocellular carcinoma and, 203,
239–240
hypertension and renal failure, 246
hyperuricemia and gout, 246

transplantation, liver (*cont.*)
  immunosuppressive agents and their
      complications, 243–244
  immunosuppressive protocols,
      common, 243*t*
  increase in patients awaiting, 215
  indications, 235–236
  infection after, 242
  intrahepatic cholangiocarcinoma, 207
  long-term complications, 245
  long-term survival, 239, 240*t*, 241
  medical complications, 245
  obesity and metabolic issues, 245–246
  operation, 241–242
  osteoporosis, 247
    malignancies, 247
  post-operative complications, 242
  primary biliary cirrhosis, 164
  PSC, 158
  psychosocial issues, 241
  recipient, evaluation of potential,
      236–241
    alternative treatment, 238
    need assessment, 236, 237*t*, 238
    operative and perioperative survival,
        238–239
    potential for success, 238–241
  renal failure after, 243
  Wilson's disease, 131, 133, 137–138
treatment studies and trials
  acute hepatitis C, 15
  alcoholic liver disease, 101, 104*f*, 108
  chronic hepatitis D, 36
  HCV/HIV-coinfected patients, 62, 63
  hepatitis C, in HIV-infected patient,
      64*t*
  Human Liver Proteome Project,
      265–266
  insulin resistance, 87
  interferon therapy, 15
  Multicenter AIDS Cohort Study, 67*f*
  NAFLD and NASH, 77–78, 84–85,
      86–87, 88–89.,
  NASH in children, 79
  weight loss medication, 200–202. *See
      also* Novel technologies, for
      studying CLDs
trientene hydrochloride, and Wilson's
    disease, 137
troglitazone, 179, 180
Tumor Necrosis Factor (TNF)-α, 257–258
Tumor Necrosis Factor (TNF)-β, 257–258
tumors of liver, benign and malignant,
    195–208
  focal nodular hyperplasia, 196–197

    clinical presentation, 197
    diagnosis, 197
    treatment, 197
  general considerations, 195
  hemangioma, 195–196
    clinical presentation, 196
    diagnosis, 196
  hepatic adenoma, 197–199
    clinical presentation, 198
    diagnosis, 198
    treatment, 199
  hepatocellular carcinoma, 199–206
    chemoembolization, 205
    clinical presentation, 203
    diagnosis, 200
    diagnosis, of small HCC, 200–202
    liver transplantation, 203
    local ablation, 205
    other therapy, 205–206
    screening, 200
    staging of, 204*f*
    surgical resection, 203–205
    treatment, 203–206
  intrahepatic cholangiocarcinoma,
      206–207
    clinical presentation, 206
    diagnosis, 206–207
    treatment, 207
  other liver tumors, 207–208
tumor markers, 207
two-dimensional polyacrylamide gel
    electrophoresis (2D-PAGE), 264,
    267, 268
type II diabetes
  NAFLD and, 77, 80
  NASH and, 79, 89
  troglitazone and, 179

ultrasonography, 81–82, 159, 196,
    200–202
  contrast-enhanced, 82, 197, 198
  endoscopic, 207
University of Toronto clinical laboratory
    index, 101–102
ursodeoxycholic acid (UDCA), 89, 163,
    163*f*, 164, 170

vaccine
  hepatitis E, 20. *See also* Immunization
variceal hemorrhage, 217–221
  gastric varices, 220–221
  management of acute, 220*f*
  prevention of recurrent bleeding,
      219–220
  primary prophylaxis, 217–218

prophylaxis of, 218*f*
prophylaxis of recurrent, 221*f*
treatment of acute, 218–219
vasculitis, 5, 52*t*, 144, 146–147
vasopressin, 219
Vitamin E, as antioxidant, 87, 88, 106, 108, 138

water contamination, and hepatitis A, 3
Wilson's disease, 131–138
  clinical presentation, 132–133
  diagnosis, 134
  diagnosis, caveats, 135*t*
  general considerations, 131
  hepatic presentations, 133
  Kayser-Fleischer rings, 132–133, 135
  less common manifestations, 134*t*
  management, 136–138
  NAFLD and, 80
  neurological disease and, 132, 137–138

other causes of low ceruloplasmin
    levels,
pathophysiology of, 131–132
pregnancy and, 138
presentations, hepatic, 133
presentations, neurological, 133
presentations, other, 134
presentations, psychiatric, 134
ruling out, 134*t*
screening, 136, 136*t*
sunflower cataracts and, 132–133
World Health Organization (WHO)
    international standard for HBV
    DNA, 29

xanthelasma, 161
xanthomata, 161

zidovudine, 64
zinc, and Wilson's disease, 137